Frontiers in Arthritis

(Volume 2)

(The Management of the Haemophilic Arthropathy)

Edited by

Christian Carulli

Orthopaedic Clinic, University of Florence, Florence, Italy

General:

1. Any dispute or claim arising out of or in connection with this License Agreement or the Work (including non-contractual disputes or claims) will be governed by and construed in accordance with the laws of the U.A.E. as applied in the Emirate of Dubai. Each party agrees that the courts of the Emirate of Dubai shall have exclusive jurisdiction to settle any dispute or claim arising out of or in connection with this License Agreement or the Work (including non-contractual disputes or claims).

2. Your rights under this License Agreement will automatically terminate without notice and without the need for a court order if at any point you breach any terms of this License Agreement. In no event will any delay or failure by Bentham Science Publishers in enforcing your compliance with this License Agreement constitute a waiver of any of its rights.

3. You acknowledge that you have read this License Agreement, and agree to be bound by its terms and conditions. To the extent that any other terms and conditions presented on any website of Bentham Science Publishers conflict with, or are inconsistent with, the terms and conditions set out in this License Agreement, you acknowledge that the terms and conditions set out in this License Agreement shall prevail.

Bentham Science Publishers Ltd.
Executive Suite Y - 2
PO Box 7917, Saif Zone
Sharjah, U.A.E.
Email: subscriptions@benthamscience.org

**BENTHAM
SCIENCE**

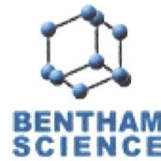

CONTENTS

To Giulia and Alessia, my Masterpieces

FOREWORD

This book is the result of 20 years of clinical activity in the management of the haemophilic arthropathy. It is based on the personal experience and on the cultural and professional aspects shared with active scientists involved in the study and treatment of Haemophilia.

My personal experience started in the '90s as a consultant at the Florence Haemophilic Service, at that moment in the vanguard as a haematologic department; however, it lacked a modern orthopaedic approach to this disease, that was then introduced. Arthroscopic and prosthetic surgery were at the beginning focused on knees and hips; subsequently other surgeons in my hospital joined and shared with me their experience in elbow, hand, and ankle surgery. Moreover, I progressively and successfully applied in haemophilic patients several principles of the regenerative medicine when indicated, in particular in cases of important bone loss.

The high expertise of eminent haematologists as Dr. Morfini initially, and Dr. Castaman later with their equipes allowed us to safely perform complex surgical procedures without complications.

Subsequently, non-operative approaches as hyaluronic acid injections and chemical synoviorthesis were largely used, and physical therapy strategies increasingly promoted.

The local health service punctually granted financial resources, and enabled me to perform surgery in patients with inhibitors too.

In addition to clinical and surgical aspects, the book offers a detailed overview of the general aspects of Haemophilia and the haemophilic arthropathy: from the definition and features of the disease to the pathogenesis of arthropathy; from the pharmacokinetics of the most important drugs to the laboratory perspective. A chapter is dedicated to the radiological findings, lifestyle recommendations, and postoperative rehabilitation. A section on the nursing of such patients is also considered.

I think that anyone wishing to approach haemophilic patients and to treat the haemophilic arthropathy will find in this volume a useful and complete guide.

Massimo Innocenti
Professor of Orthopaedics, Orthopaedic Clinic,
University of Florence,
Florence,
Italy

PREFACE

Haemophilia is one of the most common rare diseases, characterized by bleedings and haemorrhages related to an inherited deficiency of coagulative factors. For decades it has been associated with higher rates of mortality and morbidity, until clotting factor concentrates were diffused, significantly limiting most of the complications. A dramatic raise of morbidity and mortality after blood transfusions was reported when HIV and Hepatitis infections were discovered. The development of recombinant concentrates, the modern prophylactic treatment, and the multidisciplinary approach to this disease lead over the years to the reduction of such complications and improvements in the management of the related clinical settings.

Then, why another book on the management of the haemophilic arthropathy? Simply because arthropathy may be to date considered the most frequent complication of Haemophilia.

Since childhood, the first falls in the physiological development of gait ability and the high frequency of impacts during games and sports activity may induce bleedings in muscles and joints. While a haematoma in muscles usually shows a self-resolution, blood in some joints, named "target joints", may induce early negative effects, producing the so-called "arthropathy". Such degenerative and inflammatory condition finally results in a mild to severe irreversible damage, that nowadays represents not a cause of mortality but rather a source of severe disability.

Even the powerful efficacy of bleeding prophylaxis, musculoskeletal alterations are still yet highly represented. Thus, the management of the haemophilic arthropathy has gained importance being to date one of the most essential goals of the modern approach to Haemophilia. Lifestyle modifications, selected sports activity, periodic evaluations by the multidisciplinary team (haematologist, orthopaedic surgeon, skilled nurse, radiologist, physiotherapist, lab personnel, and several other figures), and tailored prophylactic treatments represent the best way to prevent articular degenerative changes or to delay the progression of the arthropathy. In cases of fair results with this approach, it is possible to adopt conservative therapies, as braces, physical therapy, and articular injections with several substances and different indications. This would mean to avoid the early recourse to surgical procedures that until a decade ago was the only choice to ensure an acceptable quality of life in young symptomatic patients. On the other hand, a significant number of patients still now found no improvements with these strategies. In such cases, surgery is mandatory. With respect to the past, knee arthroplasty, ankle fusions, and arthroscopy are not the only orthopaedic procedures useful to address a joint arthropathy. Elbow and ankle arthroscopy, hip, ankle, and elbow arthroplasty are gaining popularity given the good outcomes and high reproducibility, simultaneously with the development of modern implants and devices, less invasive techniques, and biomaterials with better tribology and performance. Nowadays, it is possible to delay a joint replacement by a minimally invasive surgery, and also to achieve a long-term survival of implant after an arthroplasty. Joint fusions are unfrequently indicated, mostly after failure of the above mentioned procedures. Amputations are to date very uncommon, and proposed only in difficult cases when no limb salvage procedures are feasible. As expected, joint replacements in young haemophilic patients will fail, and revision arthroplasty often associated with reconstructive and plastic surgery will progressively arise. Thanks to modern modular revision implants, also such challenging conditions have been well addressed. Finally, no orthopaedic procedures may produce a good result without a valid and tailored rehabilitative protocol: specific approaches under control of the multidisciplinary team now ensure an effective functional recovery, and a better feeling referred by the operated patients.

Our future target will be the prevention of arthropathy by a multimodal and multidisciplinar approach, in order to make Haemophilia an early diagnosis but no more a source of disability. In specific challenging cases, as patients with inhibitors, the goal will eventually be the limitation of the natural history of arthropathy by all conservative or minimally invasive means that are now available, more than surgical procedures.

This textbook represents an updated overview on all aspects related to Haemophilia and its orthopaedic complications; it may be considered the most multidisciplinary textbook on this topic, focusing on this disease from the bench to the surgical room.

Christian Carulli
Orthopaedic Clinic, University of Florence,
Florence,
Italy

List of Contributors

Antonio Amenta	Plastic Surgery and Reconstructive Microsurgery Unit, University of Messina, Messina, Italy
Alberto Ricciardi	Department of Orthopedics, Castelfranco Veneto General Hospital, Castelfranco Veneto, Treviso, Italy
Anna Rosa Rizzo	Orthopaedic Clinic, University of Florence, Florence, Italy
Christian Carulli	Orthopaedic Clinic, University of Florence, Florence, Italy
Caterina Martini	Orthopaedic Clinic, University of Florence, Florence, Italy
Daniela Melchiorre	Rheumatology Unit, University of Florence, Florence, Italy
Dario Melita	Plastic Surgery and Reconstructive Microsurgery Unit, University of Florence, Florence, Italy
Enrichetta Paladino	Atherotrombotic Disease Unit, Department of Heart and Vessels, AOU Careggi, Florence, Italy
Elisa Pratelli	AOU Careggi, Florence, Italy
E. Carlos Rodriguez-Merchan	Department of Orthopaedic Surgery, "La Paz" University Hospital-IdiPaz, Madrid, Spain
Federico Cipriani	Plastic Surgery and Reconstructive Microsurgery Unit, University of Florence, Florence, Italy
Francesco De Martis	Department of Heart and Vessels AOU Careggi, Center for Bleeding Disorder, Florence, Italy
Fabrizio Matassi	Orthopaedic Clinic, University of Florence, Florence, Italy
Filippo Parretti	Department of Radiology, University of Florence, Florence, Italy
Gianluigi Pasta	Fondazione IRCCS Ca' Granda Ospedale Maggiore Policlinico, Milan, Italy
Giuliana Roselli	Department of Radiology, AOU Careggi, Florence, Italy
Giorgia Saccullo	Policlinico Paolo Giaccone, Centro di Riferimento Regionale per le Coagulopatie Congenite, Palermo, Italy
Giuseppe Tagariello	Transfusion Service, Haemophilia Centre and Hematology, Castelfranco Veneto, Treviso, Italy
Giancarlo Castaman	Department of Heart and Vessels, AOU Careggi, Florence, Italy
Giovanni D'Elia	Department of Radiology, AOU Careggi, Florence, Italy
Giuseppe Mangone	AOU Careggi, Florence, Italy
Giuseppe Mazza	Institute for Liver and Digestive Health, University College of London, London, UK
Giulio Menichini	Plastic Surgery and Reconstructive Microsurgery Unit, University of Florence, Florence, Italy
Irene Felici	Orthopaedic Clinic, University of Florence, Florence, Italy
Luigi Piero Solimeno	Emergency Trauma Department, Ca' Granda Foundation, IRCCS Policlinico Hospital, Milan, Italy

Lorenzo Apicella	Physical Medicine and Rehabilitation, Aggregate Venue of Florence, University of Pisa, Florence, Italy
Marco Basso	Pharmacology and Hematology, Castelfranco Veneto, Treviso, Italy
Marco Biondi	Orthopaedic Clinic, University of Florence, Florence, Italy
Massimo Ceruso	Hand Surgery and Reconstructive Microsurgery Unit, AOU Careggi, Florence, Italy
Marco Innocenti	Plastic Surgery and Reconstructive Microsurgery Unit, University of Florence, Florence, Italy
Massimo Innocenti	Orthopaedic Clinic, University of Florence, Florence, Italy
Michael Makris	Sheffield Haemophilia and Thrombosis Centre, Royal Hallamshire Hospital, Sheffield, UK Department of Infection, Immunity and Cardiovascular Disease, University of Sheffield, Sheffield, UK
Marco Matucci-Cerinic	Rheumatology Unit, University of Florence, Florence, Italy
Maria Chiara Susini	Department of Heart and Vessels Azienda Ospedaliero, Center for Bleeding Disorders, Universitaria Careggi, Florence, Italy
Massimiliano Tani	University of Florence, Florence, Italy
Prospero Bigazzi	Hand Surgery and Reconstructive Microsurgery Unit, AOU Careggi, Florence, Italy
Pietro Pasquetti	Rehabilitation Unit, AOU Careggi, Florence, Italy
Paolo Quaglierini	University of Florence, Florence, Italy
Paolo Radossi	Transfusion Service, Haemophilia Centre and Hematology, Castelfranco Veneto, Treviso, Italy
Roberto Civinini	Orthopaedic Clinic, University of Florence, Florence, Italy
Silvia Linari	Department of Heart and Vessels, Center for Bleeding Disorder, AOU Careggi, Florence, Italy
Sandra Pfanner	Hand Surgery and Reconstructive Microsurgery Unit, AOU Careggi, Florence, Italy
Virginia Puliga	Department of Heart and Vessels Azienda Ospedaliero-Universitaria Careggi, Center for Bleeding Disorders, Florence, Italy

CHAPTER 1

Pathogenesis of the Haemophilic Arthropathy

Daniela Melchiorre[1,*], Silvia Linari[2], Fabrizio Matassi[3] and **Giancarlo Castaman[2]**

[1] *Rheumatology Unit, University of Florence, Florence, Italy*

[2] *Center for Bleeding Disorders, Azienda Ospedaliero-Universitaria Careggi, Florence, Italy*

[3] *Orthopaedic Clinic, University of Florence, Florence, Italy*

Abstract: Joint damage due to recurrent bleedings in Haemophilia is the cause for long-term disabilities. The pathogenetic mechanism of haemophilic arthropathy is multifactorial and includes inflammatory synovium-mediated and degenerative cartilage-mediated phenomenons, in addition to neoangiogenesis and bone loss. Free blood in the joint has a direct effect on cartilage and synovium, and the deposit of iron appears to play a pivotal role. Iron may promote the apoptosis of chondrocytes by catalyzing the formation of oxygen metabolites. Iron may also act on the synovial membrane by favouring its proliferation through the induction of proto-oncogenes involved in cellular proliferation and stimulation of inflammatory cytokines. Such degenerative and inflammatory processes occur concomitantly, but also independently. A reduction of bone mineralization is usually present as a part of the articular damage associated to a multifactorial mechanism: it seems that the molecular triad (osteoprotegerin/Receptor activator of nuclear factor kB/Receptor activator of nuclear factor kB ligand) probably plays a major role, inducing osteoclastic differentiation and maturation. These processes finally result in a fibrotic and irreversible altered joint, feature of haemophilic arthropathy.

Keywords: Arthropathy, Haemophilia, Haemarthrosis, Haemosiderin, Neoangio-genesis, Osteoporosis, Synovitis.

INTRODUCTION

Haemophilia A and B are rare X-linked recessive bleeding disorders characterized by the absence or functional defect of clotting factor VIII (FVIII) or factor IX (FIX) respectively. The hallmark of such disease is represented by musculoskeletal bleedings, particularly haemarthrosis, leading to orthopaedic complications. Joint bleeding is the most common and potentially most disabling manifestation of severe Haemophilia (*i.e.* plasma FVIII or FIX <1U/dL) [1]. In

[*] **Corresponding author Daniela Melchiorre:** Rheumatology Unit, University of Florence, Florence, Italy; Tel: +39 0552751688; Email: daniela.melchiorre@unifi.it

Christian Carulli (Ed.)
All rights reserved-© 2017 Bentham Science Publishers

nearly half of all children affected by severe Haemophilia, the initial haemartrosis occurs during the first year of life [2], and 90% of patients experience at least a joint bleeding before the age of 4.5 years [3]. Eighty per cent of joint bleedings involve knees, elbows, and ankles [4], and patients often develop multiple "target" joints. Although blood is rapidly cleared from the joint space also by the replacement with the missing factor, the pathologic process still continues, resulting in both clinical and radiographic changes. Recurrent bleedings cause an irreversible joint damage with progressive functional impairment [5], chronic pain [6], and heavy impact on quality of life [7]. Haemarthrosis can be prevented or controlled by the prophylactic administration of clotting factor concentrates. Compared with an on-demand treatment strategy, a primary prophylactic treatment (*i.e.* the regular continuous treatment initiated in the absence of documented osteochondral joint disease and started before the second clinically evident large joint bleed in children >3 years) leads to better musculoskeletal outcomes, as clearly established [8 - 11]. [8]. However despite such strategy, joint bleedings and related damages may recur and the haemophilic arthropathy (HA) may realize, as confirmed by the radiographic evidence by the age of 6 in some subjects who had no bleeding or few subclinical haemarthroses [11].

The mechanism of the progressive joint damage in patients with Haemophilia is still relatively unclear, but recurrence and persistence of blood into the joint cavity is the key factor responsible for synovial and cartilage changes [12, 13]. Increasing evidences of a close relationship between the type of mutation ("null" and/or "missense" mutations), bleeding, inflammatory process, and neoangiogenesis are emerging and suggesting that iron, cytokines, and neoangiogenic factors can initiate synovial and early cartilage damages with molecular changes and perpetuation of a chronic inflammatory condition [14].

From Bleeding to Synovial and Cartilage Damage

Bleeding into a joint exposes synovial cells to blood and its components including iron that plays a pivotal role in joint damage [15] (Fig. **1**). The progressive accumulation over time of iron as haemosiderin (normally removed from the by synovial macrophages) represents the trigger for synovial inflammation [16]. Haemosiderin deposits are crucial in the early stages of HA, triggering synoviocyte hypertrophy (resulting in "villi"), neoangiogenesis, and release of hydrolytic enzymes from synovial cells. Iron up-regulates the expression of proinflammatory cytokines, as interleukin-6 (IL-6), IL-1alpha, IL-1beta and tumor necrosis factor-alpha (TNF-alpha) in synovial cells and induces the regulator genes c-myc and MDM2 expression, resulting in synovial proliferation [17, 18]. Another effect of haemosiderin is the lymphocytes infiltration of the synovial membrane with subsequent inflammatory changes. Moreover, different proinflammatory cytokines released by synovial cells may inhibit the formation of human cartilage matrix [15]. Synovitis is one of the earliest macroscopic effect of a target joint and it is not always easily distinguishable from a clinical point of view from haemarthrosis. Synovitis is an inflammatory process involving synovial tissue, characterized by hypertrophy, migration of inflammatory cells, and a high degree of neoangiogenesis [18 - 22].

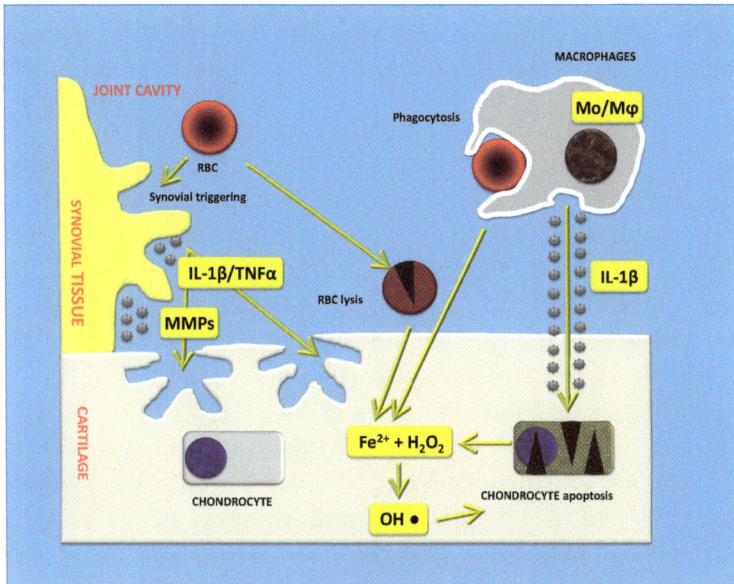

Fig. (1). Mechanisms of blood-induced joint damage in Haemophilia: the role of iron (Fe^{2+}) interacting with Hydrogen peroxide (H$_2$O$_2$), macrophages'activation (Mo/Mö), matrix metalloproteinases (MMPs), and involvement of several cytokines.

Recurrent bleedings and synovitis rapidly evolving into joint damage can be considered two different aspects of HA. Intense, chronic effusion of the affected joint after one or several haemarthrosis typically occurs in the early stages of HA [23, 24]. Synovitis can lead to further bleedings with transformation of an acute process in a chronic disease.

Also the presence of free blood in a target joint has a direct harmful effect on cartilage, resulting in adverse changes in chondrocyte activity [25]. Moreover, these alterations may occur before the synovial inflammation becomes evident. Human articular cartilage consists of a relatively small number of chondrocytes embedded in a relatively large amount of extracellular matrix that consists mainly of collagen and proteoglycans. There is a continuous turnover of these components, with a delicate balance between synthesis and breakdown [26].

A pivotal role in the whole process is played by the high-weight molecular complex called "inflammasome". The inflammasome controls the maturation and the secretion of IL-1beta by means of the activation of caspase 1. The inflammasome constituents are the pattern-recognition receptors (PRRs), including the Toll-like receptors (TLRs) and lectins (CTLs), which analyze the extracellular environment and are associated with pathogen-associated molecular patterns (PAMPs). PRRs also include the intracellular NOD-like receptors (NLR) which recognize both PAMPs that harmful signals caused by danger associated molecular patterns (DAMPs) as demonstrate by Mendonça et colleagues [27].

In vitro studies have shown that a relatively short exposure (4 days, the expected natural evacuation time of blood from a human joint) of human cartilage to whole blood in concentrations up to 50% (blood concentration during haemarthroses are expected to approach 100%) induces long-lasting damaging effects [28]. The marked inhibition of matrix formation (proteoglycan synthesis) and increased breakdown, *i.e.* release of matrix components (proteoglycan release) result in a progressive loss of matrix, caused by the induction of apoptosis of chondrocytes by hydroxyl radicals formed upon exposure to blood [29]. Hydroxyl radicals are formed when hydrogen peroxide production by chondrocytes is increased upon stimulation by pro-inflammatory cytokines, such as IL-1beta, originating from activated blood monocytes/macrophages present in the blood within the joint. Hydrogen peroxide reacts with haemoglobin-derived iron from damaged and phagocytosed red blood cells close to chondrocytes. This triggers the formation of radicals that induce apoptosis and consequently an irreversible inhibition of cartilage matrix synthesis [25, 29, 30]. Canine *in vivo* studies have corroborated these findings [31] and demonstrated that immature cartilage is more susceptible to blood-induced damage than mature cartilage [32]. Joint bleeding leads to initially independent adverse changes in synovial tissue, articular cartilage, and consequently subchondral bone. Taken together, the mechanism of blood-induced joint damage includes both degenerative (cartilage-mediated) and inflammatory (synovium-mediated) components. Although influencing each other, these processes also occur independently [33].

Neoangiogenesis

Neoangiogenesis associated with the recruitment of bone marrow-derived progenitors is a critical, independent mechanism involved in the development and maintenance of HA. Neoangiogenesis is also implicated in tumor growth and inflammatory arthritis [14, 34, 35]. The proangiogenic vascular endothelial growth factor (VEGF) is the principal signaling molecule in angiogenesis and can be induced by hypoxia and different cytokines through interaction with its receptors, VEGFR1 and 2. Similarly to other joint diseases, sharing histological similarities with HA, the synovial pannus has enhanced oxygen demand with evidence of *de novo* blood vessel formation of the synovium. A four-fold elevation in different proangiogenic factors as VEGF, stromal cell-derived factor-1 (SDF-1), and metalloproteinase 9 (MMP-9) has been recorded. Also pro-angiogenic macrophage/monocyte cells (VEGF+/CD68+ and VEGFR1+/CD11b+ and VEGF/CD68+) in synovium and peripheral blood of haemophilic subjects were observed. A significant increase of VEGFR2/AC133+ endothelial progenitor cells and CD34/ VEGFR1+ haemopoietic progenitors cells was also demonstrated [34, 36]. Human synovial cells, when incubated with haemophilic sera, up-regulated hypoxia-inducible factor 1alpha (HIF1A) mRNA, implicating hypoxia in the neoangiogenesis process [36]. Moreover, an increased microvessels density has been shown by immunofluorescence in synovial cells from patients with end-stage HA [34]. This suggests that also late stages of HA can be characterized by an active neoangiogenesis.

From Bleeding to Osteoporosis

Osteoporosis is a disorder characterized by decreased bone mass and microarchitectural deterioration, resulting in loss of bone strength and fragility fractures [37]. Such condition has been recently recognized as a severe comorbidity in Haemophilia [38, 39].

The pathogenesis of low bone mineral density in subjects with Haemophilia is multifactorial. Primary key factors include: prolonged immobilization [38 - 40]; lack of weight-bearing exercises and failure to achieve an optimal strength during growth [41]; excessive bone resorption resulting in loss of bone mass and failure to replace the lost bone due to defects in bone formation [42, 43]. Other factors such as Human Immunodeficiency Virus (HIV) or hepatitis C virus (HCV) infections, and their treatments, may be independently associated with decreased bone mineral density [38, 42, 44]. The mechanism and pathways by which blood in the joint cavity causes bone quality and quantity depletion have not been to date fully elucidated [45, 46]. However, members of the TNF receptor superfamily probably play a major role. Effectively, the molecular triad osteoprotegerin/Receptor activator of nuclear factor kB/Receptor activator of nuclear factor kB ligand (OPG/RANK/RANKL) that tightly controls the bone turnover is a crucial parameter of bone biology [47, 48]. RANKL is a transmembrane ligand mainly expressed on osteoblasts/stromal cells in the bone microenvironment. RANKL exists either as a cell-bound form or a truncated ectodomain variant derived by enzymatic cleavage of the cellular form (soluble RANKL, sRANKL). It binds to its receptor RANK expressed at cell surface of osteoclast precursor, possibly of the macrophage lineage, and induces osteoclastic differentiation and maturation, leading to bone resorption. In synovial membrane,

RANKL is expressed by fibroblast-like synoviocytes (synoviocytes type B), and by activated T cells and may induce osteoclastogenesis, through a mechanism enhanced by several cytokines (TNF-alpha, IL1, and IL17) that promote both inflammation and bone resorption [49, 50]. OPG, also a member of the TNF receptor family, acts as a decoy receptor for RANKL, and competes for binding of RANKL to RANK [51 - 53]. By this mechanism, OPG negatively regulates osteoclast differentiation, activity, and survival both *in vivo* and *in vitro* [48, 50, 53, 54]. RANKL inhibits osteoclast apoptosis whereby OPG acts as antagonist [49]. OPG is predominantly found in macrophages of the intimal synovial lining and in endothelial cells, where is complexed with von Willebrand factor within the Weibel-Palade bodies [54]. Variations in the balance between OPG and RANKL leads to pathological bone changes. Osteoclasts precursors (OCPs) are derived from haemopoietic (monocyte) progenitors in the spleen and liver migrating from blood into bone where they fuse with one another to form multinucleated osteoclasts. Blood neutrophils in the joint create an inflammatory environment that produces IL-1, IL-6, RANKL, and TNF-alpha [55, 56]. TNF increases the proliferation and differentiation of OPCs [57]. TNF also inhibits the production by bone marrow stromal cells of stromal cell-derived factor 1, which, in turn, increases the release of OPCs from the bone marrow [58]. RANKL synthesized by reactive lymphocytes in the joint binds to RANK stimulating osteoclasts to resorb bone (Fig. **2**).

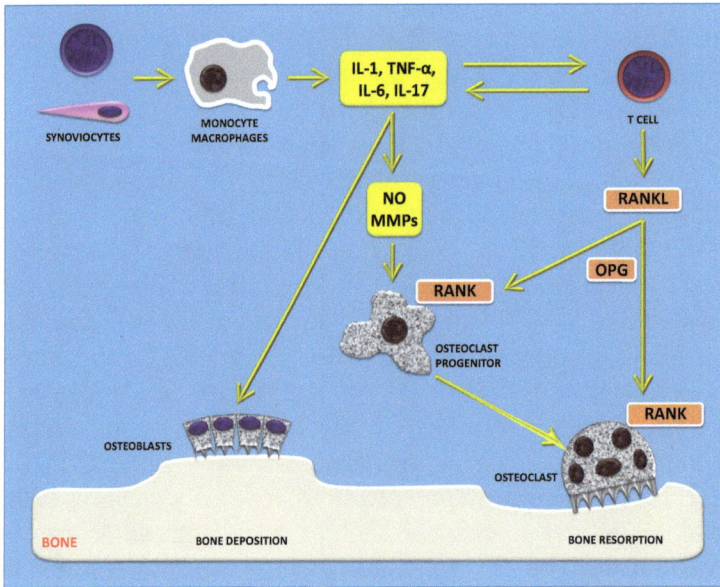

Fig. (2). The role of the molecular triad osteoprotegerin/RANK/RANKL in bone remodelling.

As key regulators of bone remodeling, serum levels of OPG/RANKL were analysed in a wide population of patients with haemophilia, together with the expression of the triad OPG/RANK/RANKL in synovial tissue of adult patients with Haemophilia, undergoing to knee replacement surgery [59]. OPG levels in all Haemophilia A patients were decreased and a strong expression of RANK and RANKL was found. A strict correlation between instrumental findings and severity of HA, according to the World Federation of Haemophilia orthopaedic joint scale (WFH score) [60], Petterson [61], and ultrasound score [62] was also observed. The biochemical markers of bone turnover in the synovial tissue of haemophiliacs indicate an osteoclastic activation, not counteracted by OPG. In fact, RANK and RANKL were found to be strongly expressed in the synovium. Instead, the expression of OPG was dramatically reduced in synovial tissue. The absence of OPG in synovial tissue suggests that the balance is shifted *versus* osteoclastic activity. In conclusion, osteoclastogenesis seems to be activated in synovial tissue of haemophilic patients, and it may be mediated by an inflammatory milieu (Fig. **3**).

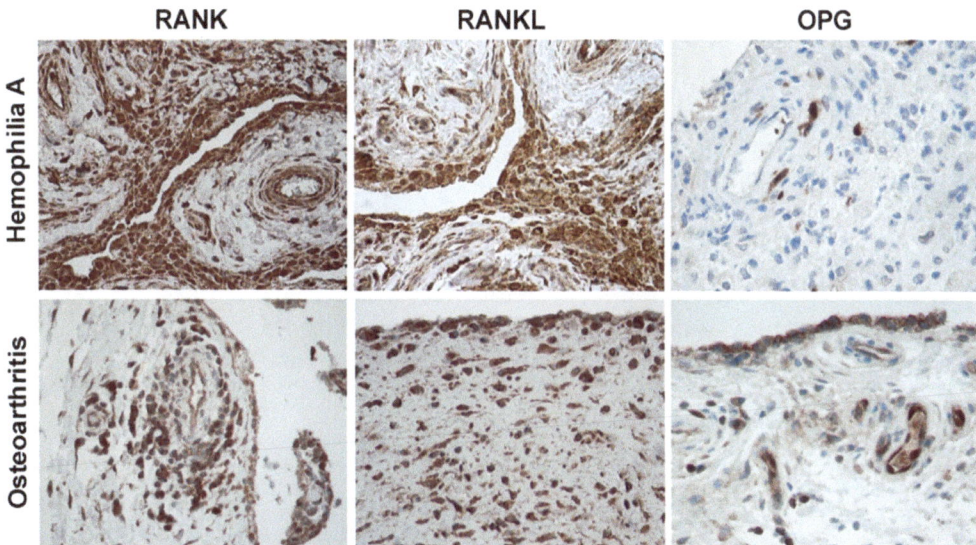

Fig. (3). Expression of receptor activator of nuclear factor-κB (RANK), RANK ligand (RANKL), and osteoprotegerin (OPG) in synovial tissue from patients with Haemophilia A and osteoarthritis. Representative microphotographs of tissue sections subjected to immunoperoxidase staining for RANK, RANKL, and OPG (brownish-red color) and counterstained with hematoxylin are shown.

Arthropathy in Haemophilia A and B: Some Differences

Haemophilia A and B are considered clinically indistinguishable, sharing recurrent joint bleeds as hallmark of a severe disease. However some evidences suggest that Haemophilia B may be less severe than Haemophilia A [1, 63 - 65].

In a recent study, a large population of patients with Haemophilia A and B was evaluated by using clinical, imaging, and biochemical markers [66]. WFH score and US score were significantly worse in patients with Haemophilia A than the others, matched for age, even with similar frequency of haemarthroses. Notwithstanding the equivalent degree of clotting deficiency, the number of haemarthroses was significantly less in Haemophilia B patients. The lower serum OPG and sRANKL levels in Haemophilia A are in keeping with more severe forms of arthropathy and clinical outcomes. Similar significance can be attributed to the reduced expression of OPG with the marked expression in the synovial tissue of RANK and RANKL in Haemophilia A. Moreover, the histological analysis in synovial tissue of patients affected by Haemophilia B underlines the differences of the expression of RANK/RANKL/OPG triad with respect to Haemophilia A. Effectively, the increased expression of OPG and the lower number of patients undergoing arthroplasty confirm that the arthropathy may be less severe.

CONCLUDING REMARKS

Joint bleeding is the most common and potentially most important long-term disabling manifestation of severe Haemophilia. Recurrent joint bleedings cause irreversible articular damages with progressive functional impairment. The subsequent release of iron from destroyed red cells has a direct pathogenetic effect on cartilage, synovium, and bone. Different cytokines play a crucial role in blood-induced arthropathy inducing an overreaction and leading to irreversible damages independent from the bleeding. These processes finally result in an altered, restructured, and not functional joint, with risk of ankylosis, feature of the classic haemophilic arthropathy that tends to be more severe in Haemophilia A than in Haemophilia B.

CONFLICT OF INTEREST

The authors confirm that they have no conflict of interest to declare for this publication.

ACKNOWLEDGEMENTS

Declared none.

REFERENCES

[1]   Bolton-Maggs PH, Pasi KJ. Haemophilias A and B. Lancet 2003; 361(9371): 1801-9. [Review]. [http://dx.doi.org/10.1016/S0140-6736(03)13405-8] [PMID: 12781551]

[2]   Pollmann H, Richter H, Ringkamp H, Jürgens H. When are children diagnosed as having severe haemophilia and when do they start to bleed? A 10-year single-centre PUP study. Eur J Pediatr 1999; 158 (Suppl. 3): S166-70.

[http://dx.doi.org/10.1007/PL00014347] [PMID: 10650861]

[3]   Fischer K, van der Bom JG, Mauser-Bunschoten EP, *et al.* The effects of postponing prophylactic treatment on long-term outcome in patients with severe hemophilia. Blood 2002; 99(7): 2337-41. [http://dx.doi.org/10.1182/blood.V99.7.2337] [PMID: 11895765]

[4]   Pergantou H, Matsinos G, Papadopoulos A, Platokouki H, Aronis S. Comparative study of validity of clinical, X-ray and magnetic resonance imaging scores in evaluation and management of haemophilic arthropathy in children. Haemophilia 2006; 12(3): 241-7. [http://dx.doi.org/10.1111/j.1365-2516.2006.01208.x] [PMID: 16643208]

[5]   Soucie JM, Cianfrini C, Janco RL, *et al.* Joint range-of-motion limitations among young males with hemophilia: prevalence and risk factors. Blood 2004; 103(7): 2467-73. [http://dx.doi.org/10.1182/blood-2003-05-1457] [PMID: 14615381]

[6]   Choinière M, Melzack R. Acute and chronic pain in hemophilia. Pain 1987; 31(3): 317-31. [http://dx.doi.org/10.1016/0304-3959(87)90161-8] [PMID: 3501097]

[7]   Klamroth R, Pollmann H, Hermans C, *et al.* The relative burden of haemophilia A and the impact of target joint development on health-related quality of life: results from the ADVATE Post-Authorization Safety Surveillance (PASS) study. Haemophilia 2011; 17(3): 412-21. [http://dx.doi.org/10.1111/j.1365-2516.2010.02435.x] [PMID: 21332888]

[8]   Fischer K, van der Bom JG, Molho P, *et al.* Prophylactic *versus* on-demand treatment strategies for severe haemophilia: a comparison of costs and long-term outcome. Haemophilia 2002; 8(6): 745-52. [http://dx.doi.org/10.1046/j.1365-2516.2002.00695.x] [PMID: 12410642]

[9]   Srivastava A, Brewer AK, Mauser-Bunschoten EP, *et al.* Guidelines for the management of hemophilia. Haemophilia 2013; 19(1): e1-e47. [http://dx.doi.org/10.1111/j.1365-2516.2012.02909.x] [PMID: 22776238]

[10]   Nilsson IM, Berntorp E, Löfqvist T, Pettersson H. Twenty-five years experience of prophylactic treatment in severe haemophilia A and B. J Intern Med 1992; 232(1): 25-32. [http://dx.doi.org/10.1111/j.1365-2796.1992.tb00546.x] [PMID: 1640190]

[11]   Manco-Johnson MJ, Abshire TC, Shapiro AD, *et al.* Prophylaxis versus episodic treatment to prevent joint disease in boys with severe hemophilia. N Engl J Med 2007; 357(6): 535-44. [http://dx.doi.org/10.1056/NEJMoa067659] [PMID: 17687129]

[12]   Roy S, Ghadially FN. Pathology of experimental haemarthrosis. Ann Rheum Dis 1966; 25(5): 402-15. [http://dx.doi.org/10.1136/ard.25.5.402] [PMID: 4161917]

[13]   Mainardi CL, Levine PH, Werb Z, Harris ED Jr. Proliferative synovitis in hemophilia: biochemical and morphologic observations. Arthritis Rheum 1978; 21(1): 137-44. [http://dx.doi.org/10.1002/art.1780210122] [PMID: 623683]

[14]   Acharya SS, Kaplan RN, Macdonald D, Fabiyi OT, DiMichele D, Lyden D. Neoangiogenesis contributes to the development of hemophilic synovitis. Blood 2011; 117(8): 2484-93. [http://dx.doi.org/10.1182/blood-2010-05-284653] [PMID: 21163925]

[15]   Morris CJ, Blake DR, Wainwright AC, Steven MM. Relationship between iron deposits and tissue damage in the synovium: an ultrastructural study. Ann Rheum Dis 1986; 45(1): 21-6. [http://dx.doi.org/10.1136/ard.45.1.21] [PMID: 3954454]

[16]   Roosendaal G, Lafeber FP. Pathogenesis of haemophilic arthropathy. Haemophilia 2006; 12 (Suppl. 3): 117-21. [http://dx.doi.org/10.1111/j.1365-2516.2006.01268.x] [PMID: 16684006]

[17]   Øvlisen K, Kristensen AT, Jensen AL, Tranholm M. IL-1 beta, IL-6, KC and MCP-1 are elevated in synovial fluid from haemophilic mice with experimentally induced haemarthrosis. Haemophilia 2009; 15(3): 802-10. [http://dx.doi.org/10.1111/j.1365-2516.2008.01973.x] [PMID: 19444976]

[18]   Gao D, Nolan DJ, Mellick AS, Bambino K, McDonnell K, Mittal V. Endothelial progenitor cells control the angiogenic switch in mouse lung metastasis. Science 2008; 319(5860): 195-8.
[http://dx.doi.org/10.1126/science.1150224] [PMID: 18187653]

[19]   Eubank TD, Galloway M, Montague CM, Waldman WJ, Marsh CB. M-CSF induces vascular endothelial growth factor production and angiogenic activity from human monocytes. J Immunol 2003; 171(5): 2637-43.
[http://dx.doi.org/10.4049/jimmunol.171.5.2637] [PMID: 12928417]

[20]   Rüger B, Giurea A, Wanivenhaus AH, *et al*. Endothelial precursor cells in the synovial tissue of patients with rheumatoid arthritis and osteoarthritis. Arthritis Rheum 2004; 50(7): 2157-66.
[http://dx.doi.org/10.1002/art.20506] [PMID: 15248213]

[21]   Maeno N, Takei S, Imanaka H, *et al*. Increased circulating vascular endothelial growth factor is correlated with disease activity in polyarticular juvenile rheumatoid arthritis. J Rheumatol 1999; 26(10): 2244-8.
[PMID: 10529148]

[22]   Busso N, Morard C, Salvi R, Péclat V, So A. Role of the tissue factor pathway in synovial inflammation. Arthritis Rheum 2003; 48(3): 651-9.
[http://dx.doi.org/10.1002/art.10869] [PMID: 12632417]

[23]   Rodríguez-Merchán EC. Pathogenesis, early diagnosis, and prophylaxis for chronic hemophilic synovitis. Clin Orthop Relat Res 1997; (343): 6-11.
[PMID: 9345198]

[24]   Rodriguez Merchant EC. Haemophilic synovitis: basic concept. Haemophilia 2007; 13 (Suppl. 3): 1-3.
[http://dx.doi.org/10.1111/j.1365-2516.2007.01532.x]

[25]   Jansen NW, Roosendaal G, Bijlsma JW, Degroot J, Lafeber FP. Exposure of human cartilage tissue to low concentrations of blood for a short period of time leads to prolonged cartilage damage: an in vitro study. Arthritis Rheum 2007; 56(1): 199-207.
[http://dx.doi.org/10.1002/art.22304] [PMID: 17195222]

[26]   Niibayashi H, Shimizu K, Suzuki K, Yamamoto S, Yasuda T, Yamamuro T. Proteoglycan degradation in hemarthrosis. Intraarticular, autologous blood injection in rat knees. Acta Orthop Scand 1995; 66(1): 73-9.
[http://dx.doi.org/10.3109/17453679508994645] [PMID: 7863774]

[27]   Mendonça R, Silveira AA, Conran N. Red cell DAMPs and inflammation. Inflamm Res 2016; 65(9): 665-78.
[http://dx.doi.org/10.1007/s00011-016-0955-9] [PMID: 27251171]

[28]   Roosendaal G, Vianen ME, van den Berg HM, Lafeber FP, Bijlsma JW. Cartilage damage as a result of hemarthrosis in a human *in vitro* model. J Rheumatol 1997; 24(7): 1350-4.
[PMID: 9228136]

[29]   Hooiveld M, Roosendaal G, Wenting M, van den Berg M, Bijlsma J, Lafeber F. Short-term exposure of cartilage to blood results in chondrocyte apoptosis. Am J Pathol 2003; 162(3): 943-51.
[http://dx.doi.org/10.1016/S0002-9440(10)63889-8] [PMID: 12598327]

[30]   Hooiveld MJ, Roosendaal G, van den Berg HM, Bijlsma JW, Lafeber FP. Haemoglobin-derived iron-dependent hydroxyl radical formation in blood-induced joint damage: an in vitro study. Rheumatology (Oxford) 2003; 42(6): 784-90.
[http://dx.doi.org/10.1093/rheumatology/keg220] [PMID: 12730540]

[31]   Roosendaal G, TeKoppele JM, Vianen ME, van den Berg HM, Lafeber FP, Bijlsma JW. Blood-induced joint damage: a canine *in vivo* study. Arthritis Rheum 1999; 42(5): 1033-9.
[http://dx.doi.org/10.1002/1529-0131(199905)42:5<1033::AID-ANR24>3.0.CO;2-#]   [PMID: 10323461]

[32] Hooiveld MJ, Roosendaal G, Vianen ME, van den Berg HM, Bijlsma JW, Lafeber FP. Immature articular cartilage is more susceptible to blood-induced damage than mature articular cartilage: an in vivo animal study. Arthritis Rheum 2003; 48(2): 396-403.
[http://dx.doi.org/10.1002/art.10769] [PMID: 12571849]

[33] Jansen NW, Roosendaal G, Lafeber FP. Understanding haemophilic arthropathy: an exploration of current open issues. Br J Haematol 2008; 143(5): 632-40.
[http://dx.doi.org/10.1111/j.1365-2141.2008.07386.x] [PMID: 18950457]

[34] Zetterberg E, Palmblad J, Wallensten R, Morfini M, Melchiorre D, Holmström M. Angiogenesis is increased in advanced haemophilic joint disease and characterised by normal pericyte coverage. Eur J Haematol 2014; 92(3): 256-62.
[http://dx.doi.org/10.1111/ejh.12227] [PMID: 24168433]

[35] Mainardi CL, Levine PH, Werb Z, Harris ED Jr. Proliferative synovitis in hemophilia: biochemical and morphologic observations. Arthritis Rheum 1978; 21(1): 137-44.
[http://dx.doi.org/10.1002/art.1780210122] [PMID: 623683]

[36] Acharya SS. Exploration of the pathogenesis of haemophilic joint arthropathy: understanding implications for optimal clinical management. Br J Haematol 2012; 156(1): 13-23.
[http://dx.doi.org/10.1111/j.1365-2141.2011.08919.x] [PMID: 22050780]

[37] NIH Consensus Development Panel on Osteoporosis Prevention, Diagnosis, and Therapy. Osteoporosis prevention, diagnosis, and therapy. JAMA 2001; 285(6): 785-95.
[http://dx.doi.org/10.1001/jama.285.6.785] [PMID: 11176917]

[38] Wallny TA, Scholz DT, Oldenburg J, et al. Osteoporosis in haemophilia - an underestimated comorbidity? Haemophilia 2007; 13(1): 79-84.
[http://dx.doi.org/10.1111/j.1365-2516.2006.01405.x] [PMID: 17212729]

[39] Gerstner G, Damiano ML, Tom A, et al. Prevalence and risk factors associated with decreased bone mineral density in patients with haemophilia. Haemophilia 2009; 15(2): 559-65.
[http://dx.doi.org/10.1111/j.1365-2516.2008.01963.x] [PMID: 19187193]

[40] Barnes C, Wong P, Egan B, et al. Reduced bone density among children with severe hemophilia. Pediatrics 2004; 114(2): e177-81.
[http://dx.doi.org/10.1542/peds.114.2.e177] [PMID: 15286254]

[41] Tlacuilo-Parra A, Morales-Zambrano R, Tostado-Rabago N, Esparza-Flores MA, Lopez-Guido B, Orozco-Alcala J. Inactivity is a risk factor for low bone mineral density among haemophilic children. Br J Haematol 2008; 140(5): 562-7.
[http://dx.doi.org/10.1111/j.1365-2141.2007.06972.x] [PMID: 18275434]

[42] Katsarou O, Terpos E, Chatzismalis P, et al. Increased bone resorption is implicated in the pathogenesis of bone loss in hemophiliacs: correlations with hemophilic arthropathy and HIV infection. Ann Hematol 2010; 89(1): 67-74.
[http://dx.doi.org/10.1007/s00277-009-0759-x] [PMID: 19488753]

[43] Christoforidis A, Economou M, Papadopoulou E, et al. Comparative study of dual energy X-ray absorptiometry and quantitative ultrasonography with the use of biochemical markers of bone turnover in boys with haemophilia. Haemophilia 2011; 17(1): e217-22.
[http://dx.doi.org/10.1111/j.1365-2516.2010.02385.x] [PMID: 20825502]

[44] Linari S, Montorzi G, Bartolozzi D, et al. Hypovitaminosis D and osteopenia/osteoporosis in a haemophilia population: a study in HCV/HIV or HCV infected patients. Haemophilia 2013; 19(1): 126-33.
[http://dx.doi.org/10.1111/j.1365-2516.2012.02899.x] [PMID: 22776099]

[45] Valentino LA. Blood-induced joint disease: the pathophysiology of hemophilic arthropathy. J Thromb Haemost 2010; 8(9): 1895-902.
[http://dx.doi.org/10.1111/j.1538-7836.2010.03962.x] [PMID: 20586922]

[46]   Hoots WK, Rodriguez N, Boggio L, Valentino LA. Pathogenesis of haemophilic synovitis: clinical aspects. Haemophilia 2007; 13 (Suppl. 3): 4-9.
[http://dx.doi.org/10.1111/j.1365-2516.2007.01533.x] [PMID: 17822514]

[47]   Boyce BF, Xing L. Biology of RANK, RANKL, and osteoprotegerin. Arthritis Res Ther 2007; 9 (Suppl. 1): S1-S23.
[http://dx.doi.org/10.1186/ar2165] [PMID: 17634140]

[48]   Vandooren B, Cantaert T, Noordenbos T, Tak PP, Baeten D. The abundant synovial expression of the RANK/RANKL/Osteoprotegerin system in peripheral spondylarthritis is partially disconnected from inflammation. Arthritis Rheum 2008; 58(3): 718-29.
[http://dx.doi.org/10.1002/art.23290] [PMID: 18311801]

[49]   Saidenberg-Kermanach N, Cohen-Solal M, Bessis N, De Vernejoul MC, Boissier MC. Role for osteoprotegerin in rheumatoid inflammation. Joint Bone Spine 2004; 71(1): 9-13.
[http://dx.doi.org/10.1016/S1297-319X(03)00131-3] [PMID: 14769514]

[50]   Lacey DL, Timms E, Tan HL, *et al.* Osteoprotegerin ligand is a cytokine that regulates osteoclast differentiation and activation. Cell 1998; 93(2): 165-76.
[http://dx.doi.org/10.1016/S0092-8674(00)81569-X] [PMID: 9568710]

[51]   Jones DH, Kong Y-Y, Penninger JM. Role of RANKL and RANK in bone loss and arthritis. Ann Rheum Dis 2002; 61 (Suppl. 2): ii32-9.
[http://dx.doi.org/10.1136/ard.61.suppl_2.ii32] [PMID: 12379618]

[52]   Hofbauer LC, Heufelder AE. Role of receptor activator of nuclear factor-kappaB ligand and osteoprotegerin in bone cell biology. J Mol Med 2001; 79(5-6): 243-53.
[http://dx.doi.org/10.1007/s001090100226] [PMID: 11485016]

[53]   Simonet WS, Lacey DL, Dunstan CR, *et al.* Osteoprotegerin: a novel secreted protein involved in the regulation of bone density. Cell 1997; 89(2): 309-19.
[http://dx.doi.org/10.1016/S0092-8674(00)80209-3] [PMID: 9108485]

[54]   Skoumal M, Kolarz G, Haberhauer G, Woloszczuk W, Hawa G, Klingler A. Osteoprotegerin and the receptor activator of NF-kappa B ligand in the serum and synovial fluid. A comparison of patients with longstanding rheumatoid arthritis and osteoarthritis. Rheumatol Int 2005; 26(1): 63-9.
[http://dx.doi.org/10.1007/s00296-004-0579-1] [PMID: 15889303]

[55]   Kawanaka N, Yamamura M, Aita T, *et al.* CD14+,CD16+ blood monocytes and joint inflammation in rheumatoid arthritis. Arthritis Rheum 2002; 46(10): 2578-86.
[http://dx.doi.org/10.1002/art.10545] [PMID: 12384915]

[56]   Lorenzo J, Horowitz M, Choi Y. Osteoimmunology: interactions of the bone and immune system. Endocr Rev 2008; 29(4): 403-40.
[http://dx.doi.org/10.1210/er.2007-0038] [PMID: 18451259]

[57]   Yao Z, Li P, Zhang Q, *et al.* Tumor necrosis factor-alpha increases circulating osteoclast precursor numbers by promoting their proliferation and differentiation in the bone marrow through up-regulation of c-Fms expression. J Biol Chem 2006; 281(17): 11846-55.
[http://dx.doi.org/10.1074/jbc.M512624200] [PMID: 16461346]

[58]   Zhang Q, Guo R, Schwarz EM, Boyce BF, Xing L. TNF inhibits production of stromal cell-derived factor 1 by bone stromal cells and increases osteoclast precursor mobilization from bone marrow to peripheral blood. Arthritis Res Ther 2008; 10(2): R37.
[http://dx.doi.org/10.1186/ar2391] [PMID: 18371213]

[59]   Melchiorre D, Milia AF, Linari S, *et al.* RANK-RANKL-OPG in hemophilic arthropathy: from clinical and imaging diagnosis to histopathology. J Rheumatol 2012; 39(8): 1678-86.
[http://dx.doi.org/10.3899/jrheum.120370] [PMID: 22753650]

[60]   Gilbert MS. Prophylaxis: musculoskeletal evaluation. Semin Hematol 1993; 30(3) (Suppl. 2): 3-6.
[PMID: 8367740]

[61]   Pettersson H, Ahlberg A, Nilsson IM. A radiologic classification of hemophilic arthropathy. Clin Orthop Relat Res 1980; (149): 153-9.
[PMID: 7408294]

[62]   Melchiorre D, Linari S, Innocenti M, *et al.* Ultrasound detects joint damage and bleeding in haemophilic arthropathy: a proposal of a score. Haemophilia 2011; 17(1): 112-7.
[http://dx.doi.org/10.1111/j.1365-2516.2010.02380.x] [PMID: 21070482]

[63]   Pavlova A, Oldenburg J. Defining severity of hemophilia: more than factor levels. Semin Thromb Hemost 2013; 39(7): 702-10.
[http://dx.doi.org/10.1055/s-0033-1354426] [PMID: 24026911]

[64]   Mannucci PM, Franchini M. Is haemophilia B less severe than haemophilia A? Haemophilia 2013; 19(4): 499-502.
[http://dx.doi.org/10.1111/hae.12133] [PMID: 23517072]

[65]   Tagariello G, Iorio A, Santagostino E, *et al.* Comparison of the rates of joint arthroplasty in patients with severe factor VIII and IX deficiency: an index of different clinical severity of the 2 coagulation disorders. Blood 2009; 114(4): 779-84.
[http://dx.doi.org/10.1182/blood-2009-01-195313] [PMID: 19357395]

[66]   Melchiorre D, Linari S, Manetti M, *et al.* Clinical, instrumental, serological and histological findings suggest that haemophilia B may be less severe than haemophilia A. Haematologica 101: 219-25.2016;

CHAPTER 2

Pharmacokinetic Approach to the Treatment of Haemophilia

Giancarlo Castaman* and Maria Chiara Susini

Center for Bleeding Disorders, Department of Oncology, Azienda Ospedaliero-Universitaria Careggi, Florence, Italy

Abstract: Pharmacokinetic (PK) has improved our knowledge about the most appropriate dosing and timing of administration of FVIII/FIX concentrates in patients with Haemophilia. However, although several studies have recently addressed the relevance of PK of clotting factors, usual practice is still mostly based on empiric approaches since individual PK estimation is difficult to obtain unless the patient is formally enrolled in a study. In fact, several plasma samples collected over several hours and/or days are required to establish a half-life curve confidently and this may be a relevant problem, especially in children. Recently however population PKs has emerged as an important tool to overcome this drawback. Targeted prophylaxis could take advantage of knowing the individual response to factor concentrate administration. On the clinical ground, age and body weight (BW) are roughly used to guide dosing because usually *in vivo* recovery is lower and clearance is faster in children than in adults.

Keywords: Factor VIII, Factor IX, Haemophilia A, Haemophilia B, Pharmacokinetics.

INTRODUCTION

Replacement treatment with clotting factor concentrates (factor VIII – FVIII or factor IX – FIX) has dramatically improved Haemophilia care and prognosis [1]. In conjunction with the evolution of products and therapeutic regimens, the important role of pharmacokinetics (PK) has been also increasingly recognized. Methods for PK evaluation have been developed, progressively becoming more and more accurate. From the 1970s, it has been clearly shown that three times per week treatment was much better than once-weekly for prevention of bleeding [2, 3]. Subsequent careful PK studies showed the benefits of PK plotting and implementation in Haemophilia prophylaxis providing hints to a personalized

---

* **Corresponding author Giancarlo Castaman:** Center for Bleeding Disorders, Department of Oncology, Azienda Ospedaliero-Universitaria Careggi, Florence, Italy; Tel: +39557947587; E-mail: castaman@aou-careggi.toscana.it

prophylaxis in an attempt to strengthen efficacy without increasing the costs [4, 5]. Substitutive treatment for haemophilia is expensive, but inadequate treatment worsens quality of life by increasing morbidity and late sequelae and eventually increasing the associated costs. As in most fields of medical treatment, variability in response among patients is critical and thus tools to optimize clotting factor usage should be always pursued. The required dose should be administered according to the clinical setting (treatment of acute bleeding, surgical prophylaxis or regular prophylaxis), the degree of the factor deficiency, the site and severity of bleeding. On this basis the application of pharmacokinetic analysis would provide the clinicians with more accurate information to tailor patient treatment [6 - 9].

Pharmacokinetics: Basic Principles

The dose–response relationship for a drug is the result of dose, route of administration, patient characteristics and drug exposure that is defined by the PK of the drug. PK evaluates the rate of absorption, distribution, metabolism and excretion of a drug and its metabolite(s), commonly referred to as ADME. It can be broadly termed as what the body does to the drug and is essentially based on measurement of plasma concentrations. Pharmacodynamics (PD) is the other major component of the dose–response relationship and it can be defined as what the drug does to the body, that is the relationship between drug concentration at the site of action and a measurable effect. Jointly, pharmacokinetics and pharmacodynamics determine the necessary dose, dosing intervals and mode of administration [10, 11]. Typically, pharmacokinetic parameters are calculated on measurements of drug concentration serially taken over time or on measurable variations induced by the drug in plasma [6]. For coagulation products, PK differs from that of most pharmaceutical drugs since bioassays of coagulation factors are used to quantify the variation rather than on plasma immunological concentration [12]. Their concentrations in plasma are expressed as level of procoagulant activities of FVIII (FVIII:C) and FIX (FIX:C) in international units (IU) per milliliter or deciliter, rather than in molar units, as direct representations of the drug effects [10, 13].

Definitions and Applications of Pharmacokinetics

The pharmacokinetic parameters or definitions traditionally used in the study of coagulation products are summarized below together with how they are derived from the plasma concentration (or F:C) vs. time curve.

• *In vivo* recovery (IVR)

In vivo recovery (IVR) of a given clotting factor and its biological half-life, have been the standards to compare different clotting factor concentrates [7]. The percentage IVR is the measured peak plasma level relative to the expected peak plasma level, where the latter is defined as the dose divided by the plasma volume of the patient and calculated on either body weight (BW) or plasma volume. Body weight is usually preferred to calculate recovery because of the variability of plasma volume calculations according to the different results obtained with the methods of estimating plasma volume, even in the same patient [6, 12, 14]. Nowadays incremental IVR is usually reported as peak level divided by dose in U/kg.

• Half-life (T½)

It can be loosely defined as the time required for plasma factor level to decrease by half during the elimination phase. Unlike the plasma clearance value, which expresses only the ability of the body to eliminate the drug, half-life expresses the overall rate of elimination process of a given factor concentrate. This overall rate of elimination depends not only on drug clearance but also on the extent of drug distribution.

• Area under the plasma concentration *vs.* time curve (AUC)

AUC (the area under the plasma concentration vs. time curve) is a measure of drug exposure and bioavailability. It is calculated as the product of plasma drug concentration and time. The AUC is used to derive many other pharmacokinetic parameters.

• Maximum plasma concentration (Cmax)

Cmax is the maximum ("peak") plasma concentration of a drug observed after its administration and before administration of a second dose. For an i.v. drug, this is usually assessed on plasma sample(s) taken very close to the end of infusion.

• Clearance (CL)

CL is the ability of the body to eliminate a substance and can be defined as the volume of plasma that is cleared of a drug in 1 min (or 1 hour). For an i.v. drug it is calculated as dose divided by AUC.

• Volume of distribution (V, VD, Vss)

Volume of distribution is the apparent volume in which a drug distributes in the body and it results from the relationship between the amount of drug in the body and the concentration of drug in plasma. Different ways to determine the volume of distribution are used and each may yield a different result, according to the drug. It can be calculated as the initial volume (VdArea), the terminal phase (Vz), or under steady-state conditions (Vss). Vss value is directly proportional to the distribution of the drug outside the plasma compartment.

• Mean residence time (MRT)

Distribution and clearance determine the mean residence time (MRT) of the drug, expressed as Vss divided by CL. After i.v. dosing, each drug molecule spends a different amount of time in the body, with some molecules being quickly eliminated after administration and others lasting longer. MRT describes the average lifetime for all the drug molecules in the body.

Pharmacokinetics parameters are per se useful to evaluate the *in vivo* behavior of FVIII and FIX and their plasma level changes at any time and thus the dosing needed to obtain a predefined target level [13]. In addition the comparison between different preparations of coagulation factors can be based on PKs principles. Vss, CL and MRT are derived from a 'model independent' method because they do not depend on the one- or two-compartment pharmacokinetic model. In such model T½ is determined by curve-fitting while Vss, CL and MRT and IVR are calculated form the data points. Of note, the *in vivo* disappearance of FVIII:C, and especially of FIX:C, shows inner different half-lives, being characterized by an early phase related to distribution and a terminal phase due to elimination. This complicates calculations when comparing factor concentrates with different initial curve shaping or the dosing schedules and it should be emphasized that a few blood sampling, especially within a short period of time, may lead to erroneous PK results. The compartment methods are based on exponential functions which describe the decay of FVIII:C or of FIX:C over time. A simple one-compartment model (the molecule remains in plasma until eliminated from the body) corresponding to the terminal elimination can typically be used for FVIII:C, while for FIX:C bi-exponential functions (corresponding to a two-compartment model) must be used [7, 12, 13].

Pharmacokinetics of Factor VIII

FVIII is a 170-280 kDa protein circulating in plasma bound to the von Willebrand factor (VWF). VWF protects FVIII from early degradation by the activated protein C system and receptor-mediated clearance [13, 15, 16]. Thus, this interaction influences significantly the circulatory half-life of FVIII. In patients with Haemophilia A, infused FVIII rapidly binds to endogenous VWF and only a small fraction of this high molecular weight complex is distributed outside the plasma space. The binding of FVIII to VWF protects FVIII. When FVIII is infused to an adult patient, plasma FVIII:C levels on average rise by 0.020–0.025 U/mL for every U/kg administered [12]. Hence an infusion of 50 U/kg usually leads to a peak plasma level of 1.0-1.3 U/mL when basal FVIII:C is < 0.01 U/mL. The plasma disappearance pattern of FVIII:C is approximately monophasic for plasma derived-FVIII (pd-FVIII) concentrates, while for the recombinant products a biphasic pattern is observed because of a rapid initial fall. The peak value usually occurs 10–15 min after the end of infusion although sometimes it can occur later (within 1-2 hours at latest) [17 - 19]. Typical pharmacokinetic values of FVIII under non-bleeding status in adult patients with Haemophilia A after a single dose of 50 U/kg can be summarized as a peak plasma level of 1.0-1.3 U/mL; a CL of 3 mL/h/kg of body weight (ranging between 1.5 and 6 mL/h/kg); a Vss similar or slightly exceeding the plasma volume (0.04-0.06 L/kg) and an elimination T½ between 8 and 23 h [4, 5, 10, 12, 13, 17, 20 - 24]. In children, T½ is shorter, CL correlates negatively and T½ positively with age [7]. Several factors contribute to the inter-patient variability in haemophilia A, including age, weight, plasma volume, blood group, VWF level, the occurrence of an active bleed, polymorphisms of receptors involved in clearance, and the presence of inhibitors to FVIII [25]. Another source of variability of FVIII kinetics can result from variations in type of preparation, including the presence of other proteins, the size and protein-binding properties of the coagulation factor. There are no major differences between plasma-derived and recombinant FVIII concentrates, apart from long-lasting modified products [13]. These products are mainly on clinical trials, but they will become rapidly available and their PK compared to the "traditional" products. Even among the various recombinant FVIII concentrates PK differences are minor and clinically not significant [7, 26 - 30]. There is some variability in FVIII kinetics correlated to endogenous VWF, even when within the normal range and not only for patients with VWD lacking VWF, as a direct consequence of the VWF stabilizing effects and the mechanisms of clearance of both factors. A significant correlation between pre-infusion VWF levels and T½ was described not only with a B-domain deleted rFVIII, but also with plasma-derived and full-length rFVIII [23, 24, 31]. Furthermore the endogenous increase of VWF in the post-operative period, as a reactive parameter, may hypothetically clear up the lower CL of FVIII observed during continuous infusion after surgery [32, 33]. Blood group could also contribute as a further explanation of VWF levels variability, as persons with blood group O have on average lower levels of VWF [15, 16, 34]. In this regard Vlot *et al.* reported a significantly shorter T½ in patients with blood group 0 than in those with blood group A [35], persisting also when adjusted for VWF levels. On the other hand other studies [31, 36] did not confirm this finding, so this correlation remains more difficult to be ascertained.

Pharmacokinetics of Factor IX

FIX has a lower molecular weight (55 kDa) compared to FVIII and circulates as a free molecule that readily distributes into extravascular spaces. It also binds rapidly and reversibly to the vascular endothelium (collagen IV), unlike the FVIII-VWF large molecular complex that distributes only in a small fraction outside the vascular system. As a consequence, FIX has a much larger initial volume of distribution than FVIII and therefore also lower IVR [12, 37 - 39]. This pattern complicates the correct PK evaluation and interpretation. FIX has a longer half-life in the circulation than FVIII, and therefore PK assessment requires longer sampling schedules [2, 7]. Furthermore, plasma-derived factor IX (pdFIX) and the only available recombinant factor IX (rFIX) show marked differences in post-translational modification of the polypeptide chain, resulting in biochemical dissimilarities which in turn lead to significant differences in the PKs properties with implications for dosing. In particular rFIX shows a higher CL but a similar terminal T1/2 and typical recovery of rFIX is around two-third that of pdFIX. Vss is on average 0.15 L/kg for plasma-derived and 0.20 L/kg for recombinant FIX. After pdFIX infusion in an adult patient, plasma FIX:C on average rises by 0.010–0.014 U/mL for every U/kg administered [13, 40]. Thus an infusion of 50 U/kg will increase FIX to a peak level of 0.5-0.7 U/mL. Interindividual variations in the FIX:C of pdFIX are not completely defined because adequate studies in this regard are rather few. In a large study on rFIX, the CL (L/h) and Vdss (L) showed a positive correlation with body weight up to adolescence while remaining constant during adulthood. On the contrary, if Cl and Vss are normalized by body weight and expressed in terms of ml/h/kg and ml/kg respectively, they are both decreasing during childhood and adolescence [41]. Such correlation was not observed for MRT and T½. A linear correlation between IVR and body weight has also been described with pdFIX, as for FVIII, probably due to the fact that plasma volume as a fraction of body weight tends to decrease with increasing body weight [7, 41, 42].

Population Pharmacokinetics

Population pharmacokinetic is the study of the sources and correlates of variability in drug concentrations among patients belonging to a target patient population [43]. This approach allows the analysis of data from a variety of studies using different designs and not uniform PK analysis. A non-linear mixed-effects modeling approach allows the analysis of data collected under less stringent and restrictive conditions. A standard two-stage approach is used in which a PK model is fitted to each subject's data in the first step and in the second step estimates of population characteristics of each parameter are computed as the empirical mean (arithmetic or geometric) and variance of the individual parameter estimates. Population PK was endorsed by the FDA in USA in 1999 and recommended as guidance for industry when testing new drugs [44]. However, this model has been rarely used in PK assessment of FVIII [20, 36, 45]. To understand the value of population PK, Björkman *et al* used a model to comprehensively evaluate the relationships of the PK of a recombinant FVIII concentrate (Advate®, Baxter AG, Vienna, Austria) with age and body weight in 152 Haemophilia A patients, aged 1-65 years enrolled in 3 different PK trials (46). In 100 adults/adolescents, 184 full PK datasets (10 post-infusion samples) were available, while 52 reduced sample PK datasets (4 post-infusion samples) were available for 52 children 1 to 6 years of age. A wide range of individually estimated body weight-adjusted clearance was observed in adults, ranging from 1.42 to 7.39 ml/hr per kg. The study confirmed that the clearance per kilogram body weight of FVIII declines markedly during growth and slightly during adulthood. Since elimination T½ is inversely related to clearance, it increases according to the age variation. The comparison of the results obtained by population PK *versus* individual PK analysis were remarkably similar, especially in adults, and fitted with the classical mean PK results obtained with FVIII in adult patients [12]. The results of this study are important because they suggest that it is possible to reduce blood sampling in PK studies, decreasing the inconvenience to the patient, especially in case of children, with the discomfort of repeated veni-punctures, and diminishing the cost of assays. By using therapeutic drug monitoring computer programs, individual PK in children and adults can be designed and will need 2 or 3 post-infusion samples, thus facilitating an individually designed treatment schedule. Perhaps, this approach should be considered also in new protocols testing novel FVIII products, which are typically demanding for the patients and the researcher. The observed changes in T½ with age will influence the dose of FVIII required to maintain a desired trough level during prophylaxis, suggesting that the dose of FVIII per kilogram BW required for adequate prophylaxis probably changes throughout a patient's life.

CONCLUDING REMARKS

PKs of FVIII and FIX are gaining wide acceptance among clinicians to guide replacement therapy, especially for prophylactic regimes. The use of population PK methodology may allow to reduce significantly the number of blood sampling, without significantly affect the estimates of the various PK parameters. The use of software with specific programs for calculation will facilitate the implementation of population PK, allowing for repeated testing when needed.

CONFLICT OF INTEREST

The authors confirm that they have no conflict of interest to declare for this publication.

ACKNOWLEDGEMENTS

Declared none.

REFERENCES

[1]   Berntorp E. Factor VIII concentrates. In: Forbes CD, Aledort L, Eds. Hemophilia. London: Chapman & Hall 1997; pp. 181-92.

[2]   Berntorp E, Dolan G, Hermans C, Laffan M, Santagostino E, Tiede A. Pharmacokinetics, phenotype and product choice in haemophilia B: how to strike a balance? Haemophilia 2014; 20 (Suppl. 7): 1-11. [http://dx.doi.org/10.1111/hae.12556] [PMID: 25370925]

[3]   Schimpf K, Fischer B, Rothmann P. Hemophilia A prophylaxis with factor VIII concentrate in a home-treatment program: a controlled study. Scand J Haematol Suppl 1977; 30: 79-80. [PMID: 327532]

[4]   Carlsson M, Berntorp E, Björkman S, Lindvall K. Pharmacokinetic dosing in prophylactic treatment of hemophilia A. Eur J Haematol 1993; 51(4): 247-52. [http://dx.doi.org/10.1111/j.1600-0609.1993.tb00638.x] [PMID: 8243614]

[5]   Collins PW, Fischer K, Morfini M, Blanchette VS, Björkman S. Implications of coagulation factor VIII and IX pharmacokinetics in the prophylactic treatment of haemophilia. Haemophilia 2011; 17(1): 2-10. [http://dx.doi.org/10.1111/j.1365-2516.2010.02370.x] [PMID: 20731726]

[6]   Shapiro AD, Korth-Bradley J, Poon MC. Use of pharmacokinetics in the coagulation factor treatment of patients with haemophilia. Haemophilia 2005; 11(6): 571-82. [http://dx.doi.org/10.1111/j.1365-2516.2005.01149.x] [PMID: 16236106]

[7]   Berntorp E, Björkman S. The pharmacokinetics of clotting factor therapy. Haemophilia 2003; 9(4): 353-9. [http://dx.doi.org/10.1046/j.1365-2516.2003.00762.x] [PMID: 12828668]

[8]   Rickard KA. Guidelines for therapy and optimal dosages of coagulation factors for treatment of bleeding and surgery in haemophilia. Haemophilia 1995; 1 (Suppl. 1): 8-13. [http://dx.doi.org/10.1111/j.1365-2516.1995.tb00104.x] [PMID: 27214734]

[9]   Roberts HR, Eberst ME. Current management of hemophilia B. Hematol Oncol Clin North Am 1993; 7(6): 1269-80. [PMID: 8294316]

[10]   Björkman S, Carlsson M. The pharmacokinetics of factor VIII and factor IX: methodology, pitfalls and applications. Haemophilia 1997; 3(1): 1-8. [http://dx.doi.org/10.1046/j.1365-2516.1997.00074.x] [PMID: 27214611]

[11]   Shargel L, Yu A. Applied Biopharmaceutics and Pharmacokinetics. Stamford, CT, USA: Appleton & Lange 1999.

[12]   Björkman S, Berntorp E. Pharmacokinetics of coagulation factors: clinical relevance for patients with haemophilia. Clin Pharmacokinet 2001; 40(11): 815-32. [http://dx.doi.org/10.2165/00003088-200140110-00003] [PMID: 11735604]

[13]   Björkman S. Pharmacokinetics. In: Berntorpp E, Hoots WK, Eds. Textbook of Hemophilia. 3rd ed. Lee, CA: Wiley Blackwell 2014; pp. 117-22.
[http://dx.doi.org/10.1002/9781118398258.ch16]

[14]   Morfini M, Lee M, Messori A. The design and analysis of half-life and recovery studies for factor VIII and factor IX. Thromb Haemost 1991; 66(3): 384-6.
[PMID: 1746011]

[15]   Terraube V, ODonnell JS, Jenkins PV. Factor VIII and von Willebrand factor interaction: biological, clinical and therapeutic importance. Haemophilia 2010; 16(1): 3-13.
[http://dx.doi.org/10.1111/j.1365-2516.2009.02005.x] [PMID: 19473409]

[16]   Lenting PJ, VAN Schooten CJ, Denis CV. Clearance mechanisms of von Willebrand factor and factor VIII. J Thromb Haemost 2007; 5(7): 1353-60.
[http://dx.doi.org/10.1111/j.1538-7836.2007.02572.x] [PMID: 17425686]

[17]   Björkman S, Carlsson M, Berntorp E, Stenberg P. Pharmacokinetics of factor VIII in humans. Obtaining clinically relevant data from comparative studies. Clin Pharmacokinet 1992; 22(5): 385-95.
[http://dx.doi.org/10.2165/00003088-199222050-00005] [PMID: 1505144]

[18]   Messori A, Longo G, Matucci M, Morfini M, Ferrini PL. Clinical pharmacokinetics of factor VIII in patients with classic haemophilia. Clin Pharmacokinet 1987; 13(6): 365-80.
[http://dx.doi.org/10.2165/00003088-198713060-00002] [PMID: 3125001]

[19]   Allain JP. Principles of in vivo recovery and survival studies of VIII:C. Scand J Haematol Suppl 1984; 41 (Suppl. 41): 123-30.
[PMID: 6440278]

[20]   Björkman S, Blanchette VS, Fischer K, *et al.* Comparative pharmacokinetics of plasma- and albumin-free recombinant factor VIII in children and adults: the influence of blood sampling schedule on observed age-related differences and implications for dose tailoring. J Thromb Haemost 2010; 8(4): 730-6.
[http://dx.doi.org/10.1111/j.1538-7836.2010.03757.x] [PMID: 20398185]

[21]   Björkman S, Oh M, Spotts G, *et al.* Population pharmacokinetics of recombinant factor VIII: the relationships of pharmacokinetics to age and body weight. Blood 2012; 119(2): 612-8.
[http://dx.doi.org/10.1182/blood-2011-07-360594] [PMID: 22042695]

[22]   Collins PW, Björkman S, Fischer K, *et al.* Factor VIII requirement to maintain a target plasma level in the prophylactic treatment of severe hemophilia A: influences of variance in pharmacokinetics and treatment regimens. J Thromb Haemost 2010; 8(2): 269-75.
[http://dx.doi.org/10.1111/j.1538-7836.2009.03703.x] [PMID: 19943875]

[23]   Fijnvandraat K, Peters M, ten Cate JW. Inter-individual variation in half-life of infused recombinant factor VIII is related to pre-infusion von Willebrand factor antigen levels. Br J Haematol 1995; 91(2): 474-6.
[http://dx.doi.org/10.1111/j.1365-2141.1995.tb05325.x] [PMID: 8547097]

[24]   van Dijk K, van der Bom JG, Lenting PJ, *et al.* Factor VIII half-life and clinical phenotype of severe hemophilia A. Haematologica 2005; 90(4): 494-8.
[PMID: 15820945]

[25]   Allain JP, Frommel D. Antibodies to factor VIII. V. Patterns of immune response to factor VIII in hemophilia A. Blood 1976; 47(6): 973-82.
[PMID: 1276479]

[26]   Schwartz RS, Abildgaard CF, Aledort LM, *et al.* Human recombinant DNA-derived antihemophilic factor (factor VIII) in the treatment of hemophilia A. N Eng. J Med 1990; 323: 1800-5.

[27]   Harrison JF, Bloom AL, Abildgaard CF. The pharmacokinetics of recombinant factor VIII. The rFactor VIII Clinical Trial Group. Semin Hematol 1991; 28(2) (Suppl. 1): 29-35.
[PMID: 1908124]

[28]　White GC II, Courter S, Bray GL, Lee M, Gomperts ED. A multicenter study of recombinant factor VIII (Recombinate) in previously treated patients with hemophilia A. Thromb Haemost 1997; 77(4): 660-7.
[PMID: 9134639]

[29]　Morfini M, Longo G, Messori A, Lee M, White G, Mannucci P. Pharmacokinetic properties of recombinant factor VIII compared with a monoclonally purified concentrate (Hemofil M). Thromb Haemost 1992; 68(4): 433-5.
[PMID: 1448776]

[30]　Fijnvandraat K, Berntorp E, ten Cate JW, *et al.* Recombinant, B-domain deleted factor VIII (r-VIII SQ): pharmacokinetics and initial safety aspects in hemophilia A patients. Thromb Haemost 1997; 77(2): 298-302.
[PMID: 9157585]

[31]　Barnes C, Lillicrap D, Pazmino-Canizares J, *et al.* Pharmacokinetics of recombinant factor VIII (Kogenate-FS) in children and causes of inter-patient pharmacokinetic variability. Haemophilia 2006; 12 (Suppl. 4): 40-9.
[http://dx.doi.org/10.1111/j.1365-2516.2006.01333.x]

[32]　Martinowitz U, Schulman S, Gitel S, Horozowski H, Heim M, Varon D. Adjusted dose continuous infusion of factor VIII in patients with haemophilia A. Br J Haematol 1992; 82(4): 729-34.
[http://dx.doi.org/10.1111/j.1365-2141.1992.tb06951.x] [PMID: 1482660]

[33]　Schulman S, Varon D, Keller N, Gitel S, Martinowitz U. Monoclonal purified F VIII for continuous infusion: stability, microbiological safety and clinical experience. Thromb Haemost 1994; 72(3): 403-7.
[PMID: 7855792]

[34]　ODonnell J, Laffan MA. The relationship between ABO histo-blood group, factor VIII and von Willebrand factor. Transfus Med 2001; 11(4): 343-51.
[http://dx.doi.org/10.1046/j.1365-3148.2001.00315.x] [PMID: 11532189]

[35]　Vlot AJ, Mauser-Bunschoten EP, Zarkova AG, *et al.* The half-life of infused factor VIII is shorter in hemophiliac patients with blood group O than in those with blood group A. Thromb Haemost 2000; 83(1): 65-9.
[PMID: 10669157]

[36]　Björkman S, Folkesson A, Jönsson S. Pharmacokinetics and dose requirements of factor VIII over age range 374 years. Eur J Clin Pharmacol 2009; 65: 989-98.
[http://dx.doi.org/10.1007/s00228-009-0676-x] [PMID: 19557401]

[37]　Miller GJ, Howarth DJ, Attfield JC, *et al.* Haemostatic factors in human peripheral afferent lymph. Thromb Haemost 2000; 83(3): 427-32.
[PMID: 10744149]

[38]　Björkman S, Carlsson M, Berntorp E. Pharmacokinetics of factor IX in patients with haemophilia B. Methodological aspects and physiological interpretation. Eur J Clin Pharmacol 1994; 46(4): 325-32.
[http://dx.doi.org/10.1007/BF00194400] [PMID: 7957517]

[39]　Thompson AR. Factor IX concentrates for clinical use. Semin Thromb Hemost 1993; 19(1): 25-36.
[http://dx.doi.org/10.1055/s-2007-994003] [PMID: 8456321]

[40]　Björkman S. A commentary on the differences in pharmacokinetics between recombinant and plasma-derived factor IX and their implications for dosing. Haemophilia 2011; 17(2): 179-84.
[http://dx.doi.org/10.1111/j.1365-2516.2010.02431.x] [PMID: 21299739]

[41]　Björkman S, Shapiro AD, Berntorp E. Pharmacokinetics of recombinant factor IX in relation to age of the patient: implications for dosing in prophylaxis. Haemophilia 2001; 7(2): 133-9.
[http://dx.doi.org/10.1046/j.1365-2516.2001.00465.x] [PMID: 11260271]

[42] White GC, Shapiro AD, Kurczynski EM, *et al.* Variability of *in vivo* recovery of factor IX concentrates in patients with hemophilia B. Thromb Haemost 1995; 73: 779-84. [PMID: 7482403]

[43] Aarons L. Population pharmacokinetics: theory and practice. Br J Clin Pharmacol 1991; 32(6): 669-70. [PMID: 1768557]

[44] FDA. Guidance for industry: population pharmacokinetics , [October 20, 2015]; Available at: http://www.fda.gov/downloads/Drugs/GuidanceComplianceRegulatoryInformation/Guidances/ucm07 2137.pdf

[45] Ruffo S, Messori A, Grasela TH, *et al.* A calculator program for clinical application of the Bayesian method of predicting plasma drug levels. Comput Programs Biomed 1985; 19(2-3): 167-77. [http://dx.doi.org/10.1016/0010-468X(85)90008-X] [PMID: 3928243]

[46] Björkman S, Oh M, Spotts G, *et al.* Population pharmacokinetics of recombinant factor VIII: the relationships of pharmacokinetics to age and body weight. Blood 2012; 119(2): 612-8. [http://dx.doi.org/10.1182/blood-2011-07-360594] [PMID: 22042695]

CHAPTER 3

Haematological Care of the Haemophilic Patient

Giancarlo Castaman[*] and Silvia Linari

Center for Bleeding Disorders and Coagulation, Department of Oncology, AOU Careggi, Florence, Italy

Abstract: Haemophilia A and B are X-linked recessive coagulation disorders resulting from the deficiency or abnormal function of either factor VIII or IX, respectively. Musculoskeletal bleedings, particularly joint bleeding, are the hallmark of severe Haemophilia. Recurrent joint bleedings lead to arthropathy and functional disability. Haemophilia can be treated either on demand to stop bleeding or with prophylaxis to prevent joint damage. A variety of high-quality clotting concentrates are available for patients with Haemophilia and long-acting concentrates are becoming available, with further improvements in the treatment of this potentially disabling disease. Also gene therapy is an impressive promise of cure for the patients, especially those with Haemophilia B. Currently, the development of alloantibodies directed against FVIII or FIX, able to neutralize their clotting activity, and making replacement therapy ineffective represents the most serious challenge of the treatment. A comprehensive care of patients with Haemophilia should be provided by a multidisciplinary team, offering the more appropriate and innovative therapies for Haemophilia and its complications.

Keywords: Factor VIII, Factor IX, Gene therapy, Haemophilia, Haemarthroses, infections, inhibitors, Prophylaxis, Replacement therapy, Target joint.

EPIDEMIOLOGY AND GENETICS

Haemophilia is the epitome of the inherited bleeding disorders, and is caused by the deficiency or functional defect of coagulation factor VIII in Haemophilia A (HA) or factor IX in Haemophilia B (HB). The incidence of HA and HB is respectively one in 5,000-10,000 and one in 30,000 – 50,000 male births regardless of ethnic and racial background [1].

The human *F8* gene comprises 186,000 base pairs while *F9* gene consists of 34,000 base pairs. These genes are located on particularly fragile portions of the X chromosome. The *F8* gene maps to the most distal band Xq28 on the long arm

[*] **Corresponding author Giancarlo Castaman:** Center for Bleeding Disorders and Coagulation, Department of Oncology, AOU Careggi, Florence, Italy; Tel: +39557947587; E-mail: castaman@aou-careggi.toscana.it

of the X chromosome and F9 gene is close to *F8* gene, on the tip of the long arm of the X chromosome at Xq27.1 [2]. Because of its greater size, *F8* gene is more susceptible to mutations resulting in the higher prevalence of HA *versus* HB (4:1).

F8 gene contains 26 exons and 25 introns, usually exon length ranges from 69 to 262 nucleotides apart from exon 14, 3,106 nucleotides long, and the last exon 26, which has 1,958 nucleotides. The spliced FVIII mRNA is approximately 9kb in length and predicts a precursor protein of 2351 amino acids. After removing peptide secretory leader sequence, mature FVIII comprises 2,332 amino acids with the domain structure A1-a1-A2-a2-B-a3-A3C1-C2 [3]. The liver appears to be the primary site of FVIII synthesis, although it is still unclear if the cells producing FVIII are hepatocytes or, more likely, liver sinusoidal endothelial cells [4]. FVIII circulates in plasma non covalently bound to von Willebrand factor (VWF), which represents 99% of the whole mass of the complex. VWF is the plasma carrier of FVIII, protecting it from proteolysis and rapid clearance. Unlike several other coagulation factors, FVIII does not have enzymatic activity, but as cofactor it accelerates the activation of FX by FIXa on a suitable phospholipid surface, thus amplifying coagulation reaction by several folds. Specific proteolytic cleavages between the domains both activate and inactivate the cofactor [5].

F8 gene mutations responsible for HA may be divided classically into several categories: gross gene rearrangements, insertions or deletions ranging from one base pair up to the entire gene, and single DNA base substitutions resulting in either amino acid replacement ("missense"), premature peptide chain termination ("nonsense" or stop mutations) or mRNA splicing defects [6]. At least 45% of severe HA cases are explained by the presence of the inversion of intron 22 in *F8* gene. The inversion occurs by the translocation and exchange of DNA between either of the two nonfunctional FVIII-related genes with intron 22 and areas of homologous DNA within the functional *F8* gene [7]. The recombination produces disjointed and inverted DNA sequences, preventing the transcription of a normal full-length FVIII molecule.

F9 gene contains 8 exons and 7 introns, the spliced FIX mRNA is about 2.8kb length and predicts a single chain glycoprotein of 415 amino acids. FIX is a vitamin-K-dependent coagulation factor; prior its secretion from hepatocytes, FIX undergoes gamma–carboxylation, O- and N-linked glycosylation, phospho-rylation, sulfation, disulfide bond formation, and beta–hydroxylation, as well as cleavage of the signal peptide to propeptide. FIX plays a critical role in blood coagulation. When activated by FXI or FVII, FIX activates FX in presence of Ca^{2+}, membrane phospholipids, and FVIII as a cofactor [8].

Missense mutations are the most frequent cause of *F9* gene mutations in HB patients, but small insertions or deletions have also been identified [9]. As a consequence, frequently these patients have immunologically detectable FIX protein in plasma, but with discrepantly lower FIX activity (Cross-Reactin-
-Material positive, CRM+). Gross genetic abnormalities as complex gene rearrangements or deletions affecting the whole, or a large part, of the gene are much more rare than HA, and account for 7% of HB cases only.

Severity of Haemophilia

Severity of Haemophilia is defined according to the level of clotting factor activity in plasma, as compared to a reference standard that is assumed to have FVIII levels of 100% or to a FVIII activity of 1.0U/mL. The FVIII level in normal population ranges from 50 to 150% (0.50-1.5U/mL). Patients with factor levels <0.01 IU/mL are classified as severe haemophiliacs, those with factor levels between 0.01 and 0.05 IU/mL as moderate and those with >0.05 to 0.4 IU/mL as mild Haemophilia [1]. This classification is in good agreement with the severity and frequency of bleeding symptoms, although some phenotypic heterogeneity can occur [10, 11] (Table **1**).

Table 1. Clinical classification of Haemophilia A and B.

Classification	FVIII or FIX Activity	Clinical Manifestations
Severe	<1% of normal (0.1 U/mL)	Spontaneous hemorrhage from early infancy Frequent spontaneous haemarthroses and hemorrhages, requiring clotting factor replacement
Moderate	1-5% of normal (0.01-0.05 U/mL)	Hemorrhage secondary to trauma or surgery Occasional spontaneous haemarthroses
Mild	>5- 40% of normal (0.05-0.40 U/mL)	Hemorrhage secondary to trauma or surgery Rare spontaneous haemarthroses

Clinical Manifestations

Historically, severe HA and HB have been considered clinically indistinguishable, with musculoskeletal bleedings, particularly in joints, as hallmark of a severe Haemophilia. Recent evidences, however, suggest that patients with severe HB may have a less severe bleeding phenotype, a lower bleeding frequency and better long-term outcomes, compared to severe HA patients [12].

Repeated haemarthroses result in chronic, crippling haemophilic arthropathy. In decreasing incidence, the most commonly involved joints are knees, elbows, ankles, shoulders, wrists, and hips [13]. The first sign of a joint bleeding is a sensation of intraarticular burning, followed by fullness, tightness, swelling, and increasing pain leading to limitation of motion. Involuntary muscle splinting due to pain induces joint immobilization and initiates a vicious cycle of atrophy and contracture. Recurrent haemarthroses result in deposition of haemosiderin, which contributes to the synovial inflammation and increased vascularity, predisposing to further bleedings. Joints with a chronically inflamed and hypertrophic synovium are referred to as "target joints", and are susceptible to recurrent bleedings unless treated [14]. Intramuscular haemorrhages are the second most common sites of bleedings in HA and HB. The site of bleeding determines the actual risk of long-term disabilities. Haemorrhages into large muscles, though extensive, generally may resolve without complications, as they are not confined. Bleeding into a closed fascial compartment can lead to compression of vital structures, resulting in a compartment syndrome characterized by ischemia, gangrene, flexion contractures, and neuropathy. Bleeding into the iliopsoas muscles and retroperitoneal space is associated with a sudden onset of inguinal pain and decreased range of motion of the ipsilateral hip, which assumes a flexed position, usually with external lateral rotation. Bleeding can be life-threatening when a large volume of blood is lost and it is not appropriately treated. In addition, femoral nerve compression can occur with permanent disability if a compartment syndrome develops. In 1-2% of patients with severe HA and HB pseudotumors may develop, that are cystic lesions in the subperiosteal area of bone or in soft tissues, produced by repetitive bleedings with enlargement and encapsulation. Pseudotumors are composed of old clots and necrotic tissues, arising after inadequate treatments. Symptoms associated with expanding pseudotumors are related to the size of the mass and the degree of damage of the integrity of the structure they are invading. Spontaneous gross haematuria can occur frequently in patients with Haemophilia and is usually painless unless intraureteral clots develop. Haematuria can be precipitated by the use of drugs, trauma or physical exercises. Often the causes of hematuria remain and no anatomical lesions are detected. Haematuria is sometimes self-limited to few days, but it may be unresponsive to replacement therapy and may recovers spontaneously. Gastrointestinal bleedings occur in 10-15% of adult haemophiliacs and anatomic lesions are frequently observed. In patients with chronic hepatitis C and cirrhosis, varices as result of portal hypertension are the leading cause of acute bleeds. Intracranial haemorrhage is the most common cause of death from bleeding in HA and HB and it can occur after a minor trauma, particularly in children, or even spontaneously. Fifty percent of patients with intracranial haemorrhage have neurological sequelae, and 30% events results in death.

Therapeutic Modalities for Haemophilia A and B

Haemophilia treatment centers (HTCs) provide comprehensive medical and psychosocial assistance to patients with inherited bleeding disorders. HTCs, consisting of multidisciplinary teams, offer to patients with Haemophilia and its complications the more appropriate and innovative treatments. In Italy only HTCs recognized at a regional level can prescribe replacement products, on the basis of individual therapeutic plans.

Clotting Factor Replacement Therapy with Coagulation Factor Concentrates

Replacement of FVIII or FIX to haemostatically adequate circulating levels for prevention or treatment of acute bleeding is the basis of the management of Haemophilia. This treatment should be administered at early onset of symptoms to limit the amount of bleeding and to prevent long-term disability. Replacement therapy should also be given immediately before surgery to prevent intraoperative bleeding complications or prophylactically to prevent chronic event arthropathy [15]. Primary prophylaxis, that is the regular continuous treatment initiated in the absence of documented osteochondral joint disease and started before the second clinically evident large joint bleed and age 3 years [16], actually represents a primary goal of FVIII and FIX replacement therapy. Primary prophylaxis is the regimen of choice for treatment of children with severe Haemophilia, with the aim of achieving FVIII and FIX levels always >1-2 IU/dL with infusion of 25-40 IU/kg concentrates twice-thrice weekly on non-consecutive days, or every other day.

FVIII and FIX replacement products may be either plasma derived or produced with recombinant DNA technology. Factor replacement products are classified based on their final purity, defined as specific activity (International Units of clotting factor activity/mg of protein). Intermediate purity products have relatively low specific activities (less than 50U/mg) because they usually contain additional plasma proteins; high-purity (more than 50U/mg) and ultra-high-purity (more than 3000U/mg for FVIII concentrates; more than 160 U/mg for FIX concentrates) products contain little or no contaminating plasma proteins other than albumin as a stabilizer. The first-generation rFVIII proteins were stabilized with bovine or human serum albumin (HSA) either in preparation or in final formulation. Thus, in second-generation therapies HSA in the final formulation has been replaced by non-protein stabilizers and third-generation products lack added bovine and/or human protein in either the cell culture procedure or in the final formulation. Albumin-free formulations of recombinant "full-length" and B-domain deleted or truncated FVIII concentrates are available. Monoclonal antibody-purified, plasma-derived FIX concentrate and recombinant FIX concentrate are free of albumin (Table **2a** and **2b**).

Table 2a. Plasma-derived and recombinant FVIII concentrates available in Italy.

Plasma-Derived FVIII Concentrates			
Drug & Company	Fractionation	Viral Inactivation	Activity IU/mg of total protein
Alphanate Grifols	Precipitation/heparin ligand chromatography	SD (TNBP/Tween80) + dry heat 80°C, 72 h	100
Beriate P CSL Behring	Ion exchange chromatography	Pasteurization at 60°, 10 h	170
Klott Kedrion	Ion exchange chromatography	SD (TNBP/Tween80) + dry heat 100°C,30 min	>80
Fandhi Grifols	Precipitation/heparin ligand chromatography	SD (TNBP/Tween80) + dry heat 80°C, 72 h	100
Octanate Octapharma	Adsorption on aluminum hydroxide gel, ion exchange chromatography, filtration	SD (TNBP/Tween80) + dry heat 100°C,30 min	>100
Haemate P CSL Behring	Multiple precipitation	Pasteurization at 60°, 10 h	38
Haemoctin Biotest AG	Precipitation on aluminum hydroxide gel, anion exchange chromatography	SD (TNBP/Tween80) + dry heat 100°C, 30min	103.5
Talate Baxalta	Ion exchange chromatography	Detergent (Polysorbate 80) + vapour heat 60°, 10h	70
Wilate Octapharma	Precipitation on aluminium hydroxide gel, ion exchange chromatography, size exclusion chromatography	SD (TNBP/Octoxynol) + dry heat 100°C, 2h	>100
Recombinant FVIII Concentrates			
Drug & Company	Fractionation	Viral Inactivation	Activity IU/mg of total protein
Kogenate Bayer Bayer	Ion exchange chromatography, MoAb affinity chromatography, metal chelate affinity chromatography, cationic exchange chromatography	SD (TNBP/Polysorbate 80)	2,600-2,800
Helixate NexGen CSL Behring	Ion exchange chromatography, MoAb affinity chromatography, metal chelate affinity chromatography, cationic exchange chromatography	SD (TNBP/Polysorbate 80)	2,600-2,800
Advate Baxalta	MoAb affinity chromatography, ion exchange chromatography	SD (TNBP/Triton X-100/Polysorbate 80)	4,000-10,000

(Table 2a) contd.....

Plasma-Derived FVIII Concentrates			
Refacto AF Pfizer	Ion exchange chromatography, hydrophobic interaction chromatography, size exclusion chromatography, affinity chromatography with a synthetic peptide (27 amino acids)	SD (TNBP/Triton X-100), nanofiltration (35 nm pore size filter)	7,600-13,800
NovoEight Novo Nordisk	Immunoaffinity chromatography with monoclonal F25 antibody against the integral A2 domain, Ion exchange chromatography, gel filtration	SD, nanofiltration (20 nm pore size filter)	8,300
Nuwiq Octapharma	Multimodal cation exchange chromatography, VIII select affinity chromatography, anion exchange chromatography, size exclusion chromatography	SD, nanofiltration (20 nm pore size filter)	9,500

Table 2b. Plasma-derived and recombinant FIX concentrates available in Italy.

Plasma-Derived FIX Concentrates			
Drug & Company	Fractionation	Viral Inactivation	Activity IU/mg of total protein
Ixed Kedrion	Ion exchange chromatography, heparin affinity chromatography, filtration	SD (TNBP/Tween80) + dry heat 100°C, 30 min	100
AlphaNine Grifols	Ion exchange chromatography, dual polysaccharide ligand chromatography	SD + nanofiltration (15 nm pore size filter)	>210
FIXNOVE Baxalta	Ion exchange chromatography, hydrophobic interaction chromatography	Detergent (Polysorbate 80) + vapour heat, 60° 10 h, 190 mbar + 80°C, 1 h, 375 mbar	100
Haemobionine Biotest	Anion exchange chromatography, MoAb affinity chromatography, hydrophobic interaction chromatography	SD (TNBP/ Polysorbate 80) + nanofiltration (15 nm pore size filter)	>100
Octanine Octapharma	Ion exchange chromatography, heparin affinity chromatography, ultrafiltration/diafiltration	SD (TNBP/ Polysorbate 80) + nanofiltration	>100
Mononine CSL Behring	MoAb affinity chromatography	Sodium thiocyanate + ultrafiltration (35 nm pore size filter)	>190
Recombinant FIX Concentrates			
Benefix Pfizer	Ion exchange chromatography, metal chelate affinity chromatography	Nanofiltration (20 nm pore size filter)	>200

All coagulation factor concentrates are subjected to different methods of viral inactivation, attenuation or elimination. This is because until the 1985, the infusion of non-virally inactivated products from single donor and plasma derived concentrates obtained from pools of thousand donors transmitted hepatitis viruses B and C (HBV, HCV) to more than 90% of patients treated with replacement therapy worldwide [17]. The epidemic spread of human immunodeficiency virus (HIV) infection affected about 30 and 70% of HA and HB patients respectively [18]. Several factors actually contribute to the viral safety of plasma derived factor concentrates, including the quarantine of plasma units used for industrial fractionation and the introduction of nucleic acid amplification testing for five viruses (HIV 1-2, HBV, HCV, hepatitis A virus and parvovirus B19) and viral inactivation techniques as dry heating, pasteurisation, vapour and solvent/detergent procedures, ultrafiltration and nanofiltration steps. Actually both plasma-derived and recombinant concentrates have a very good safety profile. The main advantage of recombinant products are viral safety, independence from plasma supply, and very small volumes. All of the commercially available FVIII concentrates appear to be equally efficacious and the choice of type of clotting factor concentrate to administer should be individualized, considering age of patient, presence HIV and HCV status and costs. According to the Italian Association of Haemophilia Centres (AICE, Associazione Italiana Centri Emofilia) recommendations [19], recombinant concentrates are the products of choice for previously untreated patients (PUPs), minimally treated patients, and those exclusively exposed to recombinant concentrates. Also in HIV-positive patients with clinical signs of immune deficiency and in patients who have not been infected by HCV or who have cleared the virus, recombinant concentrates are the treatment of choice.

The dosing of clotting factor replacement therapy in Haemophilia is based on several factors: age, patient's plasma volume, distribution of the clotting protein between the intravascular and extravascular compartments, circulating half-life of the clotting factor in the plasma, and level of activity required to achieve adequate haemostasis or prophylaxis. Dosages are calculated by assuming that 1 U/kg body weight of FVIII replacement will raise the plasma activity of FVIII by approximately 0.02 U/ml (2%), and 1U/kg of FIX concentrate, which has a larger volume of distribution, will increase plasma FIX levels by 0.01U/mL (1%). The circulating half-life for FVIII is 8 to 12 hours, and for FIX is around 18 hours. Optimal haemostatic plasma levels for FVIII and FIX depends on the clinical situation (Table **3**).

Table 3. Recommended plasma factor peak levels and duration of administrations of FVIII and FIX.

Clinical Condition	HA FVIII Desired Level (%)	HB FIX Desired Level (%)	Treatment Duration (days)
Mild/moderate haemarthroses or haematomas	40-60	40-60	1-2, longer if inadequate response
Severe haemarthroses or haematomas *Initial treatment* *Maintenance*	80-100 30-60	60-80 30-60	1-2 5-7, sometimes longer as secondary prophylaxis during physiotherapy
Central nervous system/spinal cord haemorrhage Gastrointestinal haemorrhage Throat/neck *Initial treatment* *Maintenance*	80-100 50	60-80 30	1-7 8-21
Renal haemorrhage	50	40	5-7
Moderate head injury Severe head injury	30-50 50-100	40-60 50-100	2-5 2-5
Major surgery *Pre-op* *Post-op*	80-100 60-80 40-60 30-50	60-80 40-60 30-50 20-40	1-3 4-6 7-14
Minor surgery *Pre-op* *Post-op*	50-80 30-80	50-80 30-80	1-5, depending on the type of procedure

The most serious complication of treatment with coagulation factor concentrates in Haemophilia is actually the development of alloantibodies (inhibitors) directed against FVIII or FIX, able to neutralize their clotting activity. Inhibitors makes replacement therapy ineffective, preventing patients from receiving long-term prophylaxis and exposing them to an increase risk of mortality, morbidity, and disability. Inhibitors are much less frequently encountered in HB, occurring in less than 5% of patients, but in about half of them severe allergic reactions in association with treatment further complicate the therapeutic management [1]. The cumulative incidence of inhibitor development in severe HA is in the range of 20-30% and approximately 5-10% in moderate or mild disease, usually within the first 10-15 days of exposure [20]. The inhibitor risk is significantly reduced in patients exposed to FVIII for more than 50-150 days. Several metanalysis failed to demonstrate a significant difference of inhibitor occurrence in patients treated with recombinant FVIII compared to plasmaderived products. However, very recently it has been demonstrated in a randomized prospective study that the use of recombinant products in previously untreated patients is associated with a 1.8 greater risk of inhibitor development compared to plasma-derived products [21].The pathogenesis of inhibitors is multifactorial and not fully understood, several risk factors have been identified [22, 23].Treatment of patients with inhibitors may be difficult and management of bleeding must be in consultation with an experienced center. The choice of treatment product should be based on titer of inhibitors. Patients with a low-responding inhibitor (<5 Bethesda Units) may be still treated with factor replacement at much higher doses, to neutralize the antibody and stop bleeding. On the other hand, patients with high-responding inhibitors (>5 Bethesda Units) accompanied by brisk anamnesis have to be treated with bypassing agents such as recombinant activated factor VII (rFVIIa) or activated prothrombin complex concentrates (aPCC)(Table **4**) [24, 25]. In addition to the treatment of bleeding episodes in patients with inhibitor, eradication of inhibitors by immune tolerance induction (ITI) therapy should be the primary aim in patients with a high-responding inhibitor, to restore the efficacy of FVIII replacement treatment [26]. The main candidates for ITI are children with recent onset high-responding inhibitors, when titers <10 Bethesda Units/mL are measured.

Table 4. Efficacy of treatment of bleeding in patients with inhibitor with by-passing agents.

Treatment	Effective Bleed Resolution
	% of bleeds not needing rescue medication at 9 hours
rFVIIa: 90 µg/kg x 3 every 3 hours	90.9%
rFVIIa: 270 µg/kg x 1	91.7%
pd-aPCC: 75IU/kg x 1	63.6%
	Effective or partially effective at 6 hours and 12 hours
rFVIIa: 90-120 µg/kg x 2 every 2 hours	78.7% and 84.4%
pd-aPCC: 75-100IU/kg x1	80.9% and 80.0%

An important role in the management of responsive patients with mild/moderate HA is played by DDAVP (1-deamino-8-D-arginine-vasopressin), that is an analog of the antidiuretic hormone vasopressin, V2 agonist [27]. The drug is free of risk of viral transmission and inexpensive. DDAVP produces a rise in circulating FVIII and VWF protein levels by 3-or 5-fold over the patient's native level by causing a release of FVIII/VWF from the storage sites in the vascular endothelial cells. DDAVP can be administered intravenously, subcutaneously, or intranasally. The recommended dosages are 0.3 µg/kg by slow intravenous infusion or subcutaneous injection, and fixed doses of 300 µg in adults and 150 µg in children by intranasal spray. The peak effect of intravenous infusion or subcutaneous injection is seen after 30-60 minutes, while the intranasal administration peaks in 60-90 minutes. Thus, DDAVP can be given in advance to surgical procedures, or at the time of acute spontaneous or traumatic bleeding events. DDAVP can be administered every 12 to 24 hours; however, tachyphylaxis often develops because of the depletion of FVIII/VWF from the storages. Common side effects include flushing, hypertension, and retention of free water that can induce hyponatremia, especially in infants and the elderly, and precipitate the onset of seizures. Therefore, free-water fluid intake should be restricted and serum sodium levels monitored in these subjects. There are occasional reports of arterial thrombosis during treatment, so that DDAVP should be avoided in patients with overt cardiovascular disease. Treatment with DDAVP is usually administered in association with antifibrinolytic agents. Antifibrinolytic agents are useful in the management of mucocutaneous bleeding from the gastrointestinal tract, oropharynx and nose in patients with HA and HB. Antifibrinolytics can maintain the integrity of the clot and prevent haemorrhage, by inhibiting the fibrinolysis of the thrombus by plasmin. Tranexamic acid and epsilon-aminocaproic acid can be administered intravenously, orally, or topically. These medications can be used alone or in association with coagulation factor concentrates or DDAVP for the prevention or control of bleeding. The optimum dose and duration is not well defined but tranexamic acid is dosed at 1 - 1.5 g every 8 hours for 3 to 6 days and epsilon–aminocaproic acid is given at a dose of 50mg/kg every 6 hours for 3 to 10 days. Their use during surgery is still debated, but their use tends to increase. As ancillary treatment, fibrin glues can be useful, being composed of thrombin, fibrinogen, and sometimes FXIII and antifibrinolytic agents. The major benefit are obtained when the fibrin glues are combined with continuous or bolus infusions of factor concentrate, in particular in oral surgery.

Long-acting Concentrates

New clotting factor concentrates are becoming available or are in advanced clinical studies that will significantly improve the treatment of patients with HA or HB. Different technologies are applied to extend half-life and/or allow for alternative routes of administration, as subcutaneous route. The conjugation with polyethylene glycol and the production by genetic engineering of fusion proteins containing the FVIII and FIX linked to a long-lived plasma protein such as albumin or the Fc fragment of immunoglobulin G (IgG) represent the most used strategies (Table **5**).

The results obtained with these novel rFIX concentrates are impressive with a significant half-life extension to up to 100 hours (up to 5-fold longer), allowing substitution intervals of 1-2 weeks. Due to its greater size and the dependence of the pharmacokinetics of infused FVIII on patient's endogenous vWF, the effect for rFVIII products so far is only small, as the half-life extension is limited to about 15-18 hours, approximately 1.5 fold longer [28].

Table 5. Long-acting FVIII and FIX products.

Drug Name	Description	Company	Status
rFIXFc	rFIX Fc fusion	Biogen Idec/SOBI	Approved
NN-7999	GlycoPEGylated FIX	Novo Nordisk	Phase 3 Clinical
CSL-654	rFIX albumin fusion	CSL Behring	Approved
rFVIIIFc	rFVIII Fc fusion	Biogen Idec/SOBI	Approved
BAY-94-9027	PEGylated FVIII	Bayer	Phase 3 Clinical
NN-7088	GlycoPEGylated FVIII	Novo Nordisk	Phase 3 Clinical
BAX855	PEGylated FVIII	Baxalta	Phase 3 Clinical

Expressing rFVIII in a single-chain form and from a human cell line result in molecules with a higher affinity for vWF and may enhance both pharmacokinetic and the immunogenic profile of FVIII. Long-acting coagulation factors have the potential to change current paradigms of care for HA and HB. Less frequent infusions may provide prolonged protection from bleeding and bleed resolution with fewer injections.

Gene Therapy

Since the isolation and characterization of the genes for FVIII and FIX, a long-standing goal has been development of successful gene therapy for HA and HB. Gene therapy offers a potential cure, with the possible continuous expression of a clotting factor gene following the administration of a viral vector carrying that gene. Hepatocytes, skeletal muscle cells and haemopoietic stem cells have been shown to be capable of maintaining stable clotting factor expression levels. Moreover, they are suitable target cells for gene therapy, but the gene delivery vector has been the problem of such approach. Optimal characteristics for a viral vector are the non-pathogenicity, the non-influence on innate immunity, the low prevalence of specific antibodies in HA or HB, the non-integration into host chromosomal DNA, the high replicative tendency, and the efficient transduction of target cells. Adeno-associated virus (AAV) based vectors have been shown to produce long-term expression of FIX levels. A single intravenous infusion of AAV8 vector encoding FIX under the control of a liver-restricted promoter has resulted in a dose-dependent expression of FIX at plateau levels ranging from 1% to 6%, over a median period of 3.2 years in 10 adult males with severe HB. Thus, at present, the possibility to change severe Haemophilia phenotype to a moderate one (and rarely mild) is a promising perspective for HB. This resulted in a reduction of more than 90% in both bleeding episodes and the consumption of prophylactic FIX concentrates [29].There are currently three ongoing trials of AAV-mediated gene transfer in HB all aiming to express the FIX gene from the liver. For HA the road is even more complicated and winding: generating AAV-FVIII is very challenging and currently none of the five approved human trials on gene therapy has progressed beyond phase I [30].

Haemophilia and Orthopaedic Surgery

Haemophilia care has steadily improved over the years, however there is still a group of young adults who have a severe degree of joint destruction and significant functional disability as a result of repeated articular bleeding episodes during their early years. Severe arthropathy in one or more susceptible joints (knee, elbow, ankle, hip, and shoulder) can be definitively addressed only with orthopedic surgery. Synovectomy, arthroscopy, and joint fusion have been some of the surgeries performed on haemophiliacs with acceptable outcomes in the past. However, total joint replacement is the treatment that transformed the quality of life of haemophilic patients, with significant reduction in pain and in spontaneous haemarthrosis, as improvements in measurable outcome parameters. Total joint replacement, managed in a comprehensive HTC, with the close cooperation between haematologists and orthopaedic surgeons, is a safe and effective procedure for the management of severe arthropathy to rehabilitate the patient. An accurate and timely administered factor replacement before and after surgery, an adequate hospital stay, and tailored rehabilitation protocols are required for the successful outcome of surgery when total knee [31], elbow, ankle, hip [32], or shoulder replacements are performed. Joint replacements have been successfully performed in haemophilic patients with HIV infection or those with high-responding inhibitors. In the first case, adequate antibiotic prophylaxis is mandatory; in the other, continuous infusion of rFVIIa has been demonstrated to provide stable and safe hemostatic coverage [33, 34]. Therefore also in patients with comorbidity or complications orthopedic surgery may be proposed to improve the quality of life in severe arthropathy.

CONFLICT OF INTEREST

The authors confirm that they have no conflict of interest to declare for this publication.

ACKNOWLEDGEMENTS

Declared none.

REFERENCES

[1] Bolton-Maggs PH, Pasi KJ. Haemophilias A and B. Lancet 2003; 361(9371): 1801-9.
[http://dx.doi.org/10.1016/S0140-6736(03)13405-8] [PMID: 12781551]

[2] Camerino G, Grzeschik KH, Jaye M, *et al.* Regional localization on the human X chromosome and polymorphism of the coagulation factor IX gene (hemophilia B locus). Proc Natl Acad Sci USA 1984; 81(2): 498-502.
[http://dx.doi.org/10.1073/pnas.81.2.498] [PMID: 6320191]

[3] Gitschier J, Wood WI, Goralka TM, *et al.* Characterization of the human factor VIII gene. Nature 1984; 312(5992): 326-30.
[http://dx.doi.org/10.1038/312326a0] [PMID: 6438525]

[4] Shahani T, Covens K, Lavendhomme R, *et al.* Human liver sinusoidal endothelial cells but not hepatocytes contain factor VIII. J Thromb Haemost 2014; 12(1): 36-42.
[http://dx.doi.org/10.1111/jth.12412] [PMID: 24118899]

[5] Eaton D, Rodriguez H, Vehar GA. Proteolytic processing of human factor VIII. Correlation of specific cleavages by thrombin, factor Xa, and activated protein C with activation and inactivation of factor VIII coagulant activity. Biochemistry 1986; 25(2): 505-12.
[http://dx.doi.org/10.1021/bi00350a035] [PMID: 3082357]

[6] F8 HAMSTeRS mutation database. Available at: http://europium.csc.mrc.ac.uk

[7] Antonarakis SE, Rossiter JP, Young M, *et al.* Factor VIII gene inversions in severe hemophilia A: results of an international consortium study. Blood 1995; 86(6): 2206-12.
[PMID: 7662970]

[8] Autin L, Miteva MA, Lee WH, Mertens K, Radtke KP, Villoutreix BO. Molecular models of the procoagulant factor VIIIa-factor IXa complex. J Thromb Haemost 2005; 3(9): 2044-56.
[http://dx.doi.org/10.1111/j.1538-7836.2005.01527.x] [PMID: 16102111]

[9] F9 mutation database. Available at: http://www.kcl.ac.uk/ip/petergreen/haemB-database.html

[10] Jayandharan GR, Srivastava A. The phenotypic heterogeneity of severe hemophilia. Semin Thromb Hemost 2008; 34(1): 128-41.
[http://dx.doi.org/10.1055/s-2008-1066024] [PMID: 18393149]

[11] Pavlova A, Oldenburg J. Defining severity of hemophilia: more than factor levels. Semin Thromb Hemost 2013; 39(7): 702-10.
[http://dx.doi.org/10.1055/s-0033-1354426] [PMID: 24026911]

[12] Melchiorre D, Linari S, Manetti M, *et al.* Clinical, instrumental, serological and histological findings suggest that hemophilia B may be less severe than hemophilia A. Hematologica 2016; 101(2): 219-5.

[13] Arnold WD, Hilgartner MW. Hemophilic arthropathy. Current concepts of pathogenesis and management. J Bone Joint Surg Am 1977; 59(3): 287-305.
[http://dx.doi.org/10.2106/00004623-197759030-00001] [PMID: 849938]

[14] Melchiorre D, Milia AF, Linari S, *et al.* RANK-RANKL-OPG in hemophilic arthropathy: from clinical and imaging diagnosis to histopathology. J Rheumatol 2012; 39(8): 1678-86.
[http://dx.doi.org/10.3899/jrheum.120370] [PMID: 22753650]

[15] Manco-Johnson MJ, Abshire TC, Shapiro AD, *et al.* Prophylaxis versus episodic treatment to prevent joint disease in boys with severe hemophilia. N Engl J Med 2007; 357(6): 535-44.
[http://dx.doi.org/10.1056/NEJMoa067659] [PMID: 17687129]

[16] Srivastava A, Brewer AK, Mauser-Bunschoten EP, *et al.* Treatment Guidelines Working Group on Behalf of The World Federation Of Hemophilia. Guidelines for the management of hemophilia. Haemophilia 2013; 19(1): e1-e47.
[http://dx.doi.org/10.1111/j.1365-2516.2012.02909.x] [PMID: 22776238]

[17]   Goedert JJ, Chen BE, Preiss L, Aledort LM, Rosenberg PS. Reconstruction of the hepatitis C virus epidemic in the US hemophilia population, 19401990. Am J Epidemiol 2007; 165(12): 1443-53.
[http://dx.doi.org/10.1093/aje/kwm030] [PMID: 17379617]

[18]   Ragni MV, Tegtmeier GE, Levy JA, *et al.* AIDS retrovirus antibodies in hemophiliacs treated with factor VIII or factor IX concentrates, cryoprecipitate, or fresh frozen plasma: prevalence, seroconversion rate, and clinical correlations. Blood 1986; 67(3): 592-5.
[PMID: 3081062]

[19]   Rocino A, Coppola A, Franchini M, *et al.* Italian Association of Haemophilia Centres (AICE) Working Party. Principles of treatment and update of recommendations for the management of haemophilia and congenital bleeding disorders in Italy. Blood Transfus 2014; 12(4): 575-98.
[PMID: 25350962]

[20]   Astermark J, Altisent C, Batorova A, *et al.* European Haemophilia Therapy Standardisation Board. Non-genetic risk factors and the development of inhibitors in haemophilia: a comprehensive review and consensus report. Haemophilia 2010; 16(5): 747-66.
[http://dx.doi.org/10.1111/j.1365-2516.2010.02231.x] [PMID: 20398077]

[21]   Peyvandi F, Mannucci PM, Garagiola I, *et al.* A Randomized Trial of Factor VIII and Neutralizing Antibodies in Hemophilia A. N Engl J Med 2016; 374(21): 2054-64.
[http://dx.doi.org/10.1056/NEJMoa1516437] [PMID: 27223147]

[22]   Astermark J. Inhibitor development: patient-determined risk factors. Haemophilia 2010; 16(102): 66-70.
[http://dx.doi.org/10.1111/j.1365-2516.2008.01923.x] [PMID: 19298384]

[23]   Santagostino E, Mancuso ME, Rocino A, *et al.* Environmental risk factors for inhibitor development in children with haemophilia A: a case-control study. Br J Haematol 2005; 130(3): 422-7.
[http://dx.doi.org/10.1111/j.1365-2141.2005.05605.x] [PMID: 16042693]

[24]   Young G, Shafer FE, Rojas P, Seremetis S. Single 270 microg kg(-1)-dose rFVIIa vs. standard 90 microg kg(-1)-dose rFVIIa and APCC for home treatment of joint bleeds in haemophilia patients with inhibitors: a randomized comparison. Haemophilia 2008; 14(2): 287-94.
[http://dx.doi.org/10.1111/j.1365-2516.2007.01601.x] [PMID: 18081834]

[25]   Astermark J, Donfield SM, DiMichele DM, *et al.* FENOC Study Group. A randomized comparison of bypassing agents in hemophilia complicated by an inhibitor: the FEIBA NovoSeven Comparative (FENOC) Study. Blood 2007; 109(2): 546-51.
[http://dx.doi.org/10.1182/blood-2006-04-017988] [PMID: 16990605]

[26]   Oldenburg J, Austin SK, Kessler CM. ITI choice for the optimal management of inhibitor patients - from a clinical and pharmacoeconomic perspective. Haemophilia 2014; 20 (Suppl. 6): 17-26.
[http://dx.doi.org/10.1111/hae.12466] [PMID: 24975701]

[27]   Castaman G. Desmopressin for the treatment of haemophilia. Haemophilia 2008; 14 (Suppl. 1): 15-20.
[http://dx.doi.org/10.1111/j.1365-2516.2007.01606.x] [PMID: 18173690]

[28]   Oldenburg J, Albert T. Novel products for haemostasis - current status. Haemophilia 2014; 20 (Suppl. 4): 23-8.
[http://dx.doi.org/10.1111/hae.12428] [PMID: 24762271]

[29]   Nathwani AC, Reiss UM, Tuddenham EG, *et al.* Long-term safety and efficacy of factor IX gene therapy in hemophilia B. N Engl J Med 2014; 371(21): 1994-2004.
[http://dx.doi.org/10.1056/NEJMoa1407309] [PMID: 25409372]

[30]   High KH, Nathwani A, Spencer T, Lillicrap D. Current status of haemophilia gene therapy. Haemophilia 2014; 20 (Suppl. 4): 43-9.
[http://dx.doi.org/10.1111/hae.12411] [PMID: 24762274]

[31]   Innocenti M, Civinini R, Carulli C, Villano M, Linari S, Morfini M. A modular total knee arthroplasty in haemophilic arthropathy. Knee 2007; 14(4): 264-8.
[http://dx.doi.org/10.1016/j.knee.2007.05.001] [PMID: 17601738]

[32]   Carulli C, Felici I, Martini C, *et al.* Total hip arthroplasty in haemophilic patients with modern cementless implants. J Arthroplasty 2015; 30(10): 1757-60.
[http://dx.doi.org/10.1016/j.arth.2015.04.035] [PMID: 25998131]

[33]   Valentino LA, Cooper DL, Goldstein B. Surgical experience with rFVIIa (NovoSeven) in congenital haemophilia A and B patients with inhibitors to factors VIII or IX. Haemophilia 2011; 17(4): 579-89.
[http://dx.doi.org/10.1111/j.1365-2516.2010.02460.x] [PMID: 21294815]

[34]   Caviglia H, Candela M, Galatro G, Neme D, Moretti N, Bianco RP. Elective orthopaedic surgery for haemophilia patients with inhibitors: single centre experience of 40 procedures and review of the literature. Haemophilia 2011; 17(6): 910-9.
[http://dx.doi.org/10.1111/j.1365-2516.2011.02504.x] [PMID: 21342367]

CHAPTER 4

Laboratory Aspects

Enrichetta Paladino[1,*], Maria Chiara Susini[1], Giuseppe Mazza[2], Paolo Quaglierini[3] and Giancarlo Castaman[1]

[1] *Center for Bleeding Disorders, Department of Oncology, AOU Careggi, Florence, Italy*

[2] *University College of London, Institute for Liver and Digestive Health, London, UK*

[3] *University of Florence, Florence, Italy*

Abstract: The haemostatic process is characterized by a series of biochemical reactions aiming at preventing blood loss through blood clot formation. This latter process is mediated by the interaction of platelets on the surface of the injured vessel wall which in turn induces the coagulative phase requiring the activation of inactive zymogen into active proteases.

Haemophilia A and B are rare disorders in which the coagulation cascade is affected due to the lack of blood clotting FVIII and FIX, respectively.

In order to provide the appropriate therapy for patients with these bleeding disorders, several laboratory tests have to be performed. The initial screening is conducted by screening global tests such as prothrombin time (PT) and activated partial thromboplastin time (aPTT) but only this latter is prolonged in hemophilia. Next, the measurement of factor activity is required for the diagnostic assessment and classification of the disease severity. Three methods can be performed for evaluating FVIII activity including one-stage, two-stage and chromogenic assays.

Approximately 30% of severe Haemophilia patients develop FVIII inhibitors which neutralize the clotting activity. The most common assay employed for the detection of inhibitors is the Bethesda assay that combines plasma containing normal amount of FVIII with same volume of patient plasma.

Problems in Haemophilia diagnosis or inhibitor detection can occur at any stage in the clinical diagnosis/laboratory phase, from the pre-analytical to the analytical to post-analytical. Therefore, the aim of this chapter is to summarize the diagnostic approaches, pitfalls and interpretation of coagulation assay in Haemophilia.

Keywords: Clotting factor, Haemostasis, Haemophilia, Inhibitors assays, Laboratory test.

---

[*] **Corresponding author Enrichetta Paladino:** Center for Bleeding Disorders, Department of Oncology, AOU Careggi, Florence, Italy; Tel: +39-55-7947587; E-mail: paladinoe@aou-careggi.toscana.it

Christian Carulli (Ed.)

INTRODUCTION

A sequence of biochemical and cellular reactions leads to haemostasis which is aimed to preventing blood leakage from the vascular lumen while maintaining blood within the vasculature in a fluid state, and protecting the integrity of vessels.

After injury to the integrity of vessel wall, the hemostatic process begins with an early vascular phase characterized by a vaso-constriction with reduction of the vessel lumen. This is followed by a platelet-subendothelium interaction mediated by von Willebrand factor (VWF) and subendothelial collagen and glycoprotein Ib on platelet surface. This interaction leads to the formation of a platelet plug (primary haemostasis). The simultaneous activation of clotting system eventually produces the formation of the fibrin clot (secondary haemostasis).

The coagulative or plasmatic phase, deficient in Haemophilia, comprises a series of proteolytic reactions, where an inactive precursor (zymogen) is converted into the active form (protease). This is in turn able to activate the next protease until fibrinogen, a soluble adhesive protein present in large amounts in the bloodstream, is transformed in a dense insoluble fibrin clot that completely covers the site of vessel injury.

In order to simplify and schematize the enzymatic activities of multiple molecules involved in the coagulation phase, a "cascade" model was developed. It is characterized by the sequence and by the specificity of events: for example, the first protein activates the second but can not instead activate the third, as showed in Fig. (**1**) and Table **1**.

Table 1. Nomenclature of coagulative factors.

Factor	Name	Pathway
Prekallikrein	Fletcher factor	Intrinsic
High molecular weight kininogen (HMWK)	Fitzgerald factor	Intrinsic
I	Fibrinogen	Common
II	Protrombin	Common
III	Tissue Factor	Extrinsic
IV	Calcium	Common
V	Proaccelerin	Common
VII	Proconvertin	Extrinsic
VIII	Antihemophilic factor A	Intrinsic
IX	Christmas-Factor Antihemophilic factor B	Intrinsic

(Table 1) contd.....

Factor	Name	Pathway
X	Stuart Factor	Common
XI	Plasma Thromboplastin Antecedent (PTA)	Intrinsic
XII	Hageman Factor	Intrinsic
XIII	Transglutaminase, fibrin stabilizing factor	Common

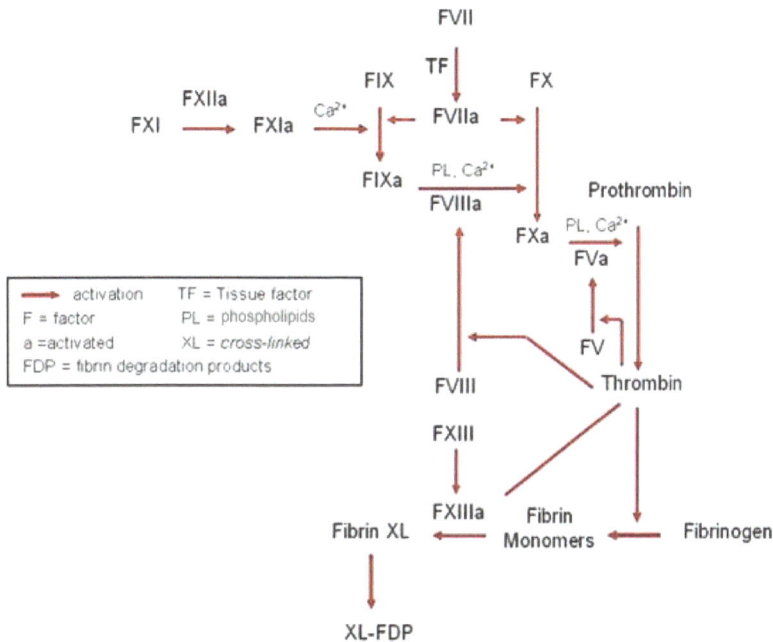

Fig. (1). Proposed mechanism of coagulation system (by courtesy of G.Castaman).

At variance with other coagulative factors, that are serine protease present in blood in the form of zymogens, tissue factor (TF), factor V and factor VIII (cofactors), and fibrinogen have no enzymatic activity. Within this sequence of events, also calcium ions and phospholipids of cell membranes, especially those of the platelet surface (PF3), critically intervene in the coagulation process, providing an appropriate cellular surface on which the coagulative process takes place.

Indeed, a series of complex events occurs to start, amplify, and propagate clotting response to the injury.

It is therefore considered that *in vivo* activation of coagulation is triggered when damage to the vessel wall allows subendothelium to take contact with the blood stream. Thereby TF, normally located outside the bloodstream, binds to factor VII which is converted to FVIIa, the complex TF / FVIIa activates FIX and FX, the FXa binds to its cofactor FVa, forming the "prothrombinase" complex that generate a small amount of thrombin (initial phase). During the subsequent *amplification* phase, small amounts of thrombin are able to first activate platelets and subsequently also FVIII, FV, and FXI which in turn activates FIX.

In the third phase, also called the *propagation* phase, the "tenase" complex, constituted by FVIIIa / FIXa, activates FX on the surface of activated platelets. Then, FXa in association with FVa converts large amounts of prothrombin to thrombin, which in turn leads to the formation of a fibrin clot that is stabilized by the intervention of FXIII, activated to FXIIIa by thrombin itself in the presence of calcium ions.

In the light of this "cellular" coagulation model, it appears that in Haemophilia A the first stages of coagulation are normal, while the propagation phase is impaired, with delayed or absent activation of FX on platelets, leading to a delayed or absent production of thrombin and then of the clot.

On the other hand in Haemophilia B the alterations affect either the early stages of the coagulation, resulting in reduced production of the first small amount of thrombin, or the propagation phase due to the reduced activation of FX on platelets.

The Preanalytical Phase

The laboratory of hemostasis is undoubtedly important for the diagnosis of bleeding disorders and for therapeutic drug monitoring. In recent years the growing request and the evolution of technology has led to the development of increasingly automated techniques that has allowed a better standardization of coagulation testing thus facilitating inter-laboratories comparison. In this context appropriate procedures for collection, separation, and storage of the sample are of great importance [1, 2].

Blood drawing for coagulation tests should be carried out by clean venopuncture. Venous stasis should be reduced to a minimum in order to avoid variations of pH and increase in CO_2 with loss of FV. Stasis also causes tissue damages with release of TF and activation of the FVII. Fasting is not strictly required, but previous strenuous exercise should be avoided before since it could produce an elevation of FVIII and von Willebrand factor.

The needle should have a diameter of 21-gauge (21g), but of course a minor calibre is used for children.

"Vacutainer" tubes containing sodium citrate at a concentration of 0.109M (3.2%) must be used and after sampling the tube should be inverted gently 3-4 times avoiding vigorous shaking that could induce hemolysis.

Of great importance is the sample filling that if not correct can alter the blood/citrate ratio which must be of 9:1. In fact an excess of anticoagulant leads to a spurious prolongation of clotting times of both the screening and the specific tests; in contrast under-filling of the test tube leads to a shortening of clotting time [3].

Since the anticoagulant is mixed with the plasma, it becomes important to calculate the concentration in case of haematocrit above 55% or below 25%, according to Table **2**.

Table 2. Influence of haematocrit on the appropriate addition of anticoagulant in the blood tube.

Hematocrit	Volume of Anticoagulant	Volume of Blood
60%	0.4 ml	4.6 ml
70%	0.25 ml	4.75 ml
80%	0.2 ml	4.8 ml
20%	0.7 ml	4.3 ml

The volume of anticoagulant should also be maintained to 0.5 ml, while the volume of blood should be adjusted depending on haematocrit. The volume of blood to be added to 0.5 ml of citrate 109M is [60: (100-Hct)] x 4.5 [3].

The test tube should not be stored at 2-8° since this can cause a loss of FVIII activity. When arriving in the laboratory it should be checked carefully to assess the correct filling and exclude the possible presence of clots. Then it has to be centrifuged at room temperature or in any case at a temperature not exceeding 25°C at 2000xg for at least 10 minutes to obtain a platelet-poor plasma (PPP) to be used for coagulation tests.

Samples with evidence of hemolysis after centrifuging must be discarded due to a possible activation of coagulation factors, even high concentrations of bilirubin or triglycerides can cause variation in the results for an erroneous clot detection [4].

Coagulative tests should be performed as soon as possible and not later than 60 minutes by centrifugation. If this is not possible, plasma should be stored in plastic tubes (not in glass that activates clotting) and stored at -20°C for 3-4 weeks, while at -80°C over 6 months. Prior to analysis, frozen samples must be thawed rapidly at 37°C for 3–5 minutes and then discarded after using.

The pre-analytical phase is a milestone for the accuracy of the results as recommended by international organizations such as:

NCCLS (National Committee for Clinical Laboratory Standards), ECCLS (European Committee for Clinical Laboratory Standards), and ECAT (European Concerted Action on Thrombosis and Disabilities of the Commission of The European Communities) [1 - 6].

Coagulation Screening Tests

Screening tests are simple and rapid evaluations performed on plasma of patients presenting with an active bleeding or awaiting for surgery to identify or exclude a Coagulation defect [7 - 9].

Prothrombin time (PT) is the time in seconds that a citrated plasma sample spends to clot when a thromboplastin (phospholipids + TF) and $CaCl_2$ are added to plasma.

PT identifies congenital or acquired deficiency of factors of the extrinsic and common pathway and is abnormal in vitamin K deficiency, liver disease, and disseminated intravascular coagulation (DIC). Isolated PT prolongation is a clue for FVII deficiency.

The variability of the test depends on the thromboplastin used, which can be recombinant or extractive from different tissues such as rabbit brain or human placenta. In order to limit the variability between laboratories, especially for the control of the therapy with oral anticoagulants, the International Normalized Ratio (INR) has been developed. It has been obtained by the ratio between the patient PT (in seconds) and the control PT (in seconds) raised to the international sensitivity index (ISI) that is determined by comparing each reagent with the reference WHO thromboplastin.

The time interval of PT is very short, ranging usually from 11 to 14 seconds and values of INR (0.85-1.2) are obtained from it. On the other hand, the prothrombin activity, whose reference values range from 70 to 130%, is determined by a specific calibration curve with controls of known concentrations.

The prothrombin activity is normal in Haemophilia patients not affected by other disorders (*e.g.*, liver disease).

The *activated partial thromboplastin time (*aPTT*)* is the time in seconds that a citrated plasma sample takes to clot after the addition of the activator of the contact phase (kaolin, silica, ellagic acid), phospholipids that substitute for the platelet membranes (partial thromboplastin, *i.e.* without TF) and $CaCl_2$.

The reagents for the aPTT are not as standardized as the PT ones, and this causes a variation of the sensitivity of the test.

Each laboratory, according to its needs must carefully consider the choice of reagents and instrumentation. Usually, a reagent that is as sensitive as possible to factor deficiencies rather than to interfering inhibitors lupus-type should be preferred.

It is valid the sensitivity of a reagent able to detect deficiencies factor of around 40%, thus it is relevant in the diagnosis of mild deficiencies that otherwise could go undiagnosed.

As for PT, also for aPTT the ratio between the seconds of the sample and the seconds of the control should be used to compare results obtained in different laboratories: a ratio between 0.8 – 1.2 is usually considered normal.

aPTT is prolonged in deficiencies of factors of the intrinsic and common pathways, in presence of heparin, and in patients affected by Lupus anticoagulant or acquired Haemophilia. In patients with Haemophilia A and B, its prolongation is usually directly related to the severity of the factor deficiency.

Another test that should never be omitted in a coagulation screening is the functional activity of fibrinogen, as PT and aPTT are altered for fibrinogen <100mg/dl. The reference values of fibrinogen range from 150 to 400mg/dl.

In case of prolonged aPTT in the suspicion of Haemophilia, mixing studies can be performed by a 50:50 mixture of the test sample with pooled normal plasma. If aPTT is corrected, factor deficiency is highly likely since adding 50% of the factor levels from normal plasma is sufficient to achieve the correction of the test. On the contrary, if aPTT of the sample is not corrected by the addition of normal plasma, it excludes the factor deficiency and the presence of interfering inhibitors of Lupus anticoagulant should be sought (Table **3**).

Table 3. Identification of lupus anticoagulant in the test sample.

Pool	Sample	Mix 50:50	Results
35 sec	60 sec	42 sec	Correction
35 sec	60 sec	52 sec	No correction (LA)

Thus, abnormalities of coagulation screening tests direct the specific research of the factors (Table **4**).

Table 4. Coagulation abnormalities suspected according to screening assays and clinical history.

PT	aPTT	Clinical Presentation	Abnormality
Prolonged	Normal	Bleeding	FVII
Normal	Prolonged	Bleeding	FVIII/FIX/FXI
Normal	Prolonged	Asymtpomatic	FXII/PK/HMWK
Prolonged	Prolonged	Bleeding	Fibrinogen/FII/FV/FX
Normal	Prolonged	Asymptomatic	LAC/CITRATE
Normal	Normal	Bleeding	FXIII/PLATELET DISORDERS

Clotting Factor Assay

Mixing study is a quick and easy way to suspect or rule out a factor deficiency (Haemophilia). For the diagnostic assessment and determination of the severity of the disease, measurement of factor activity in patient's plasma is required. Since Haemophilia A is 4-5 times more frequent than Haemophilia B, usually FVIII assay comes first.

The laboratory has a role of crucial importance for a precise and accurate measurement of circulating factor levels that significantly correlate with the severity of the clinical manifestations.

Severe Haemophilia A or B are defined by values of factor VIII or factor IX, respectively, less than 1 U/dL, moderate Haemophilia by values between 1 and <5 U/dL and mild Haemophilia by values between 5 and 40U/dL.

Even patients who have factor activity of around 30-40 U/dL are at risk of bleeding if undergoing surgery without the appropriate prophylaxis.

Factor VIII circulates in the plasma bound to the VWF, an adhesive glycoprotein which stabilizes it preventing its inactivation by the protein C system. The laboratory has a central role in the distinction of the type 3 or type 2N (Normandy) von Willebrand disease (VWD) from Haemophilia A, as in both cases of VWD the factor VIII activity is very low. For this reason the diagnosis of Haemophilia A must always be accompanied by the dosage of the antigen von Willebrand that is normal in Haemophilia subjects. However, only the assay of VWF:FVIII binding, and eventually screening for mutation either in FVIII or VWF gene can provide the final diagnosis

The differential diagnosis of Haemophilia A and VWD is outlined in Table **5**.

Table 5. Differential diagnosis between Haemophilia A and von Willebrand disease.

Test	HaemophiliaA	Von Willebrand Disease
aPTT	Prolonged	Normal/ Prolonged
FVIII	Low	Normal/Low
VWF	Normal	VariablyReduced
Bleeding Time	Normal	Prolonged /Normal in mild cases and Type 2N

FVIII assay can be performed by three methods [10].

1) The *one-stage assay* measures the ability of a sample containing the factor under investigation to correct or shorten the aPTT of a plasma of a severe Haemophilia A patient, after activation of the contact phase and recalcification.

This test therefore needs a plasma totally deficient in FVIII and normal levels of all other relevant clotting factors so that the FVIII content in the sample is the only variable limiting the reaction rate.

A completely FVIII deficient plasma can be obtained from patients with severe Haemophilia A without inhibitors that have received no infusions within 72 hours, or from commercial plasmas undergoing immunoadsorption of the factor through the use of specific antibodies [11].

Owing to the extensive use of the prophylactic regimens in patients with severe Haemophilia it is difficult to obtain large amount of natural deficient plasmas, so that lyophilized immunoadsorbed plasmas where FVIII is completely absent or lower than 1 U/dL are used, while VWF and all other components are in optimal quantities and fibrinogen is greater than 100 mg/dl [12].

Since this method is based on the determination of aPTT, all other used reagents are the same of aPTT assay, *i.e.* activators (especially *microsilica*, that is more sensitive to deficiencies compared to ellagic acid), phospholipids, that may have different origin both vegetable and animal, and calcium ions.

2) The *two-stage* assay, based on the optical detection of the clot, is based on the generation of activated factor X and involves two separate reactions. In the first phase, factor II, VII, IX, and X are removed from the sample test and, after appropriate dilution, incubated with a mixture of FV, activated FIX, FX, phospholipids, and calcium. In the second phase, normal plasma containing fibrinogen, FII and calcium ions are added, so that the time of clot formation will depend on the amount of activated FX formed in the first stage which is proportional to the activity of the FVIII in the sample test.

This method is not practical and cumbersome and it is no more used in the routine laboratory: it has been recently replaced by the chromogenic assay is based on the same principle.

3) In the *chromogenic assay*, the sample test is added to a mixture containing activated FIX, calcium, and phospholipids so that the only limiting factor is the amount of FVIII of the sample. The activated FX formed in the mixture is detected using a substrate (S-2765) containing a chromophore group whose hydrolysis forms the para-nitroaniline (pNA) measured by absorbance at 405 nm by a spectrophotometer.

The chromogenic assay has the advantage that it is not influenced by the presence of heparin or antiphospholipid antibodies.

Due to the simple and rapid execution in addition to the low cost, the one-stage assay is the most widely used in the routine laboratory practice. However, regardless of the method employed, results should overlap and, above all, there must be correspondence between the *in vitro* results and the real *in vivo* hemostatic efficacy.

Discrepancies between the one-stage and chromogenic assays, especially in mild or moderate Haemophilia, may be observed according to the type of FVIII mutation. Recent evidences suggest that both methods should be used at diagnosis in patients with Haemophilia A to identify these variants since it has been suggested that the chromogenic assay could be more sensitive in defining the bleeding risk of such patients. However, the chromogenic method is yet less used than the one-stage assay, also because more expensive.

Reference Curve

FVIII activity of a sample is expressed as a percentage in comparison to a standard or reference curve. The test must be specific and sensitive, with a high specificity. The reference curve must exhibit a high slope and all of these features depend on the reagents and the used instrumentation.

For the setup of the calibration curve, at least six dilutions of a reference standard plasma or of a pooled normal plasma are performed, values obtained are plotted on a log-linear diagram where the abscissa shows the percentage of FVIII activity and the ordinate represent the time in seconds in order to get a straight line on which the dosages of the samples under examination are calculated [13, 14].

When the level of factor VIII activity in the sample is low, the assay is repeated on scalar dilutions in buffer or in physiological solution, so the presence of a real deficiency instead of the interference of LA inhibitors can be check out. In fact the interference of these inhibitors decreases with the dilution of the sample.

The time in seconds obtained is reported on the reference curve. If the points are equally spaced along the whole length, the two curves are parallel and this point out that we are in the presence of a factor deficiency [15, 16] .

If, on the contrary, the curve of the plasma of the patient is not placed parallel to the calibration curve it indicates the presence of interfering inhibitor as Lupus anticoagulant, as reported in the graphic drawn from our instrument Fig. (**2**).

The parallelism of curves is automatically done by most coagulometers. If it is not possible, the factor activity of dilutions should be observed: if they match with the result obtained on undiluted plasma it indicates a factor deficiency, if they increased proportionally to the dilution we are in the presence of inhibitors that are moved away from dilution so the normalization of the factorial activity is achieved.

FVIII activity is expressed as percentage or as U/ml compared to a reference sample with known activity. The reference values (RV) range from 60 to 150%.

Each laboratory define its own reference intervals by performing at least twenty determinations on samples of healthy people repeated on different days. RVs are obtained from the average of these determinations +/- 2SD thus encompassing 95% of the results, since a normal distribution of data is represented by a Gaussian curve.

Another important parameter is the coefficient of variation (CV) which is the SD expressed as a percentage of the mean (CV=SD/mean x 100).

For the dosage of FVIII, a CV below 10% is considered acceptable. Relevant issues also concern the selection of the reagents, the appropriate calibration of the reference plasma, and the correct use of the laboratory equipment that must be maintained in perfect efficiency by following the instructions provided in the manufacturers manuals.

Before starting an analytic session it should be verified if the controls provided by manufacturers are lyophilized within the acceptable range.

Moreover the internal quality controls (ICQ) evaluate the accuracy of the method, the external quality controls (ECQ) assess the accuracy of results and they are used to examine the validity of individual laboratories.

Quantitative Assays for Detecting Specific Factor Inhibitors

Inhibitors are acquired antibodies (alloantibodies) targeted against a specific clotting factor, and in particular against FVIII or FIX. They are mainly a mixture of IgG4 and IgG1 immunoglobulins with the following peculiarities: specific, activity-neutralizing, time-depending, temperature depending, pH depending, specie-specific and not-precipitating [17, 18].

More frequently these alloantibodies are directed against functional epitopes of FVIII domains A2 and C2. Approximately 30% of severe Haemophilia A patients develop inhibitors. Inhibitors are far less common in moderate and mild Haemophilia A (~10% of cases) and in severe Haemophilia B (less than 5%).

Inhibitors of congenital Haemophilia are alloantibodies stimulated by infusion of exogenous factor, these antibodies complicate the treatment or prevention of bleeding, because they bind and inactivate infused factor or occasionally accelerate its clearance, often rendering standard factor replacement therapy ineffective. Management of patients with inhibitors is the most important present challenge in Haemophilia treatment, which can become very expensive (see Chapter 18).

FVIII Inhibitors

Factor VIII Inhibitors (activity-neutralizing antibodies) are classically divided into types I or II depending upon the kinetics of the inhibitor. Type I FVIII inhibitors exhibit linear inhibition kinetics [first-order kinetics], that are both time and concentration dependent. There is a linear relationship between the logarithm of residual FVIII:C and antibody concentration. Alloantibodies developing in individuals with severe Haemophilia in response to treatment, classically demonstrate type I kinetics, with the complete inhibition of FVIII activity.

In contrast, type II inhibitors show more complex kinetics [second-order kinetics] and commonly are seen with in previously healthy patients developing autoantibodies against FVIII (acquired Haemophilia A). Type II inhibitors are unable to completely inactivate FVIII:C even at maximum antibody concentration undiluted Fig. (**2**). This may explain why in some patients with an acquired FVIII inhibitor small amounts of FVIII may be detectable.

A   **B**

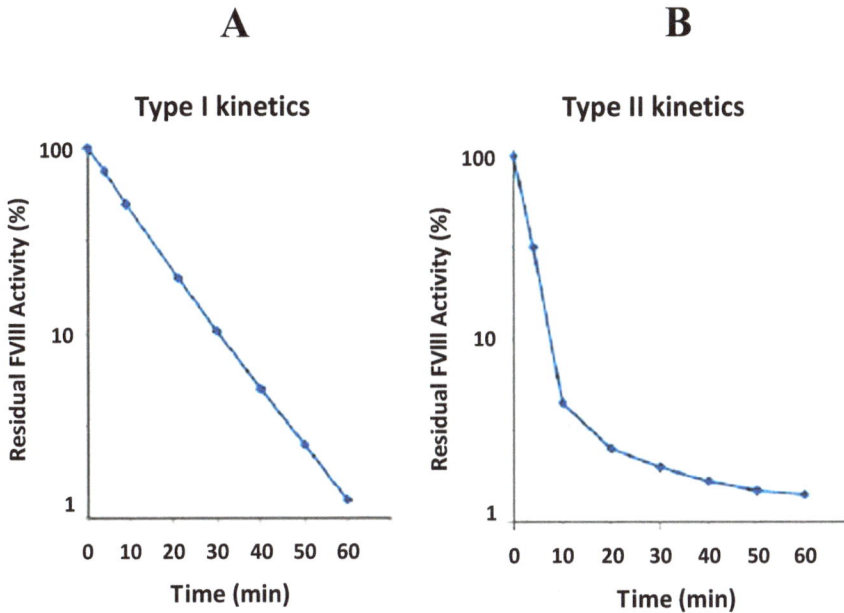

Fig. (2). Different kinetics of FVIII inhibition in congenital Haemophilia with inhibitor. (type I, panel A) and acquired Haemophilia A (type II, panel B).

Bethesda (Nijemegen) Assay for Inhibitors

Bethesda-type assays (or its modification, the Nijmegen assay) can be employed to test for inhibitors to factors. Although predominantly used for FVIII inhibitors, these assays can be adapted to detect any factor inhibitor [19, 20].

In a Bethesda assay, patient plasma is incubated in a 50/50 volume with a source of factor (usually pooled normal plasma) for 2 hours at 37°. Residual factor activity then is measured and compared with a control mixture. Usually in case of measurable amount of factor, citrated plasma test is incubated 30 minutes at 56°C to denature proteins except antibodies and the consequent factor-free supernatant is employed as sample.

One Bethesda Unit (BU) is defined as the amount of inhibitor that neutralizes 50% of 1 unit of FVIII:C in normal plasma after 120 minutes incubation at 37°C.

Principle of Assay

As factor VIII inhibitors are time-dependent, if exogenous factor VIII is added to the patient's plasma and the mixture is incubated, the added factor VIII will be progressively neutralized. If the amount of factor VIII added and the duration of incubation are standardized then the strength or concentration of the inhibitor may be measured in units according to how much of the added factor VIII is destroyed. The source of factor VIII is pooled normal plasma (PNP). The Nijmegen modification of factor VIII inhibitor assay involves buffering the normal plasma with 0.1M imidazole buffer at pH 7.4 and using immunodepleted factor VIII deficient plasma in the control mixture. At low inhibitor titres (<1 BU) the classical Bethesda assay can result in false positives whereas the Nijmegen modified assays would give zero levels of inhibition. The stabilization of ph values in the mixtures reduces the variability of assay during incubation phase [21, 22].

The assay can also be modified to use factor VIII concentrates and the incubation time can be increased to 4 hours.

The Bethesda Assay [21 - 26]

1. Doubling dilutions of test plasma in imidazole buffer are incubated with an equal volume of the normal plasma pool at 37°C. In a plasma sample with an unknown value for the inhibitor a series of dilutions are to be made.
2. PNP will normally contain 1 U/mL of factor VIII by definition.
3. A control consisting of an equal volume of normal plasma mixed with buffer (or in the case of the Nijmegen modification, immunodepleted factor VIII deficient plasma) is taken to represent the 100% value. This mixture actually has a starting concentration of 50% factor VIII (because a 50/50 dilution with buffer has been made) but this does not matter because the same source and volume is added to all incubation mixtures.
4. At the end of the incubation period the residual factor VIII is assayed using a standard one-stage APTT-based assay with the control representing the 100% standard.
5. The inhibitor concentration is calculated from a graph of residual factor VIII activity *versus* inhibitor units. The dilution of test plasma that gives a residual factor VIII nearest to 50% but within the range 30-60% is chosen for calculation of the inhibitor. It is also possible to calculate the inhibitor titer for each dilution and take the average.
6. If the residual factor VIII activity is between 80-100% the sample does not contain an inhibitor.
7. The inhibitor titer from the graph will be multiplied by the dilution to give the final titer. A positive control plasma of known inhibitor titer should be included.
8. When plotting the residual FVIII against the BU titer – the Y axis is a log scale and the X axis is linear. Residual FVIII is plotted on the Y Log axis and BU titer on the linear X axis Fig. (**3**).

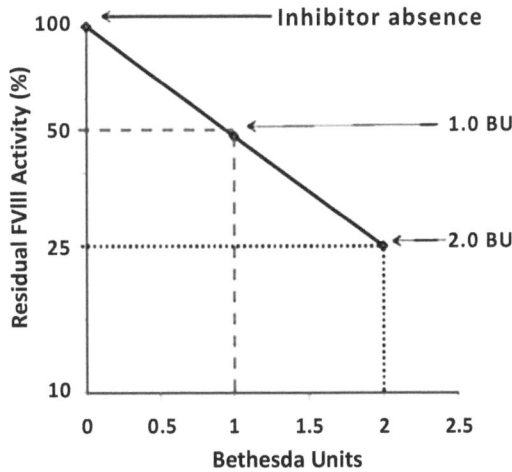

Fig. (3). Residual FVIII activity (log) *vs.* inhibitors concentration (lin): inverse.

In Table **6** three plasma samples with varying dilutions have been assayed and the inhibitor titer in Bethesda Units [BU] calculated. For example, if the dilution is 1:8 and the residual FVIII is 50% then the value of 1BU must be multiplied by 8 to give the actual inhibitor titer within the plasma sample of 8 BU.

Table 6. Calculation examples of three different positive samples for inhibitors presence.

Plasma Sample	Dilution	Residual FVIII Activity (%)	BU x Dilution	BU Titer
1	1:8	50%	1 x 8	8 BU
2	1:16	25%	2 x 16	32 BU
3	1:32	12.5%	3 x 32	96 BU

Data Interpretation

1. The Bethesda assay can give false positives at low inhibitor levels (<1 BU) whereas the Nijmegen modification would give zero levels. Changes in pH and protein concentration can affect the stability of FVIII and its inactivation increases as the pH increases and at low protein concentration. By buffering the normal plasma and using FVIII deficient plasma these variables are minimised/eliminated. The Nijmegen modification of FVIII inhibitor assay involves buffering the normal plasma with 0.1M imidazole buffer at pH 7.4, and using immunodepleted factor VIII deficient plasma in the control mixture.
2. The Bethesda assay was designed to measure FVIII inhibitors in patients with Haemophilia A or FIX inhibitors in patients with Haemophilia B.
3. In patients with complex inhibitor kinetics as commonly seen in patients with

acquired FVIII inhibitors the calculated inhibitor titer may increase as the dilutions increase [25].

CONCLUDING REMARKS

The role of laboratory is of utmost importance in the correct classification of the severity of Haemophilia A and B, thus providing a prognostic perspective in any new patient identified. The quantitation of inhibitor titer against FVIII and FIX is important not only for diagnostic purposes but also in monitoring the efficacy of immunotolerance regimes in eradicating the inhibitor. Accurate assessment of pre-analytical and analytical variables should always carefully pursued to assure the quality of the results.

CONFLICT OF INTEREST

The authors confirm that they have no conflict of interest to declare for this publication.

ACKNOWLEDGEMENTS

Declared none.

REFERENCES

[1]   National Committee for Clinical Laboratory Standards (NCCLS). Collection, transport and processing of blood specimens for coagulation testing and general performance of coagulation assays-Approved guideline H21-A3. Villanova, PA: NCCLS 1998.

[2]   CLSI. Collection, transport, and processing of blood specimens for testing plasma-based coagulation assays and molecular hemostasis assays: approved guideline. 2008.

[3]   Adcock DM, Kressin DC, Marlar RA. Minimum specimen volume requirements for routine coagulation testing: dependence on citrate concentration. Am J Clin Pathol 1998; 109(5): 595-9. [http://dx.doi.org/10.1093/ajcp/109.5.595] [PMID: 9576579]

[4]   Grafmeyer D, Bondon M, Machon M, Levillain R. The influence of bilirubin, haemolysis and turbidity on 20 analytical tests performed on automatic analyzers. Eur J Clin Chem Biochem 1995; 33: 31-52.

[5]   Danielson CF, Davis K, Jones G, Benson J, Arney K, Martin J. Effect of citrate concentration in specimen collection tubes on the International Normalized Ratio. Arch Pathol Lab Med 1997; 121(9): 956-9.
[PMID: 9302927]

[6]   Chantarangkul V, Tripodi A, Clerici M, Negri B, Mannucci PM. Assessment of the influence of citrate concentration on the International Normalized Ratio (INR) determined with twelve reagent-instrument combinations. Thromb Haemost 1998; 80(2): 258-62.
[PMID: 9716149]

[7]   Kitchen S, McCraw A, Echenagucia M. WFH Laboratory Sciences Committee. Diagnosis of Haemophilia and Other Bleeding Disorders A laboratory manual. Montreal, Canada: WFH 2000.

[8]   Greaves M, Watson HG. Approach to the diagnosis and management of mild bleeding disorders. J Thromb Haemost 2007; 5 (Suppl. 1): 167-74.
[http://dx.doi.org/10.1111/j.1538-7836.2007.02495.x] [PMID: 17635723]

[9]   Bolton-Maggs PH, Perry DJ, Chalmers EA, *et al.* The rare coagulation disorders review with guidelines for management from the United Kingdom Haemophilia Centre Doctors Organisation. Haemophilia 2004; 10(5): 593-628.
        [http://dx.doi.org/10.1111/j.1365-2516.2004.00944.x] [PMID: 15357789]

[10]   Morfini M, Cinotti S, Bellatreccia A, Paladino E, Gringeri A, Mannucci PM. ReFacto-AICE Study Group. A multicenter pharmacokinetic study of the B-domain deleted recombinant factor VIII concentrate using different assays and standards. J Thromb Haemost 2003; 1(11): 2283-9.
        [http://dx.doi.org/10.1046/j.1538-7836.2003.00481.x] [PMID: 14629459]

[11]   Cinotti S, Paladino E, Morfini M. Accuracy of FVIII: C assay by one-stage method can be improved using hemophilic plasma as diluent. J Thromb Haemost 2006; 4(4): 828-33.
        [http://dx.doi.org/10.1111/j.1538-7836.2006.01880.x] [PMID: 16634753]

[12]   Verbruggen B, Meijer P, Nováková I, Van Heerde W. Diagnosis of factor VIII deficiency. Haemophilia 2008; 14 (Suppl. 3): 76-82.
        [http://dx.doi.org/10.1111/j.1365-2516.2008.01715.x] [PMID: 18510526]

[13]   Hubbard AR, Bevan SA, Weller LJ. Potency estimation of recombinant factor VIII: effect of assay method and standard. Br J Haematol 2001; 113(2): 533-6.
        [http://dx.doi.org/10.1046/j.1365-2141.2001.02761.x] [PMID: 11380427]

[14]   Mikaelsson M, Oswaldsson U. Assaying the circulating factor VIII activity in hemophilia A patients treated with recombinant factor VIII products. Semin Thromb Hemost 2002; 28(3): 257-64.
        [http://dx.doi.org/10.1055/s-2002-32659] [PMID: 12098085]

[15]   Wagenman BL, Townsend KT, Mathew P, Crookston KP. The laboratory approach to inherited and acquired coagulation factor deficiencies. Clin Lab Med 2009; 29(2): 229-52.
        [http://dx.doi.org/10.1016/j.cll.2009.04.002] [PMID: 19665676]

[16]   Morfini M, Marchesini E, Paladino E, Santoro C, Zanon E, Iorio A. Pharmacokinetics of plasma-derived *vs.* recombinant FVIII concentrates: a comparative study. Haemophilia 2015; 21(2): 204-9.
        [http://dx.doi.org/10.1111/hae.12550] [PMID: 25274155]

[17]   Rocino A, Coppola A, Franchini M, *et al.* Italian Association of Haemophilia Centres (AICE) Working Party. Principles of treatment and update of recommendations for the management of haemophilia and congenital bleeding disorders in Italy. Blood Transfus 2014; 12(4): 575-98.
        [PMID: 25350962]

[18]   Hay CR, Palmer BP, Chalmers EA, *et al.* The incidence of factor VIII inhibitors in severe haemophilia A following a major switch from full-length to B-domain-deleted factor VIII: a prospective cohort comparison. Haemophilia 2015; 21(2): 219-26.
        [http://dx.doi.org/10.1111/hae.12563] [PMID: 25382829]

[19]   Giles AR, Verbruggen B, Rivard GE, Teitel J, Walker I. Association of Hemophilia Centre Directors of Canada. Factor VIII/IX Subcommittee of Scientific and Standardization Committee of International Society on Thrombosis and Haemostasis. A detailed comparison of the performance of the standard *versus* the Nijmegen modification of the Bethesda assay in detecting factor VIII:C inhibitors in the haemophilia A population of Canada. Thromb Haemost 1998; 79(4): 872-5.
        [PMID: 9569207]

[20]   Reber G, Aurousseau MH, Dreyfus M, *et al.* Inter-laboratory variability of the measurement of low titer factor VIII:C inhibitor in haemophiliacs: improvement by the Nijmegen modification of the Bethesda assay and the use of common lyophilized plasmas. Haemophilia 1999; 5(4): 292-3.
        [http://dx.doi.org/10.1046/j.1365-2516.1999.00329.x] [PMID: 10469186]

[21]   Verbruggen B, Giles A, Samis J, Verbeek K, Mensink E, Nováková I. The type of factor VIII deficient plasma used influences the performance of the Nijmegen modification of the Bethesda assay for factor VIII inhibitors. Thromb Haemost 2001; 86(6): 1435-9.
        [PMID: 11776311]

[22]   Verbruggen B, Novakova I, Wessels H, Boezeman J, van den Berg M, Mauser-Bunschoten E. The Nijmegen modification of the Bethesda assay for factor VIII:C inhibitors: improved specificity and reliability. Thromb Haemost 1995; 73(2): 247-51.
[PMID: 7792738]

[23]   Keeling D, Beavis J, Sukhu K. A simple inhibitor screen is more sensitive than a Bethesda assay in monitoring for the development of inhibitors in haemophilia A and B. Br J Haematol 2005; 128(6): 885.
[http://dx.doi.org/10.1111/j.1365-2141.2005.05399.x] [PMID: 15755295]

[24]   Verbruggen B, Dardikh M, Polenewen R, van Duren C, Meijer P. The factor VIII inhibitor assays can be standardized: results of a workshop. J Thromb Haemost 2011; 9(10): 2003-8.
[http://dx.doi.org/10.1111/j.1538-7836.2011.04479.x] [PMID: 21854536]

[25]   Collins PW. Management of acquired haemophilia A. J Thromb Haemost 2011; 9 (Suppl. 1): 226-35.
[http://dx.doi.org/10.1111/j.1538-7836.2011.04309.x] [PMID: 21781259]

[26]   Goodeve AC, Williams I, Bray GL, Peake IR. Recombinate PUP Study Group. Relationship between factor VIII mutation type and inhibitor development in a cohort of previously untreated patients treated with recombinant factor VIII (Recombinate). Thromb Haemost 2000; 83(6): 844-8.
[PMID: 10896236]

CHAPTER 5

Nursing of Patients with Haemophilia

Maria Virginia Puliga[*]

Center for Bleeding Disorders, Department of Oncology, Azienda Ospedaliero-Universitaria Careggi, Florence, Italy

Abstract: The management of nursing consists in the performance of leadership functions of governance and decision-making within organizations employing nurses. It includes many processes common to all management as planning, organizing, directing, and controlling. In case of rare bleeding disorders, nurses may encounter patients who are experiencing acute bleedings or receiving treatments for another condition. In Haemophilia, the nurse is not only a professional figure but also a teacher of daily actions, as self-injections of substitutive factors, and a confidant reference point for patients and their family.

Keywords: Carrier, Caregiver, Haemophilia, Home treatment, Nursing, Replacement therapy.

INTRODUCTION

As nurses, we know that every patient is special for his past and present clinical history, and that management can be complicated by the association of several other conditions. As the general population ages, our patients will have longer lists of chronic disorders and related medications, and their nursing care will become even more complex. Moreover, life-long lasting genetic disorders are usually characterized by a multidisciplinary approach: nurses play a relevant role being the link between specialists involved in the management of all medical aspects related to the disease.

Haemophilia is an inherited bleeding disorder requiring specifically complex, life-long care [1]. At variance with the very frequent inherited thrombophilic syndromes, inherited bleeding disorders are uncommon, and most nurses have generally little experience and know-how to manage such patients. Unlike the diagnosis and treatment of thromboembolic disorders, which many nurses encounter on every shift, bleeding disorders rarely come up in shift report. Patients with Haemophilia

---

[*] **Corresponding author Maria Virginia Puliga:** Center for Bleeding Disorders, Department of Oncology, Azienda Ospedaliero-Universitaria, Careggi, Florence, Italy; Tel: 00390557947587; Email: puligamv@aou-careggi.toscana.it

Christian Carulli (Ed.)

and their parents are usually well informed and self-trained about their disorders, and able to quickly catch a caregivers' lack of knowledge. Such situation makes them uncomfortable, particularly in pediatric age. Thus, nurses should be trained and educated about all aspects of bleeding disorders. In this way, learning and teaching about bleeding disorders can vastly improve the provided care, thus increasing patients' trusting in the system of care.

Bleedings have multiple inherited and acquired causes. This chapter will discuss Haemophilia A and B related conditions and needs from the nurse perspective. Other coagulation factor deficiencies or platelet disorders, including von Willebrand disease which is the most common hereditary bleeding disorder, will not be dealt with for their milder bleeding tendency and pathophysiological complexity.

Treatment

For many years, blood or plasma transfusions were the main treatment for Haemophilia. In the 1970s, development of factor replacement products from plasma donations enlarged treatment options and changed the lives of such patients [2].

In this way, in order to stop bleedings, they could receive the required factor in a small fluid volume at home by a short infusion with a small butterfly needle Fig. **(1)**.

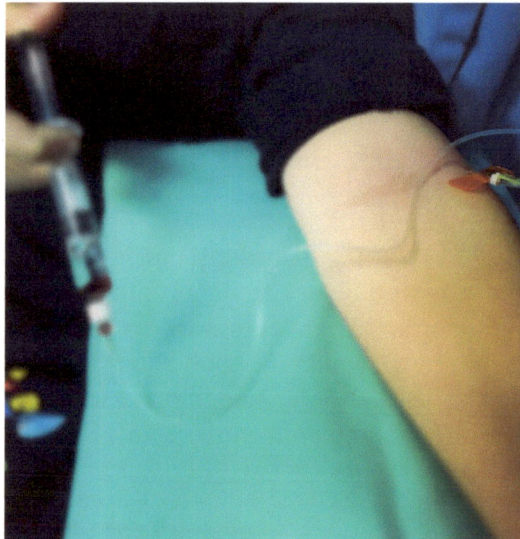

Fig. (1). Example of recombinant factor infusion.

Until not long ago, many people with Haemophilia suffered a joint damage due to recurrent bleedings [3]. Because of the further risk of haemoartrosis during and after surgery, many orthopaedic procedures were addressed as very difficult. The large availability of factor replacement products now makes such type of surgery more feasible, improving the quality of life of haemophiliacs in terms of pain reduction and functional recovery.

Although replacement factors have brought Haemophilia one step closer to a cure, the promise of a definitive therapy was clouded in the '80s by the discovery of HIV and other blood-borne diseases. Unlikely, many people with Haemophilia contracted HIV, hepatitis C, or both from transfusions and first generation factor concentrates.

Given the critical concern on the safety of those concentrates, pharmaceutical companies soon developed virucidal methods that associated with safer blood donor screening procedures, virtually abolished the risk of infectious disease transmission [4]. Eventually, factor products without the use of human plasma were developed. Today, most factor products are recombinant and not processed from human plasma.

Recombinant Factor Products

Several recombinant factor VIII or factor IX products are now available. Dosing varies with the type of bleeding, and haematologists determine the right dosage. Each vial of concentrate is labeled with the total number of units expressed as International Units (IU). Vials range from 250 to 3000 units per bottle. Dose calculations can rarely be exact due to the variability in lot yields. It is not essential to administer exact doses; doses within 10% above the ordered number of units are usually acceptable.

Practical Nursing Recommendations

1. When administering factor products, make sure to give the right one for your patient's type of Haemophilia. Further, be aware that all factor products must be reconstituted immediately before administration. They are packaged in kits that include a vial of factor (powder), a vial of diluent, and a mixing device. Most mixing devices have a built-in filter. Swirl (do not shake) the medication when mixing.
2. Never waste factor concentrate by using a portion of a vial and discarding the rest. The full vial should be used, as overdosing is not an issue. A vial size that is as close as possible to the desired dose should be chosen, but it should be always round up to the nearest whole vial size.
3. Infuse the factor by slow intravenous push as soon as possible after

reconstitution. Infusion times vary by product and volume, so always follow the recommendations of the package insert to reconstitute and administer the product correctly.

4. When infusing a child, try to get always the parents collaboration. The room should be comfortable, without relevant noise. A toy could be useful to lessen the attention of the child to the needle. Some anaesthetic cream preparations are available, and used to lessen pain or discomfort at venipuncture.

5. Be careful that peripheral venous access is carefully managed and surveyed.

Inhibitors

Some patients with Haemophilia develop inhibitors (See Chapter 18), making harder to stop a bleeding episode. When this occurs, the treatment must be adjusted. The patient may require a higher dosage of replacement factor or factor VIIa, or a bypassing agent that allows clotting to occur even without factor VIII or XI [5]. The haematologist determines suitable treatment, as well as informing the nurse.

Adverse Reaction

The administration of factor concentrate products will occasionally cause reactions including stuffy nose, itching, hives, shortness of breath, chest pain, temperature elevation, headache, dizziness, palpitation, mild chills, nausea, or stinging at the infusion site. Reactions can occur during an infusion or one to two hours after. As well as, anaphylactic reactions have been reported in patients with inhibitors to factor IX. Because of these potential severe reactions, most Haemophilia Treatment Centres (HTCs) administer initial FIX dose to Haemophilia B patients in a controlled clinical setting, and many recommend that the first 10-20 doses of factor IX be given at the HTC or a clinical infusion centre where resuscitation equipment is quickly available Figs. (**2** and **3**).

Of noting is the fact that most patients with anaphylaxis to FIX products have large or total deletions of their FIX gene. So, early genotyping may identify subjects at greater risk for this complication in a way that appropriate precautions can be taken when administering FIX concentrates to these patients.

Hormone Therapy

Hormone therapy is used to treat heavy menses in Haemophilia carriers or female patients with other bleeding disorders. Hormone manipulation may raise factor levels in mild deficiency and reduces bleedings in the affected women.

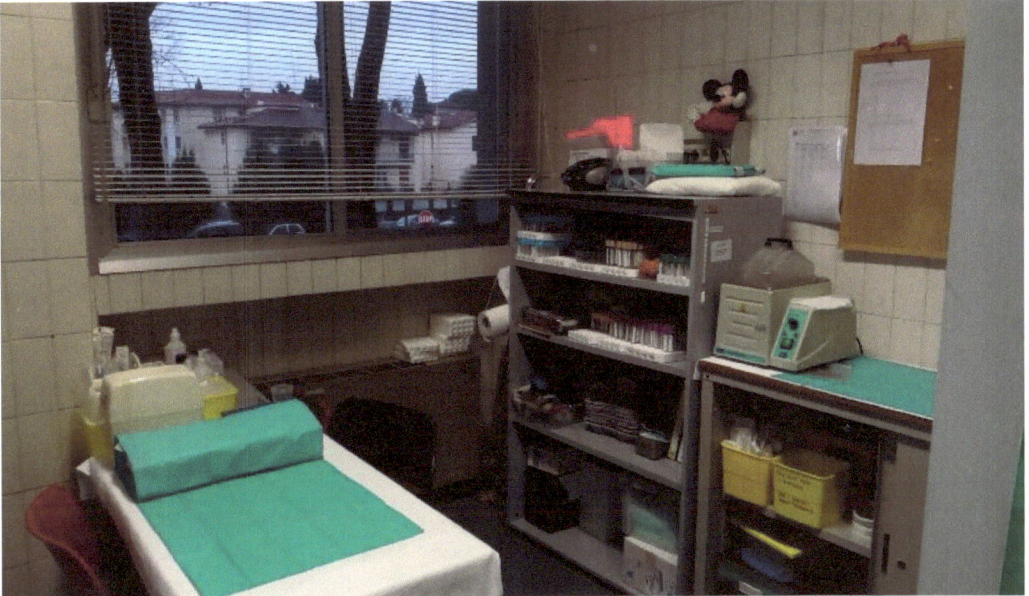

Fig. (2). Materials and equipment of a Haemophilia centre.

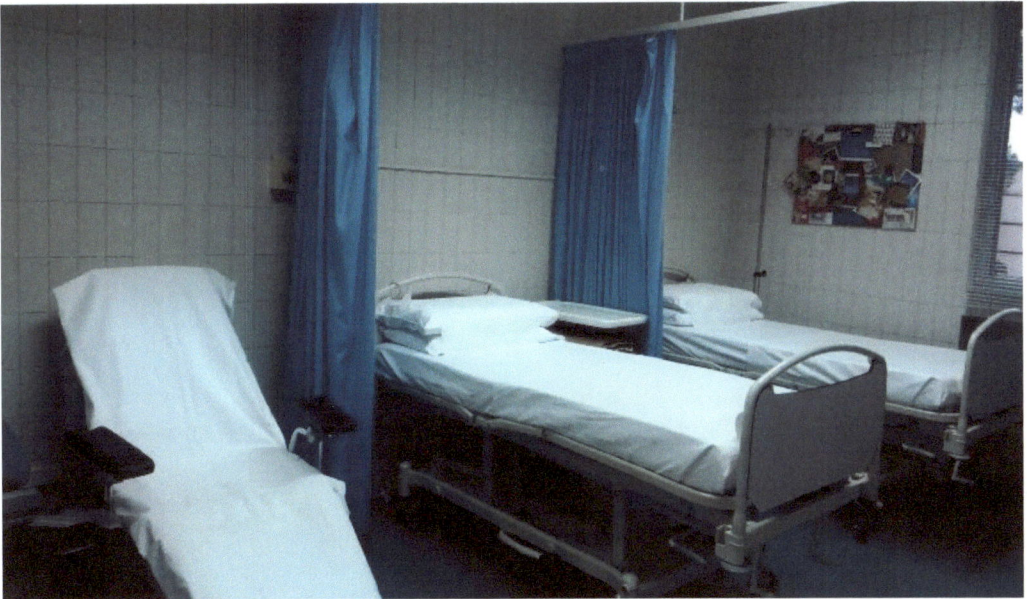

Fig. (3). Aspect of a room of a Haemophilia centre.

A gynaecological evaluation should be always performed to suggest and monitor the most appropriate hormonal treatment [6].

Other Non-Transfusional Modalities

Desmopressin (DDAVP), a synthetic vasopressin, is used to treat mild Haemophilia A or carriers of Haemophilia A with low FVIII. It is absolutely ineffective in Haemophilia B. The compound is available for IV administration or as a concentrated formulation for subcutaneous injection, as well as a nasal spray.

Desmopressin triggers the release of von Willebrand factor and FVIII endothelial cells into the bloodstream, temporarily increasing factor levels, and stopping or preventing bleeding.

Since the drug is not similarly effective in every patient, subjects should undergo a test-infusion trial with a blood sampling taken up to 4 hours to assess the magnitude and duration of FVIII increase.

Short-term headaches, facial flushing, nausea, and abdominal cramps have been noted with the administration of DDAVP. These symptoms usually disappear by slowing the infusion rate, and are lower when using subcutaneous route. Transient hypertension or hypotension may also be a side effect. DDAVP should be used with caution in patients with a history of deep venous thrombosis or cardiac disease, as there have been a few reports of thrombotic events [7].

Nursing Consideration

Blood pressure and pulse should be monitored during infusions. If used preoperatively, DDAVP should be administered 30 minutes prior to the scheduled procedure. DDAVP maintains an anti-diuretic agent. The HTC staff should alert all operating room personnel that the administration of unrestricted IV fluids may result in a syndrome of hyponatremia due to excessive water resorption from kidneys (*water intoxication*).

The rise in FVIII plasma levels after DDAVP is rapid. Peak values are reached within 30 to 45 minutes, but it may require as much as an hour to achieve them. A second dose may be given 24 hours after the initial one. However, the increase in FVIII activity may be less than the initial peak due to the relatively slow synthesis and release from the endothelial cells. A repeated administration after 48 hours generally reproduces the original response.

The nurse should document the following:

1. Date and time of infusion or administration;
2. Rate of infusion;
3. Dose infused or administered;

4. Site of infusion;
5. Blood pressure;
6. Infusion complications and reactions: last mentioned can occur during an infusion or one to two hours following an infusion;
7. Fluid restriction education;
8. DDAVP education for home use should include: indications for use, steps for administration, frequency of administration, home documentation, fluid restriction and adverse events;
9. Patient response to treatment (it may not be immediately evident): provide a phone follow-up.

Other Medications

Tranexamic acid is used to treat mucosal bleedings. As an antifibrinolytic, it prevents lysis of clots until the damaged area has completely healed. Available as oral and IV formulation, it is often used for epistaxis after dental surgery, or even heavy menses.

Discouraged Drugs

Be aware that some drugs, such as aspirin and other nonsteroidal anti-inflammatory drugs, are usually not appropriate for patients with bleeding disorders given the increased risk of bleedings. Patients should always be informed about allowed or contraindicated drugs.

Nursing Considerations

Nursing considerations for hospitalised patients with Haemophilia vary with the reason for admission so it is very important to stay alert for bleedings.

Monitor the patient for signs and symptoms of bleeding, and listen carefully as your patient describes symptoms. Typically, patients experience bleeding symptoms before signs become apparent. Pain is among the first symptoms of a joint or soft-tissue bleeding. Patients may complain of pain in a localized area, but lack outward signs of bleeding.

As the bleeding progresses without treatment, increase of pain and joint damage may occur. Finally, a bleeding causes warmth, redness, and swelling. As ordered, promptly administer the replacement factor and use ice, compression, rest and elevation protocols. Once the bleeding stops, be aware that pain may persist until the blood is fully reabsorbed.

Precautions for Patients Undergoing Invasive Procedures

Haemophilia patients undergoing surgery require a close monitoring, a factor administration before the procedure and for days/weeks postoperatively depending on the type and relevance of surgery, and consideration for deep vein thrombosis prophylaxis. As needed, arrange for follow-up care at discharge. After major surgery, many patients require multiple infusions; unless these infusions are arranged before discharge, patients may require readmission for postoperative bleedings, due may not receive a proper treatment.

Other invasive procedures requiring a previous treatment with medication are usually represented by: dental procedures, arthrocentesis, steroid injections, biopsy, and colonoscopy. It is reasonable to consult a haematologist if a patient with a bleeding disorder requires one of these procedures. Pre-treatment infusion can prevent severe complications. Also, be sure to hold the pressure after blood draws, arterial sticks, or IV line removal.

Home Treatment

Many patients with Haemophilia and their families receive a comprehensive care through a Haemophilia treatment centre that is part of a national network of family-centred Haemophilia treatment centres. One of the primary goals of these centres is to educate patients and families about the disorder [8]. These centres can find such resources as classes, camps, home-care nurses, scholarships, and other programs specially designed for such patients and families. In these organizations, caregivers closely follow patients giving useful information regarding the patient's care.

Most patients with bleeding disorders know a large deal about their disorder. At young age, they are taught to recognize symptoms. They learn to understand that a prompt and appropriate treatment is necessary after an injury, with the aim of stopping bleeding and improve their quality of life. Most have learned to advocate for themselves and seek quick treatment.

Furthermore, many patients infuse their own replacement factor at home. In many children ports or other devices (tunneled or non-tunneled intravenous catheter) for an easier administration are generally implanted. Children as young as age 6 are taught how to use a butterfly needle to infuse factors. They cannot complete the process on their own at this age, but early starting these steps would promote a later independence. In most cases, parents are taught on how to administer factor infusions when their children are infants.

Most children and many adults with severe Haemophilia treat themselves prophylactically with two or three weekly infusions in order to maintain a trough level high enough to prevent spontaneous bleedings and joint damages [9]. In these day and age, young people can participate in sports and physical activities that their grandfathers could only watch from the sidelines.

However, be aware that contact sports are still discouraged for such patients.

Nursing Considerations

The nurse should document the following data regarding home treatments:

1. Date and time of infusion;
2. Manufacturer/brand, lot number, and expiration date of factor;
3. Total dose infused;
4. Rate of infusion;
5. Site of infusion;
6. Infusion reactions or complications;
7. Pre-treatment medications (if required);
8. Response or reaction to treatment; response may not be immediately evident;
9. Follow-up instructions and recommendations.

CONCLUDING REMARKS

Patients who treat themselves at home generally do well. When they require additional treatments, they need healthcare providers who are knowledgeable about their disorder. Having accurate, up-to-date information about signs, symptoms, treatments, and nursing implications of bleeding disorders helps to ensure a proper care of patients: this will result in a better confidence in their care providers. As with all chronic disorders, even if you don't remember everything about the disorder, you can improve the care you provide by listening to the patient, and finding appropriate resources.

CONFLICT OF INTEREST

The authors confirm that they have no conflict of interest to declare for this publication.

ACKNOWLEDGEMENTS

Prof. G. Castaman is acknowledged for his helpful advice. Dr. S. Linari is acknowledged for her teachings and for always being an example of dedication.

This chapter is especially dedicated to my patients. Each page I have written represents the time spent together with them.

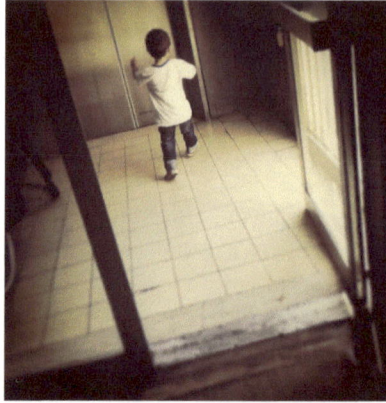

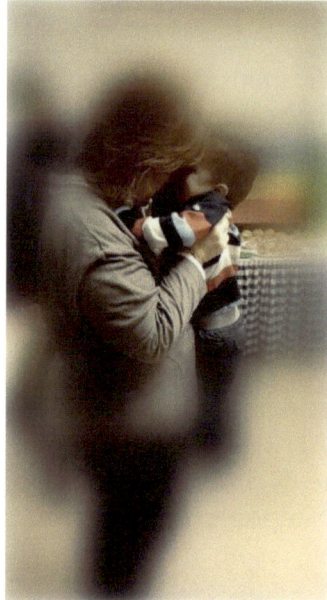

REFERENCES

[1]   Castoldi Gianluigi, Liso Vincenzo. Malattie del sangue e degli organi ematopoietici. 5th., Mc Graw-Hill 2007.

[2]   Jones Peter. Living with Haemophilia. 5th., Oxford University Press 2002.

[3]   Mauser-Bunschoten EP, De Knecht-Van Eekelen A, Smit C. Aging with Haemophilia: medical and psychological impact. Van Creveldklinick-Haematology Utrecht 2007.

[4]   Vanderhave KL, Caird MS, Hake M, *et al.* Musculoskeletal care of the hemophiliac patient. J Am Acad Orthop Surg 2012; 20(9): 553-63.
[PMID: 22941798]

[5]   Centers for Disease Control and Prevention. Hemophilia: Data and statistics , [May 4, 2015];2011 Available at: www.cdc.gov/ncbddd/hemophilia/data.html

[6]   Centers for Disease Control and Prevention. Hemophilia: Information for women , [April 15, 2015]; 2011 Available at: www.cdc.gov/ncbddd/hemophilia/women.html

[7]   Hemophilia of Georgia. Protocols for the treatment of hemophilia and von Willebrand disease , 2012 [April 15, 2015]; Available at: www.hog.org/publications/page/protocols-for-the-treatment- of-hemophilia-and-von-willebrand-disease-2

[8]   Manco-Johnson MJ, Abshire TC, Shapiro AD, *et al.* Prophylaxis *versus* episodic treatment to prevent joint disease in boys with severe hemophilia. N Engl J Med 2007; 357(6): 535-44. [http://dx.doi.org/10.1056/NEJMoa067659] [PMID: 17687129]

[9]   Medical and Scientific Advisory Council. MASAC recommendations concerning products licensed for the treatment of hemophilia and other bleeding disorders. New York: National Hemophilia Foundation 2013 2013. MASAC Document 217

CHAPTER 6

Imaging of Haemophilic Arthropathy

Giuliana Roselli[*], **Giovanni D'Elia** and **Filippo Parretti**

Department of Radiology, Azienda Ospedaliero-Universitaria Careggi, Florence, Italy

Abstract: Haemophilic arthropathy one of the most severe cause of disability in patients affected by severe Haemophilia. The identification of early signs of arthropathy and the assessment of osteochondral damage is fundamental in the management of such patients. Different imaging modalities can be useful to detect haemophilic arthropathy at various stages. Conventional radiography demonstrates bone alterations and indirectly osteochondral damages, and still remains the basis to plan a surgical treatment. Magnetic resonance imaging better detects soft tissues and cartilage abnormalities at every stages, while ultrasonography especially by the color-power Doppler modality has became crucial for the monitoring of underage subjects and for the clinical follow-up. Computed tomography is nowadays just used for the detection of invading pseudotumors, bone erosions, and some extra-musculoskeletal complications of Haemophilia.

Keywords: Computed tomography, Haemophilia, Haemophilic arthropathy, Imaging technique, Magnetic resonance imaging, Radiography, Ultrasonography.

INTRODUCTION

Haemophilia is characterized by recurrent haemorragic episodes in joints inducing an irreversible arthropathy, initially caused by inflammatory proliferation of synovial cells. Such changes may lead over several stages and in case of recurrent bleedings to cartilage and subchondral bone damages with final joint destruction, anatomical compromission, and ankyloses. A delayed haematological treatment increases the risk of arthropathy. The detection of early changes and stages of haemophilic arthropathy is thus crucial to avoid its natural history [1]. The identification of initial signs of haemophilic arthropathy is therefore fundamental and is carried out by various imaging techniques.

For over a century and until the end of 1970s conventional radiography has been used for diagnostic purposes; it still remains the standard tool of diagnosis for

[*] **Corresponding author Giuliana Roselli:** Department of Radiology, AOU Careggi, Florence, Italy; Tel: 0039 055 794 8286; E-mail: rosellig@aou-careggi.toscana.it

haemophilic arthropathy and has a central role for the planning of any orthopaedic treatment [1 - 9].

In the 1980s Magnetic Resonance Imaging (MRI) became a useful diagnostic technique for the assessment of several stages of arthropathy, and its importance progressively increased over the last years. This imaging modality has shown a considerable accuracy in assessing early soft tissues and cartilage changes, adding high levels of details with respect to x-rays [6 - 14].

Since the 1950s ultrasonography (US) was supposed to be an important technique for the clinical practice. In the last decades, its development by the use of linear high-resolution probes and dedicated software has enabled to visualize almost all musculoskeletal structures with less costs and an easier accessibility [1, 5, 12, 15, 16]. In addition, color and power Doppler modalities have been recently introduced in order to assess the synovial vascularity in case of arthropathy [17].

Finally, Computed Tomography (CT) commonly performed in the last decades and now progressively underused, is indicated to assess abnormal bone changes. It is very useful to evaluate alterations as erosions, cysts, and particularly indicated to characterize chronic encapsulated fluid structures as pseudotumors, or spontaneous or posttraumatic haemorragic episodes in other non-musculoskeletal sites [1, 16, 18 - 20].

The following is an overview of the diagnostic techniques useful to assess the diagnosis and the evolution of the haemophilic arthropathy and its related clinical issues.

CONVENTIONAL RADIOGRAPHY

For many decades the diagnosis of haemophilic arthropathy has been done by plain radiographs: radiography still nowadays represents the gold standard diagnostic tool for the clinical practice [1,13,21-23]. However, it is not properly indicated to detect early articular changes particularly in children. So, even if it represents the best examination in adults, especially before and after surgery it is often associated with US for the periodic assessment of target joints in underage patients and for follow-up evaluations after conservative treatments (see chapter 8)[15].

As mentioned in chapter 1, arthropathy usually starts from the first haemarthrosis in several target joints [1] Fig. (**1**). Knees are the most affected joints, given their high amount of synovial tissue. In children, x-rays may show the following common changes: epiphyseal overgrowth, widening of intercondylar notch, and squaring of the patella [5, 6] Fig. (**2**). Progressively, limb malalignment, and length discrepancy may develop. In adults and later stages of haemophilic arthropathy conventional plain radiographs may demonstrate loss of joint space, bone erosions, osteophytes, subchondral cysts, and even ankyloses [2,23] Figs. (**3** and **4**).

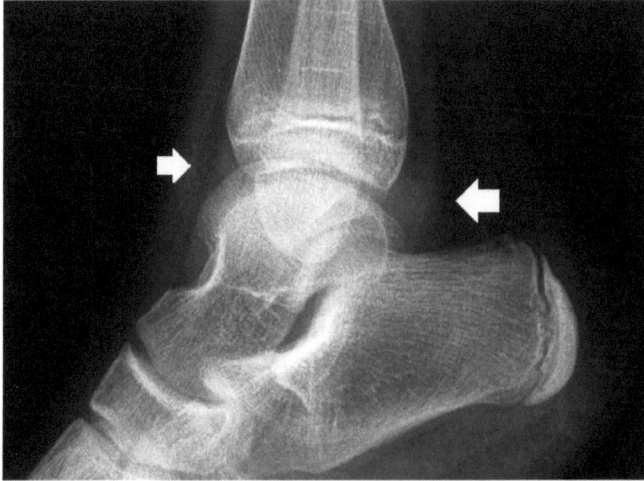

Fig. (1). Right ankle of a 11-years old child at his first episode of haemarthrosis. Note the slight swelling of articular soft tissue prevalent in the back seat due to bleeding (arrows).

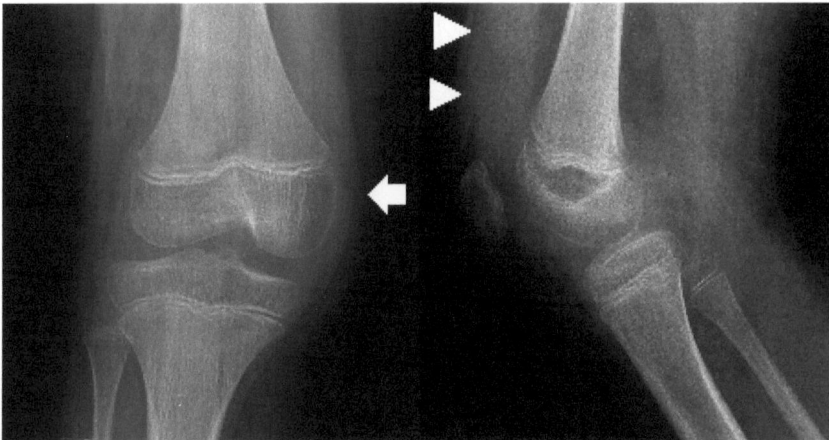

Fig. (2). Right knee of a 12-years old child with typical signs of the progression of the disease. Local osteoporosis at the medial condyle and growth of the trochlea femoral epiphysis with widening of the intercondylar notch (arrow), and effusion in the suprapatellar recess (arrow heads).

In order to quantify the severity of arthropathy, several x-rays based scores have been proposed. The most used classifications are the Arnold-Hilgartner (1977) and the Pettersson score (1980).

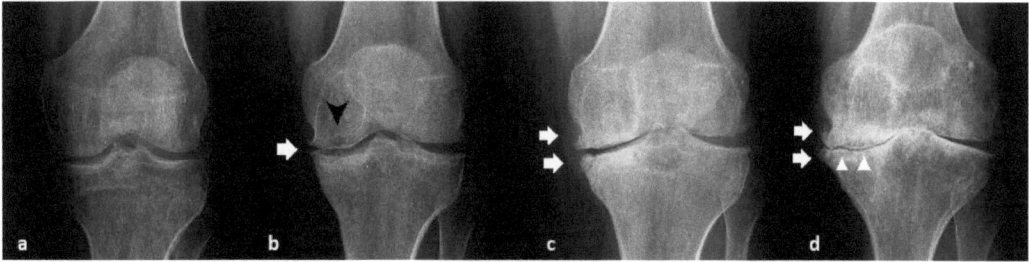

Fig. (3). Various stages of arthropathy in knees of different haemophilic patients. Early stage of disease with osteoporosis (a); initial joint space narrowing (arrow), and subchondral cysts (black arrow)(b); progressive reduction of the joint space with erosions of cartilage and soft tissue swelling (arrows)(c); late stage with subtotal loss of joint space, an indirect sign of cartilage loss (arrow heads), osteophytes (arrows), and evident varus deformity (d).

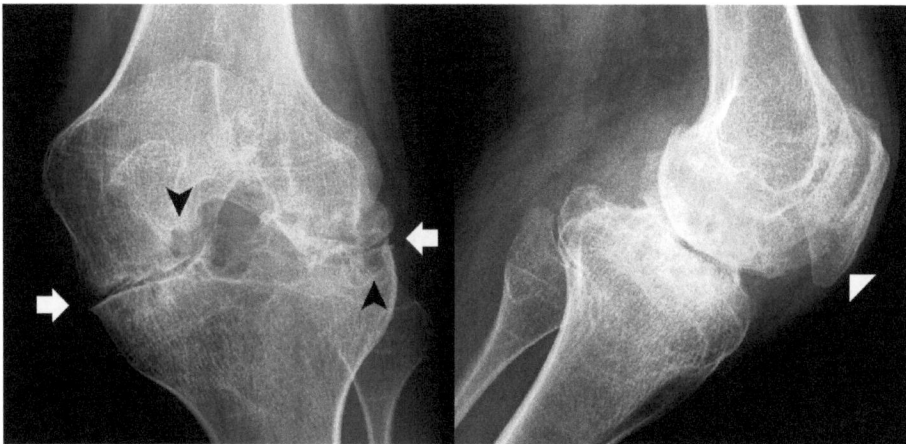

Fig. (4). Advanced stage of arthropathy in a young subject with all the characteristic patterns. Epiphyseal overgrowth, widening of the intercondylar notch, squaring of the patella (arrow head); subchondral cysts (black arrows); cartilage erosion with subtotal joint space loss and ankyloses (arrows).

The Arnold-Hilgartner score consists in the evaluation of soft tissues and osteochondral changes on a 0-5 grading system (Table **1**). Stage 0 is then assigned to the articulation defined as "normal". Stage 1 is characterized by the presence of soft tissue swelling due to haemarthrosis or bleeding in periarticular soft tissue, without however evidence of skeletal abnormalities. Stage 2 instead presents some initial skeletal manifestations such as osteopenia and excessive epiphyseal growth. Stage 3 is characterized by the presence of subchondral cysts, squaring of the profile of the patella, widening of intercondilar notch, however with a maintained cartilage thickness, unlike the next stage where we find an erosion of the cartilage with consequent reduction of the joint space. Finally, the stage 5 is the most advanced stage of the disease, where we can recognize a substantial subversion of the joint structures Fig. (**5**).

Table 1. Arnold-Hilgartner classification (1977) *modified*.

Stage	Radiographic Sign
0	"NORMAL" JOINT
1	SOFT TISSUE SWELLING PRESENT
2	OVERGROW EPIPHYSIS,WITHOUT EROSIONS OSTEOPOROSIS
3	SUBCHONDRAL CYSTS, SQUARING OF PATELLA,WIDENING OF INTERCONDILAR NOTCH(HUMERUS AND DISTAL FEMUR),CARTILAGE SPACE MAINTAINED
4	WORSENING OF STAGE 3 WITH EROSIONS AND NARROWING OF CARTILAGE SPACE
5	LOSS OF JOINT SPACE, MARKED ENLARGMENT OF EPIPHYSIS, SUBSTANCIAL STRUCTURE ABNORMALITY OF JOINT, FIBROUS JOINT CONCTRACTURE

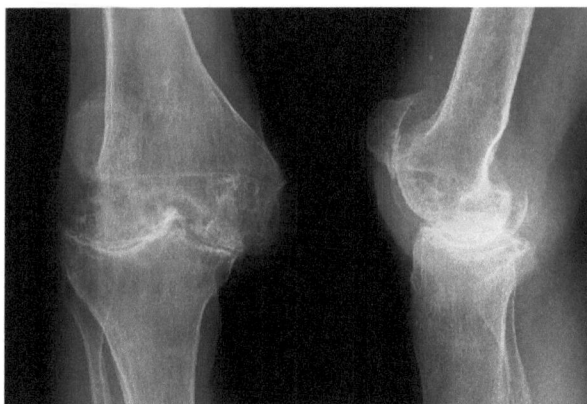

Fig. (5). Stage 5 according to Arnold-Hilgartner. Advanced degree of arthropathy with a general subversion of the joint and a complete loss of the joint space.

A further modified version of the classification of Arnold-Hilgartner provides for the presence of only 4 stages, as a result of the elimination of the original stage 2, which in clinical practice are rarely distinguished as a separate stage and presents no specific implications in terms of therapeutic treatment [2].

The Pettersson score (1980) is instead a detailed classification of joints that allows an estimation of the degree of radiographic alterations of joints. Eight different radiographic parameters are evaluated. The normal joint has a score of 0, while the score related to the maximum degree of gravity is 13. One point is assigned in case of presence of abnormalities such as osteoporosis, excessive growth of the epiphyseal cartilage, and erosion. One or two points will be awarded, depending on the degree of gravity, in presence of signs as irregular subchondral bone, incongruity of the articular surfaces, subchondral cysts, joint space narrowing, and bone remodelling (Table **2**)[7] Figs. (**6** and **7**).

Table 2. Pettersson score (1980) *modified.*

Radiographic Sign		Score
Osteoporosis	Absent	0
	Present	1
Enlarged epiphysis	Absent	0
	Present	1
Cartilage erosion at joint margins	Absent	0
	Present	1
Irregular subchondral surface	Absent	0
	Slight	1
	Pronounced	2
Inconsistency articular surfaces	Absent	0
	Slight	1
	Pronounced	2
Subchondral cysts	Absent	0
	1 Cyst	1
	>1 Cyst	2
Reduction in joint space	Absent	0
	<50%	1
	>50%	2
Deformity (angle or displacement of the joint)	Absent	0
	Slight	1
	Pronounced	2

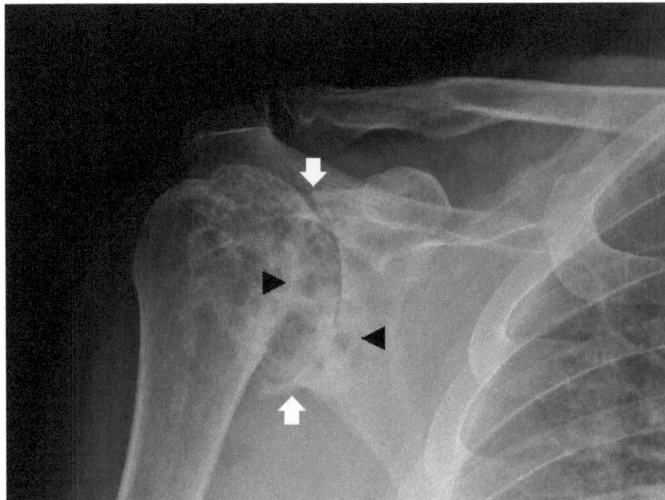

Fig. (6). Right shoulder of an adult patient affected by Haemophilia. Pettersson score: 9. Moderate degrees of cartilage erosion, slight irregular subchondral surface, subchondral cysts (black arrows), marked reduction of the joint space (arrows).

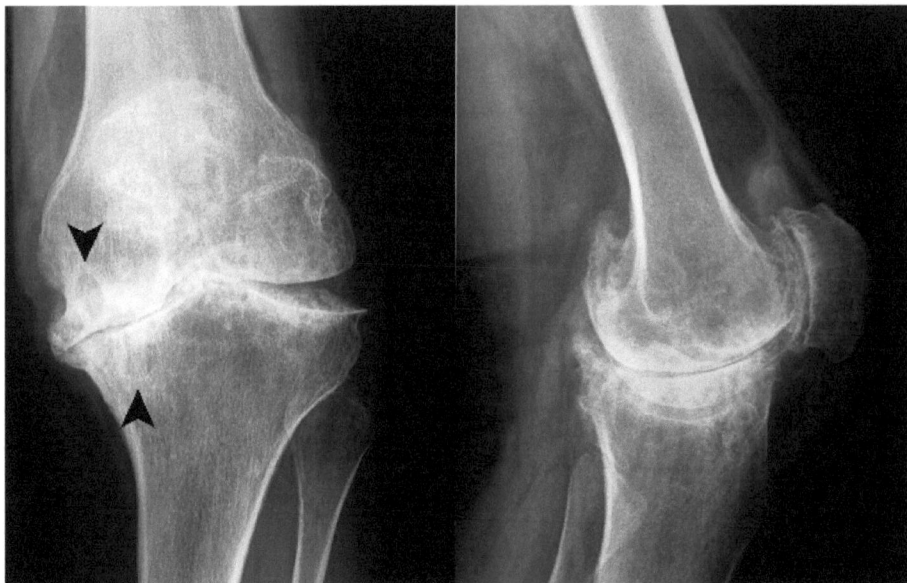

Fig. (7). Left knee of a haemophilic patient. Pettersson score: 9. Of noting the presence of an advanced degree of bone deformity (2 pts), and a marked reduction of the joint space (2 pts); also present some subchondral cysts (2 pts) (black arrows) with cartilage erosion (1 pt), and subchondral bone irregularities (2 pts).

Several differences exist between these two scores. The Arnold-Hilgartner classification is simple and easier to be interpreted, and represents a progressive scale. The Pettersson score is an additive scale with a higher complexity but better precision in the evaluation of a stage of arthropathy [3, 7]. Specifically, the Arnold-Hilgartner scale classifies as "non-specific" the typical pathological changes in haemophilic arthropathy such as joint effusion, synovial hypertrophy, hemosyderin deposits, and periarticular oedema. In addition, cartilage destruction can be indirectly assessed by the joint space narrowing on plain radiographs. On the other hand, the Pettersson score does not consider soft tissues changes. Even if such limitations, the Pettersson score has been recommended by the World Federation of Haemophilia (WFH) [7,8].

In conclusion, the detection of radiographic signs usually corresponds to moderate to severe stages of arthropathy: it means that such method may not be considered the best choice to plan a modern prevention strategy or establish the efficacy of early conservative or minimally invasive treatments. Nowadays early synovial and chondral alterations are better detected by US and MRI, and x-rays may add some informations in adult patients [11]. Despite these pitfalls, conventional radiography plays a role of paramount importance in the surgical planning for joint fusions or joint replacement (Figs. **8** and **9**).

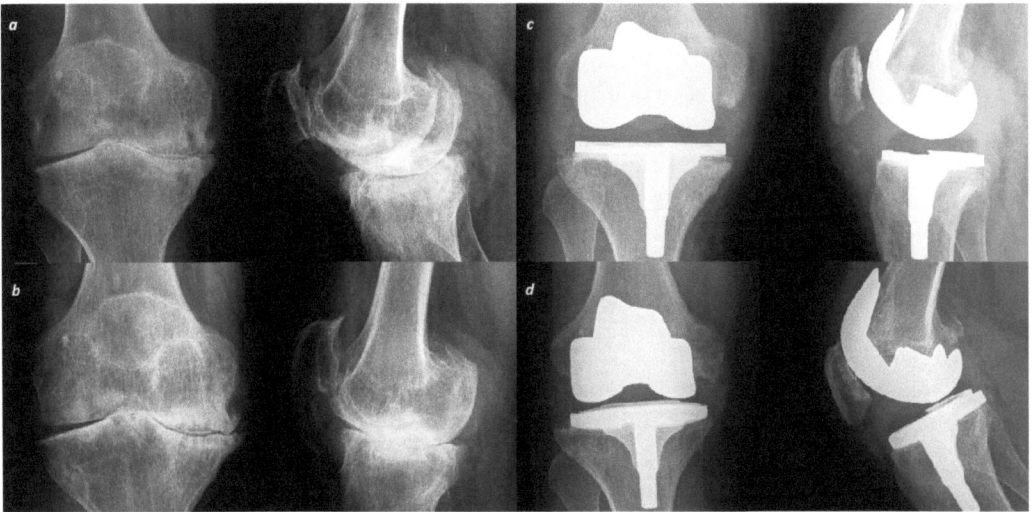

Fig. (8). Right knee of a 50-years old haemophiliac (a). A radiographic follow-up after two years shows the progression of the arthropathy with almost complete loss of the joint space (b). Immediate postoperative x-rays (c) and 5-years follow-up after total knee replacement (d).

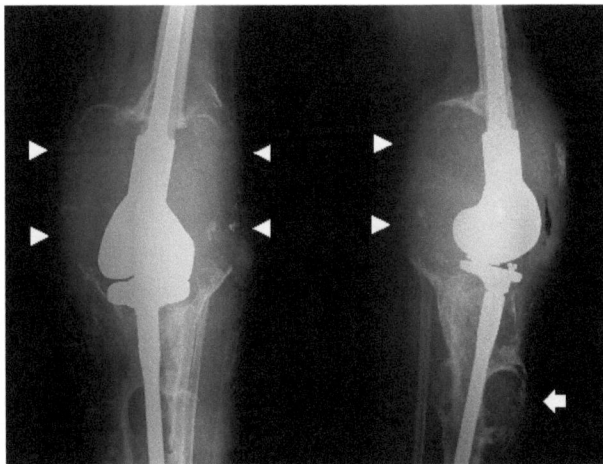

Fig. (9). Radiographic follow-up in a hemophiliac patient previously treated by a revision knee replacement. Note the progression of the arthropathy with marked periprosthetic bone erosions, formation of a large pseudotumor in the distal femur and proximal tibia.

MAGNETIC RESONANCE IMAGING

MRI has become the modality of choice for the evaluation of articular disorders [5, 8, 11]. In the diagnostic pathway of haemophilic arthropathy MRI has increasingly been used due to its superior soft-tissues contrast resolution, identifying all key pathologic features of this disease in all stages and patients [5,14].

MRI is a precise and non-invasive tool for the detection of joint effusions, haemarthrosis, synovial proliferation, chondral and subchondral abnormalities, ligaments, muscles, and juxtarticular soft tissues [10, 11, 24, 25]. It is particularly sensitive for the assessment of early preclinical stages of arthropathy still undetectable by conventional radiography, and has demonstrated high accuracy in determining the presence of deep seated haemartroses or muscle bleedings.

Moreover, the emerging main role of MRI is the evaluation of those changes of haemophilic arthropathy that may aid in the selection of patients who may benefit from a secondary haematological prophylaxis.

As mentioned in chapter 1, knees, ankles, and elbows are the most commonly affected joints [6, 26]. A bilateral involvement is frequent, but acute bleedings usually regard a single target joint. Recurrent bleedings progressively induce synovial hyperplasia, chronic inflammatory changes, fibrosis, and haemosiderin deposits in synovial membranes.

Synovial membranes and articular cartilages are the initially damaged structures: such alterations are undetectable by radiography and CT, thus MRI is the most sensitive radiological technique for their evaluation due to its inherent features [26, 27] (Fig. **10**).

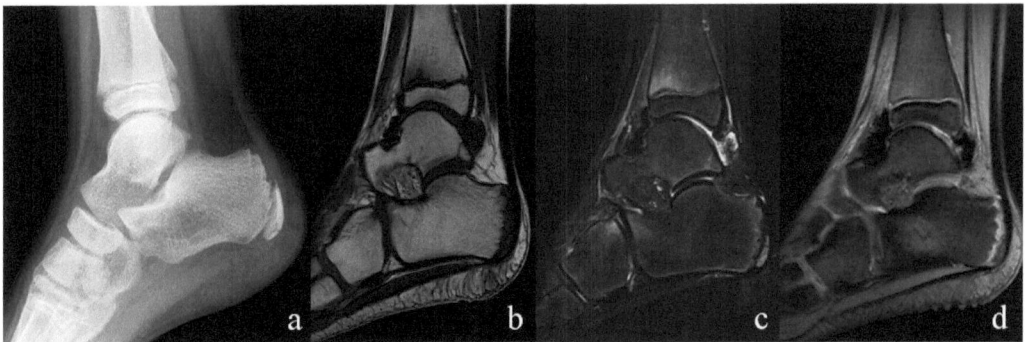

Fig. (10).   Left ankle of a 12-years old haemophilic patient. X-rays (a) does not show any skeletal alterations despite Sagittal TSET1-w (b), STIR (c), and GE T2* (d) MRI sequences reveal the synovial proliferation in the anterior and posterior recesses of the tibio-talar joint. It appears as a low signal on all sequences due to the haemosiderin deposition, associated with articular effusion and marrow oedema within the anterior tibial metaphysis, close to the growth plate.

As for other diagnostic tools, several MRI scoring systems have been proposed in the last years [10, 12, 14, 27 - 32].

The first MRI scoring method was developed in Denver in 1992, and considered the prototype of scoring systems [10, 28]. It is based on an additive score related to the severity of detected alterations, with a maximum value of 10. The Denver scale consists in the evaluation of several parameters, as effusion, haemarthrosis, synovial hyperplasia, haemosiderin, cysts, erosion, and cartilage loss (Table **3**).

Table 3. The Denver magnetic resonance imaging score *modified*.

0	Normal joint
	Effusion/haemarthrosis
1	Small
2	Moderate
3	Large
	Synovial hyperplasia/haemosiderin
4	Small
5	Moderate
6	Large
	Cyst/erosion
7	1 cyst or partial surface erosion
8	>1 cyst or full surface erosion
	Cartilage loss
9	<50%
10	≥50%

Later another MRI classification was released in Europe [27], providing a more complex additive scoring scale in the format A (e,s,h), a scheme that allows separation of different pathological components of the haemophilic arthropathy [28]. Factor A indicates the sum of scores for subchondral cysts (maximum value 6), irregularity/erosion of subchondral zone (maximum 4), and chondral destruction (maximum 6). In these three categories each statement is evaluated as true or false, and each true statement adds one point to the A component. E, s, and h parameters represent effusion/haemarthrosis, synovial hypertrophy and haemosiderin deposition respectively, and they are independently evaluated according to a five-grade scale (by values of 0 to 4) (Table **4**).

Table 4. The European magnetic resonance imaging score (*modified*).

Subchondral Cysts (part a)	
Present in at least one bone	1
Present in at least two bones	2
More than three cysts in at least one bone	3
More than three cysts in at least two bones	4

(Table 4) contd.....

Subchondral Cysts (part a)	
Largest size more than 4 mm in at least one bone	5
Largest size more than 4 mm in at least two bones	6
Irregularity/Erosion of Subchondral Cortex (part a)	
Present in at least one bone	1
Present in at least two bones	2
Involves more than half of joint surface in at least one bone	3
Involves more than half of joint surface in at least two bones	4
Chondral Destruction (part a)	
Present in at least one bone	1
Present in at least two bones	2
Full-thickness defect in at least one bone	3
Full-thickness defect in at least two bones	4
Full-thickness defect involves more than one-third of joint surface in at least one bone	5
Full-thickness defect involves more than one-third of joint surface in at least two bones	6
Effusion/Haemarthrosis (e)	0/4
Hypertrophic Sinovia (s)	0/4
Haemosiderin (h)	0/4

Both Denver and Lundin MRI classifications are the most common scores used in literature [29], even the presence of evident pitfalls. For these reasons, further systems have been proposed in the clinical practice, characterized by a higher complexity: the Compatible MRI scale [30] and the International Prophylaxis Study Group (IPSG) MRI scale [31, 32].

The Compatible MRI scale is a scoring system that includes both a 10-step progressive (*P-scale*) and a 20-step additive (*A-scale*) components. It may reveal the most severe joint changes as well as to appreciate the severity of single findings. The IPSG MRI scale is an additive scale suitable for the assessment of patients with early or moderate joint changes: the total score represents the sum of various subscores for soft tissues and osteochondral changes [14].

Whatever the method of evaluation a MRI study has to be performed using specific features. A basic MRI protocol should include: acquisitions in three planes as coronal or sagittal T1- weighted spin-echo and axial T1-weighted sequences; long axis STIR or PD fat sat, axial T2-weighted, coronal or sagittal GE-T2 sequence (GE-T2*) sequences. It is suggested to complete the analysis by acquisition of T1-weighted sequences (with and without fat saturation) before and after the intravenous contrast administration [26, 33, 34].

Synovial tissue physiologically lining joint spaces, bursae, and tendinous sheaths are usually too thin to be evaluated on MRI. After few episodes of bleedings, the deposition of haemosiderin in the superficial and deeper layers of the synovial membrane causes a proliferation of synovial fibroblasts and vascular cells [24]. The thickening of the synovial membrane results in frond-like projections along the articular surfaces leading to mechanical impingement and recurrent bleedings due to vascular disruptions. Synovitis caused by inflammatory process and characterized by increased synovial fluid volume shows intermediate/low signal intensity on T1-weighted images and intermediate/high signal intensity on T2-weighted images in relation to the percentage of its thickness and increased water content.

Usually fat suppressed T2-weighted images or short-tau inversion recovery (STIR) images show hypertrophic synovial tissues with high signal intensity and more clearly delineate extension. It may be occasionally difficult to differentiate synovitis from joint fluid on unenhanced MR images. In such cases heavily T2-weighted images can be helpful in demonstrating synovitis which has a lower signal intensity with respect to effusion. The use of intravenous contrast material may play an important role in the detection and characterization of synovitis compared to joint effusion since synovitis shows a clear enhancement after contrast medium administration [24]. In some cases, the increased synovial uptake of gadolinium makes possible to quantify the degree of synovitis [35].

Quantitative methods of evaluation of the synovial hypertrophy usually consist in the drawing of an area ("region of interest") on a given MRI slice and to repeat this procedure on contiguous slices [11, 36]. Even it is not easy, each area is then summed to obtain a quantifiable volume [5].

Alternatively, the Denver system uses a semiquantitative analysis in order to classify the synovial proliferation as: absent, small, moderate, or large. Intravenous gadolinium can aid to detect the activity of synovial tissues but it is not accurate as the quantitative method. On the other hand, the routinary use of gadolinium is discussed and not generally recommended for children, high costs, and examination time, as well as due to the risk of allergic reactions [37].

Otherwise hypertrophic synovial membrane due to repeated haemarthrosis has a characteristic low signal intensity in all pulse sequences due to the iron deposition: especially GE sequences secondary are enhanced due to the magnetic susceptibility effect caused by haemosiderin [5,38] (Fig. **11**).

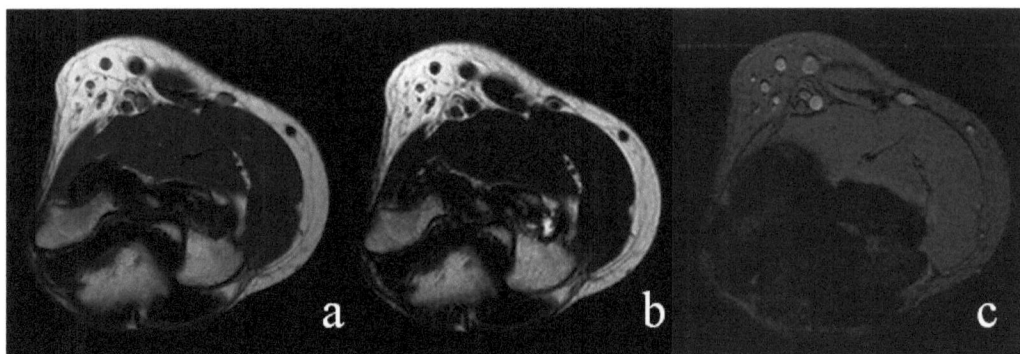

Fig. (11). Right elbow of a 24-years old patient. Axial TSET1-w (a), TSET2-w (b), and GE T2* (c) showing hypertrophic synovial membrane with the characteristic low signal intensity on all pulse sequences due to the iron deposition as result of repeated haemarthroses. The magnetic susceptibility artefacts of the GE image hamper the visualization of soft tissues resulting in an overestimation synovial proliferation.

GE-T2* is considered the most sensitive and specific sequence in the assessment of blood-derived products given its ability to demonstrate very small haemosiderin deposits characterized by a low signal. Haemosiderin depositions within the synovial membrane in patients with chronic haemarthrosis displays a low signal intensity in both GE-T2* and in the T1- and T2-weighted sequences. At the same time GE-T2* does not allow an optimal evaluation of the synovial hypertrophy because artefacts alter the visualization of soft tissues, particularly in cases of higher haemosiderin deposition and resulting in an overestimation synovial proliferation [38] (Fig. **12**).

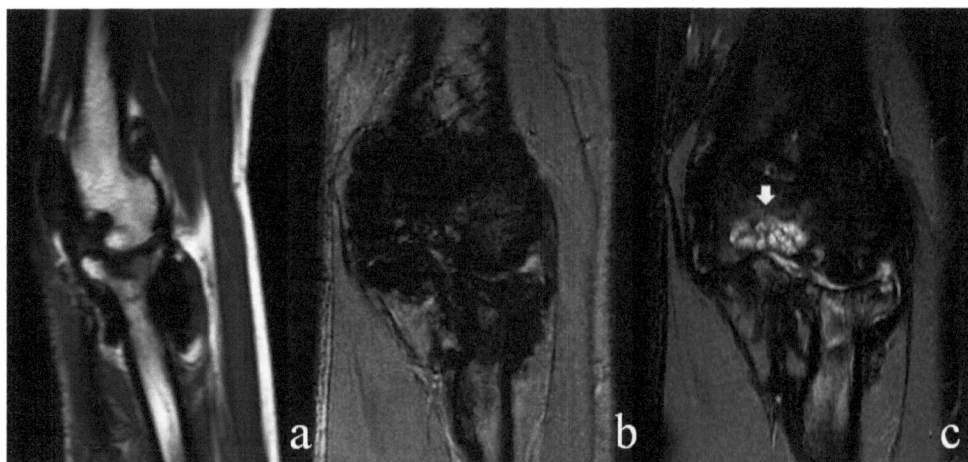

Fig. (12). Sagittal TSET1-w (a), coronal GET2* (b), and coronal STIR (c) sequences of the right elbow of the same patient in Fig. (**11**) demonstrating: lobulated low-signal haemosiderin deposits, cartilage loss, joint space thinning, subchondral irregularities, and high-signal cysts of the distal humerus (arrow). Of noting, also the marrow oedema in the proximal radius.

GE images allow also a good visualization of the articular cartilage owing its adequate spatial detection and the optimal contrast resolution: such parameter is crucial to evaluate the severity of arthropathy. Fast spin echo (FSE) sequences, gradient recalled echo acquisitions, and three dimensional SE e GRE sequences are available to assess the structure of the cartilage. These modalities provide accurate informations and allow the detection of morphologic defects such as fissuration, focal, diffuse partial or full-thickness cartilage loss. They are commonly used for semiquantitative and quantitative assessments of cartilage. There are also other techniques such as T2 mapping, delayed gadolinium-enhanced MR imaging of cartilage, T1ρ imaging, sodium imaging, and diffusion imaging that allow to evaluate the collagen network and proteoglycan content in the cartilage matrix [1, 39 - 43].

These sequences may be used in various combinations to improve the characterization of chondral alterations but require high magnetic field strengths. The field strength of 1.5 Tesla is at least recommended for morphologic assessment of cartilage, widely available and used in most centres. A field strength of 3.0 T allows better morphologic evaluation of cartilage than 1.5 T as the signal noise ratio (SNR) is roughly twice, improving image quality and spatial resolution within the same or lesser time acquisition [42,44]. However, it should be taken into account that as magnetic field strength increases the magnetic susceptibility in tissue is emphasized: thus, images are more sensitive to flow artefacts and chemical shift effects enhance. Therefore, articular blood and haemosiderin deposits in haemophilic patients may alter the image quality at higher magnetic fields. Despite such improvements, the evaluation of the chondral damage at early stages of the disease are very difficult to be estimated in small joints in which cartilage lining is very thin. The same Denver MRI score that defines as "cartilage loss" less than 50% loss of the expected height of the joint space on a coronal image of the joint for a moderate change, and 50% or greater loss for severe change can be difficult to apply [10].

Recurrent bleedings in target joints may produce a focal destruction of articular cartilage and erosions of subchondral bone: MRI is able to detect bone erosions definitely better than conventional radiography especially in the earlier stages [13]. Erosions consist of a break in cortical bones overlying a region of altered signal intensity with definite margins. Erosions may be difficult to distinguish from focal regions of bone marrow oedema, mainly on T1-weighted images, in which both appear as hypointense. High signal intensity on fat suppressed images and enhancement after the administration of gadolinium-based contrast material are the modality to ascertain such alterations. Erosions have more defined margins and clear cortical break, making it difficult to differentiate if bone marrow oedema is associated in GE-T2 sequences. Otherwise bone marrow oedema alone described in many forms of arthritis is recognized as an area in the subcortical bone with increased signal on STIR, T2-weigthed FS and post contrast T1-weighted with FS, but the post-contrast enhancement is less than the pannus [11, 13, 45] (Fig. **13**).

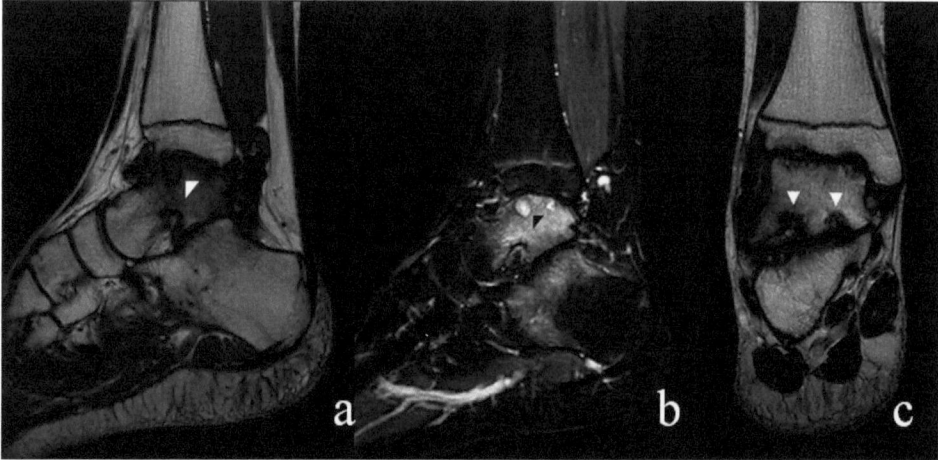

Fig. (13). Right ankle of a 34-years old patient. Sagittal TSET1-w (a), sagittal STIR (b), and coronal TSET2-w (c) MRI sequences showing: loss of joint space, cortical and subchondral irregularities, erosions and cysts of the talar dome and posterior subtalar joint (arrow heads). At this level it may be also observed a marked marrow oedema within the talus and calcaneus.

MRI easily demonstrates subchondral bone cysts which may be seen as low signal intensity area on T1-weighted images and low to high signal intensity on T2-weighted images depending on the characteristics of the extruded synovial tissue within the subchondral defects (Fig. **14**).

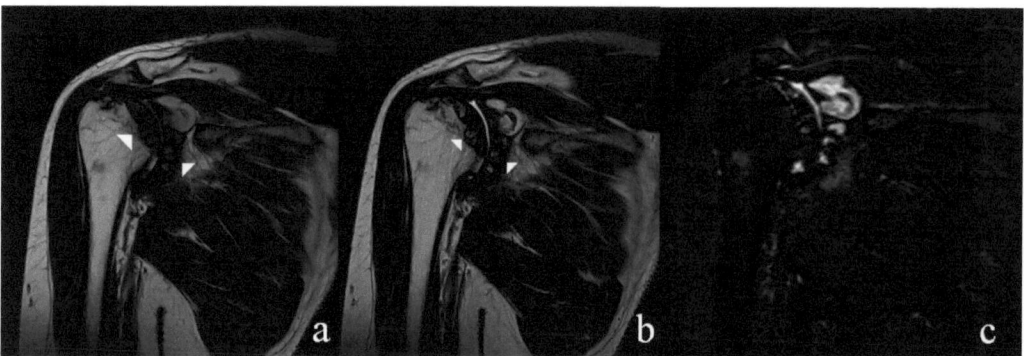

Fig. (14). Right shoulder of a 48-years old patient. Coronal TSET1-w (a), TSET2-w (b), and STIR (c) images displaying multiple subchondral cysts of the humeral epiphysis and glenoid, with intermediate/low signal contents suggestive of extruded fibrotic synovium (arrow heads). Moderate joint effusion in the supraspinous fossa with haemarthrosis visible as hyperintensity on T1 images.

The signal intensity may indicate the presence of synovial tissue with haemosiderin (low signal intensity on T2-weighted images), poorly hydrated soft tissues (intermediate signal intensity), or fluid (high signal intensity) (Fig. **15**).

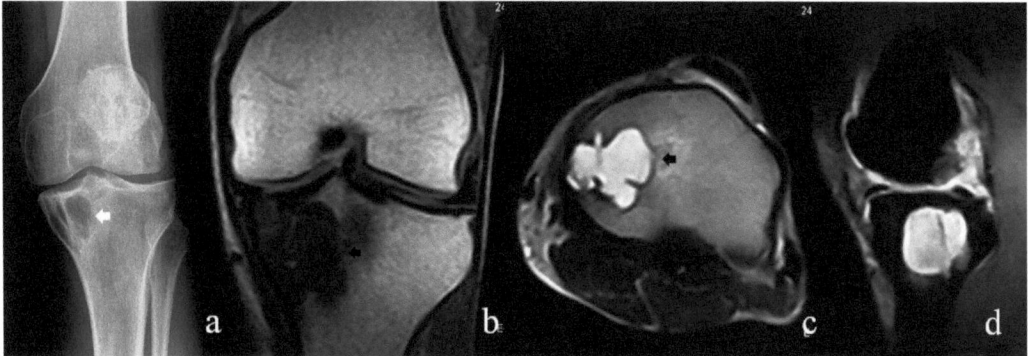

Fig. (15). Left knee of a 38-years old haemophilic patient. X-rays (a) show a large multilobulated lesion in the medial condyle of the left proximal tibia with well-defined margins (arrows). At MRI study, low signal intensity on coronal T1-w (b) and high signal on the axial T2-w (c), and sagittal STIR (d) images reflecting the presence of synovial fluid.

Some of these may be "non-enhancing" following contrast injection, if they contain fibrous tissue rather than inflammatory pannus and be relatively "inactive" [45].

Joint effusions typically display MR signal characteristics of synovial fluid, with low signal intensity on T1-weighted images and high signal intensity on T2-weighted images, or STIR and FS T2-weighted sequences. The presence of blood in the joint fluid causes a decrease of the signal intensity on T2 images, particularly in GE-T2*. These sequences enhance the signal of intraarticular bleeding and its metabolites, allowing to distinguish blood from non-haemorragic synovial fluid.

Acute or subacute and chronic types of haemarthrosis may show different aspects in signal intensity of intra-articular fluid depending on the age of bleeding. They may also have high signal on both T1 and T2 weighted spin-echo images if fluid and extracellular metahaemoglobin are together represented into the joint. Sometimes it is possible to appreciate the image of "fluid-fluid" level in the joint due to sedimentation of blood products [24].

The clinical meaning of joint effusion in haemophilic patients is unclear because several authors have found that it is not directly related to arthropathy. Moreover, it can be a transient finding frequently observed in joints of healthy subjects. Therefore it may be preferable to exclude an effusion in the scoring system for the assessment of haemophilic arthropathy [33].

In late stages, MRI may be useful to display advanced bony changes, as marked cortical irregularities, marginal osteophytes, focal subchondral necrosis, joint deformity, and finally ankyloses. However, x-rays and CT are considered most useful to plan surgery.

It appears clear that homogeneous MRI criteria for the evaluation of joint damage in haemophiliacs still lack of global consensus: however MRI is a powerful tool for diagnosis and crucial to assess specific treatments in early stages and in underage subjects, that represent the target of the future preventive strategies to limit the clinical issues related to Haemophilia [46 - 49].

Pseudotumor and Haematoma

Pseudotumors are typical complications of Haemophilia developing as a result of recurrent bleedings. They occur in 1-2% of patients with severe coagulation disorders and can be classified as subcutaneous, intramuscular, interfascial, subperiosteal, or intraosseus depending on the site of development [16, 18, 50 - 56] (Fig. **16**).

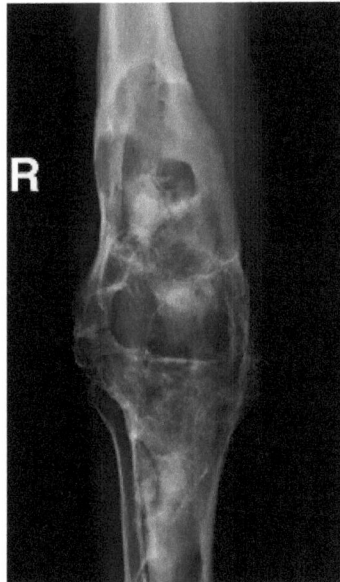

Fig. (16). X-rays of the result of a knee fusion for a severe arthropathy with large and confluent pseudo-tumors.

Usually they present as intramuscular hematomas, while less frequently haemorrhages result in bone pseudotumors or subperiosteal haematomas. Some muscles are most frequently affected, as the iliopsoas, vastus lateralis, and soleus [50] (Fig. **17**).

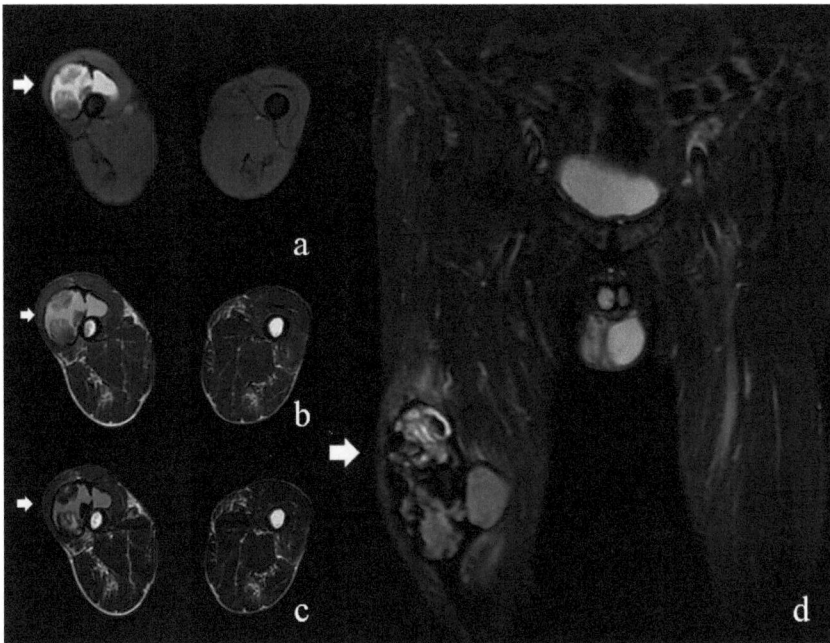

Fig. (17). MRI of a 60-years old patient. Axial TSET1-w images with (a) and without (b) fat saturation, axial TSET2-w (c), and coronal STIR (d) sequences reveal a haematoma of the vastus intermedius muscle in the right quadriceps femoris. Peculiar is the elliptical shape and different combinations of signal intensity within the lesion indicating variable stages of haemorrhage. Multiple nodules with lobulated margins are seen to attach to the capsule, exhibiting heterogeneous signal intensity compatible with blood clots in various stages of evolution (arrows).

Pseudotumors generally present as slowly expanding masses, surrounded by a fibrous wall, and may appear to be multilobulated. If recurrent bleedings realize into deeply situated muscles the diagnosis may be very difficult [50].

Proximal pseudotumors around femur and pelvis probably arise from soft tissues and secondarily erode bones from outside.

Pseudotumors of the ilium may cause significant bony erosion or even bone destruction (Fig. **18**).

Distal pseudotumors are most frequent in children and adolescents and are generally the result of a direct trauma. They are most likely secondary to an intraosseus haemorrhage and are frequently seen in small cancellous bones (carpal and tarsal bones).

MRI and CT may help to define the extent of the pseudotumor, and detecting eventual relationships with surrounding structures, joints, and neurovascular bundle.

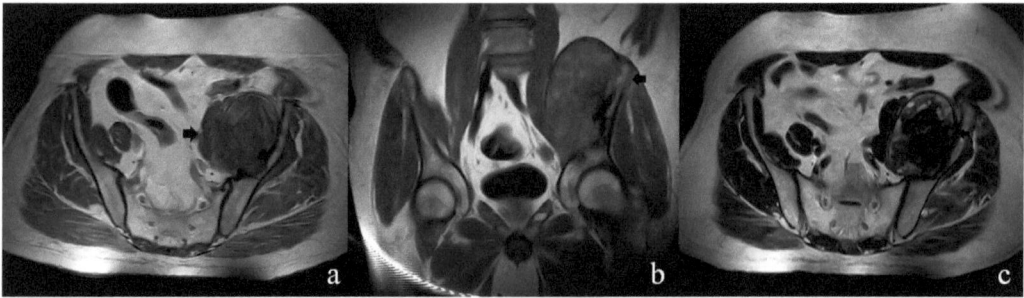

Fig. (18). Haemophilic subject of 64 years. MRI images of the pelvis demonstrating a large pseudotumour in the iliac muscle involving the left iliac bone (arrows). Most of the mass demonstrates a mixed signal on both TSET1-weighted (a,b) and TSET2-weighted images (c), compatible with blood in various stages of evolution. The peripheral capsule of the mass presents a low signal on all sequences due to the presence of haemosiderin.

MRI is however superior to CT to assess the extent in soft tissues and intramedullary spaces as well as monitoring the therapeutic response, given its better contrast resolution.

MRI aspect of a haematoma depends on its stage and it is strongly influenced by the presence of haemoglobin breakdown products [51, 55]. MRI pattern of an acute haematoma (1-3 days after bleeding) is characterized by isointensity as compared to the adjacent muscle on T1-weighted sequence, and hypointense on T2 images due to the presence of deoxyhaemoglobin. In the early subacute phase (4-7 days) metahaemoglobin is observed at the periphery of a haematoma, and produces the "concentric ring" sign, peripheral high T1 signal intensity [18, 51]. In the late subacute phase (1-4 weeks) a haematoma typically displays high signal intensity from the periphery to the center on T1 images, while may be hypointense (due to intracellular metahaemoglobin) or hyperintense (due to extracellular metahaemoglobin) on the T2-weighted sequences. As red cells lysis takes place their water content increases and in the chronic phase the final degradation product, haemosiderin, is formed peripherally. A low signal intensity on all pulse sequences will be then evaluable. A peripheral dark signal rim appearing on the T2-weighted images in the extra-articular musculoskeletal system bleeding has to be referred to a fibrous capsule of haemosiderin. Serum fluid may show a low signal intensity on T1-weighted and high signal intensity on T2-weighted images. Gradient recalled echo sequences are particularly useful for the evaluation of a hematoma characterizing haemosiderin deposits and enhancing the low signal of the fibrous capsule [51].

In some cases, it may be difficult to differentiate pseudotumors from haemorr-hagic tumors in subjects affected by chronic bleedings in soft tissue masses. Despite MRI may help to characterize a malignant mass it should not be considered as fully diagnostic: so as for non haemophilic patients, a prudent diagnostic approach should be performed.

A haematoma in muscles can have variable aspects on MRI according to the duration of bleeding. The use of contrast material helps in the exclusion of a neoplasm when the lesion does not exhibit any enhancement. Conversely, the presence of an enhancing nodule in a "pseudomass" suggests the diagnosis of a neoplasm. In any case a percutaneous biopsy with a core biopsy needle or an open biopsy should be carried out to make a diagnosis of a pseudotumor and rule out any malignancy [56].

Pseudotumors occurring in deeply situated muscles can remain within the muscle or may dissect along it inducing bone deformity and erosions, periosteal reactions, or medullary destruction [5, 53]. A great help may be deserved by conventional radiology. The aspect at MRI analysis is that of an intramedullary cystic lesion or a discrete mass confined to the subperiosteal space, extending also to the intramedullary portion or juxtaskeletal soft tissues. Frequently it shows signals compatible with the chronic stage of a bleeding. So different combinations of signal intensity may be observed: areas with low, intermediate, or high signal intensity on both T1 and T2 sequences representing blood products in various stages of resorption or activity (Fig. **19**).

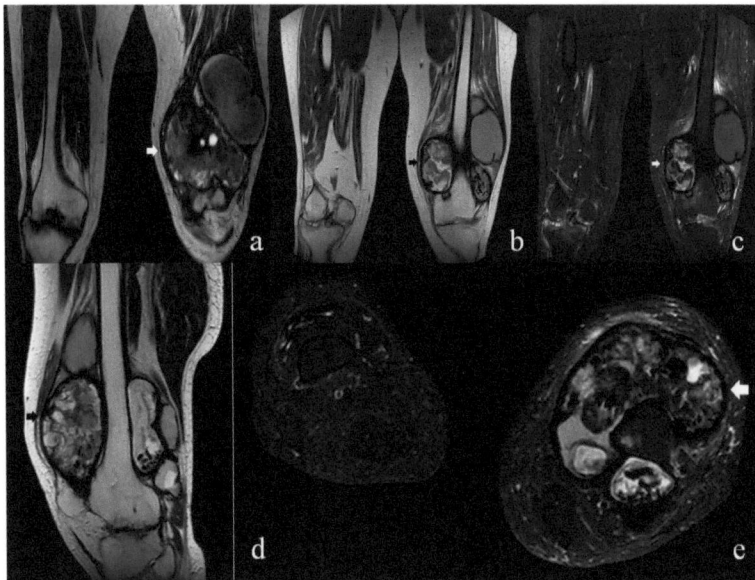

Fig. (19). Patient of 58 years. Coronal TSET1-w (a), TSET2-w (b), coronal STIR (c), sagittal TSET2-w (d), and axial STIR (e) images reveal a lobulated lesion with an internal septation in the left thigh causing bone erosions in the femoral diaphysis (arrows). Various signal intensities are related to blood products in different stages of organization.

MRI is of paramount importance when a postoperative follow-up is performed after a surgical treatment of such alterations, evaluating the signal intensity and the size of the treated lesions, also detecting further or recent bleedings into such areas [18].

COMPUTED TOMOGRAPHY

Since its development, CT has been used to detect abnormalities in joints affected by arthropathy, ensuring the evaluation of different aspects and additional informations to those obtained from MRI and radiography. Specifically, CT may identify epiphyseal overgrowth, joint space narrowing, bone erosions and cysts, and intercondylar notch widening in knees better than x-rays and similarly to MRI [16] (Figs. **20** and **21**).

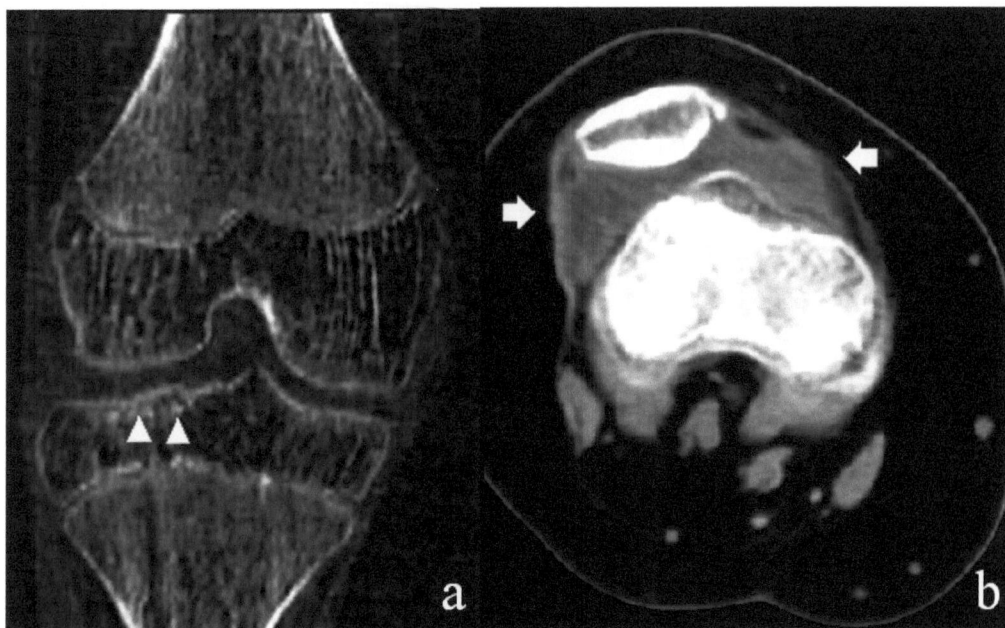

Fig. (20). Coronal and axial CT images showing fair irregularities of the articular surfaces (arrow heads) and the presence of an intraarticular effusion (arrows). These correspond to early signs of joint arthropathy hardly noticeable with traditional radiologic study.

Other aspects still lack of good visualization by CT: abnormal changes or tears of anterior and posterior cruciate ligaments tears, synovial hypertrophy, and bone marrow oedema are better evaluated by MRI. However, CT is a panoramic technique with more accessibility and better patient cooperation than MRI.

The main purpose of CT in haemophilic patients on the other hand is to detect intra- and extra-muscular pseudotumours, and extra-musculoskeletal alterations as spontaneous or posttraumatic bleedings (e.g. intracranial intraperitoneal and intramural small bowel hemorrhages) [16, 18, 57] (Fig. **22**).

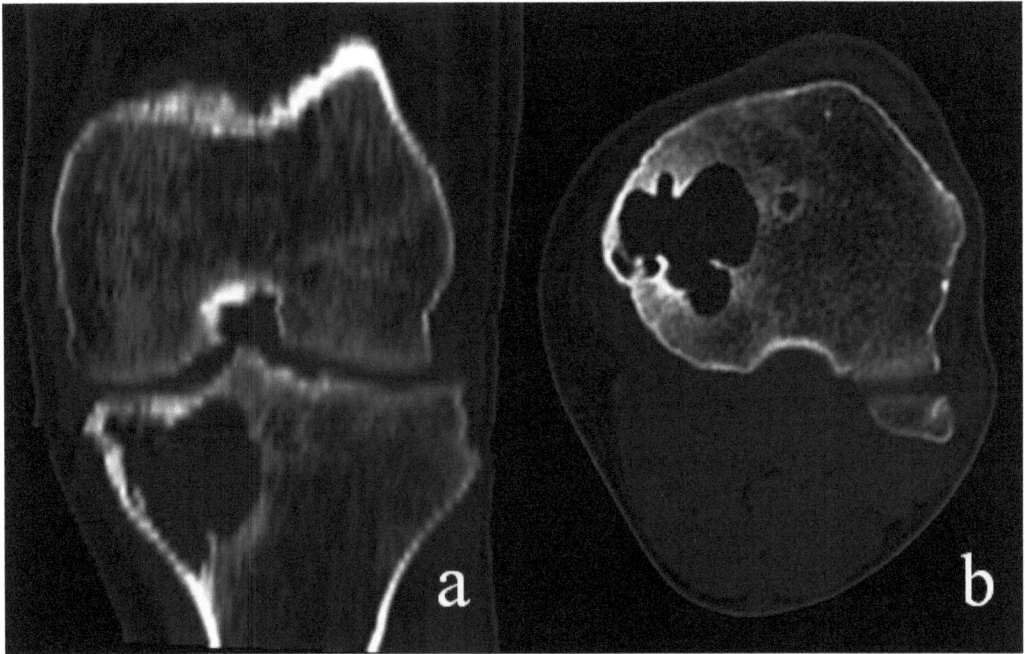

Fig. (21). CT images of the same patient in Fig. (**15**) that show the presence of some multilobulated cysts in the proximal tibial epiphysis.

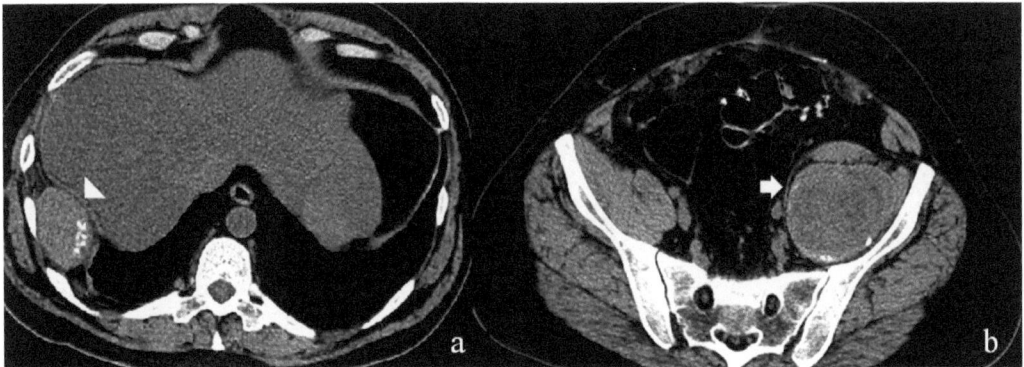

Fig. (22). CT images that demonstrate the presence of recurrent bleedings with peripheral calcifications, localized in the framework of the thoracic wall (a) and in the left iliacus muscle (b).

As mentioned before, pseudotumors are slowly expanding encapsulated haematomas. They may realize in bones, subperiosteal sites, but also in some muscles, causing compartment syndromes and neurologic and/or vascular complications. Common clinical settings are represented by periprosthetic pesudotumors or iliopsoas muscle organized haematoma, simulating infective abscesses or benign or malignant tumours. Contrast-enhanced CT imaging may assess the presence of a fibrous capsule and the density of blood-derived products at different stages of haemorrhage. In acute stages, the center of the pseudotumour is hypodense, but the periphery is isodense and indistinguishable from surrounding muscles [18, 50].

In conclusion CT is an accurate technique for detection of pseudotumours and haematomas, and their characterization in haemophiliacs. Moreover, despite a less use with respect to the past it has a high potential in the differential diagnosis between pathologic fractures and bone alterations related to bleedings.

CONCLUDING REMARKS

Imaging is an important tool for the diagnosis, evaluation of complications, and follow-up of the haemophilic arthropathy.

Conventional radiography may provide combined informations about functional ability, anatomical conditions, and bone changes but is inadequate for evaluating the efficacy of the early treatment. However, to date it remains the essential tool for the surgical planning and the follow-up of the orthopaedic treatment.

Although it shows to have a superiority with respect to standard radiology in the evaluation of the arthropathy, CT in Haemophilia is the best imaging modality for the assessment of spontaneous and posttraumatic bleedings and non musculoskeletal complications. It also plays an important role in the postoperative follow-up in association with conventional radiography.

MRI study is the most appropriate technique to assess the status of any haemophilic joint, even if it has higher costs and more difficult access. Periodic MRI studies may provide qualitative or semiquantitative assessments of pathological alterations in the altered joints.

The development of more specific imaging techniques and software allowing quantitative measures of alterations and more accurate scoring methods is nowadays the target of radiologists in Haemophilia centers.

CONFLICT OF INTEREST

The authors confirm that they have no conflict of interest to declare for this publication.

ACKNOWLEDGEMENTS

Declared none.

REFERENCES

[1] Doria AS. State-of-the-art imaging techniques for the evaluation of haemophilic arthropathy: present and future. Haemophilia 2010; 16 (Suppl. 5): 107-14.
[http://dx.doi.org/10.1111/j.1365-2516.2010.02307.x] [PMID: 20590865]

[2] Wood K, Omer A, Shaw MT. Haemophilic arthropathy. A combined radiological and clinical study. Br J Radiol 1969; 42(499): 498-505.
[http://dx.doi.org/10.1259/0007-1285-42-499-498] [PMID: 5788058]

[3] Arnold WD, Hilgartner MW. Hemophilic arthropathy. Current concepts of pathogenesis and management. J Bone Joint Surg Am 1977; 59(3): 287-305.
[http://dx.doi.org/10.2106/00004623-197759030-00001] [PMID: 849938]

[4] Kilcoyne RF, Nuss R. Radiological evaluation of hemophilic arthropathy. Semin Thromb Hemost 2003; 29(1): 43-8.
[http://dx.doi.org/10.1055/s-2003-37970] [PMID: 12640564]

[5] Maclachlan J, Gough-Palmer A, Hargunani R, Farrant J, Holloway B. Haemophilia imaging: a review. Skeletal Radiol 2009; 38(10): 949-57.
[http://dx.doi.org/10.1007/s00256-008-0586-5] [PMID: 18807029]

[6] Pergantou H, Matsinos G, Papadopoulos A, Platokouki H, Aronis S. Comparative study of validity of clinical, X-ray and magnetic resonance imaging scores in evaluation and management of haemophilic arthropathy in children. Haemophilia 2006; 12(3): 241-7.
[http://dx.doi.org/10.1111/j.1365-2516.2006.01208.x] [PMID: 16643208]

[7] Pettersson H, Ahlberg A, Nilsson IM. A radiologic classification of hemophilic arthropathy. Clin Orthop Relat Res 1980; (149): 153-9.
[PMID: 7408294]

[8] Petterson H. Modern Radiologic Evaluation and Follow-up of Hemophilic Arthropathy. New York: The National Hemophilia Foundation 1986.

[9] Roosendaal G, Van Den Berg HM, Lafeber FP, Bijlsma JW. Blood-induced joint damage: an overview of musculoskeletal research in haemophilia in Musculoskeletal aspect of Haemophilia In: Rodriguez-Merchan EC, Goddard NJ, Lee CA, Eds. Blackwell Science Ltd 2000.

[10] Nuss R, Kilcoyne RF, Geraghty S, *et al.* MRI findings in haemophilic joints treated with radiosynoviorthesis with development of an MRI scale of joint damage. Haemophilia 2000; 6(3): 162-9.
[http://dx.doi.org/10.1046/j.1365-2516.2000.00383.x] [PMID: 10792474]

[11] Dobón M, Lucía JF, Aguilar C, *et al.* Value of magnetic resonance imaging for the diagnosis and follow-up of haemophilic arthropathy. Haemophilia 2003; 9(1): 76-85.
[http://dx.doi.org/10.1046/j.1365-2516.2003.00702.x] [PMID: 12558783]

[12] Sierra Aisa C, Lucía Cuesta JF, Rubio Martínez A, *et al.* Comparison of ultrasound and magnetic resonance imaging for diagnosis and follow-up of joint lesions in patients with haemophilia. Haemophilia 2014; 20(1): e51-7.
[http://dx.doi.org/10.1111/hae.12268] [PMID: 24112687]

[13] Kilcoyne RF, Nuss R. Radiological assessment of haemophilic arthropathy with emphasis on MRI findings. Haemophilia 2003; 9 (Suppl. 1): 57-63.
[http://dx.doi.org/10.1046/j.1365-2516.9.s1.11.x] [PMID: 12709039]

[14] Chan MW, Leckie A, Xavier F, *et al*. A systematic review of MR imaging as a tool for evaluating haemophilic arthropathy in children. Haemophilia 2013; 19(6): e324-34.
[http://dx.doi.org/10.1111/hae.12248] [PMID: 23919318]

[15] Wilson DJ, McLardy-Smith PD, Woodham CH, MacLarnon JC. Diagnostic ultrasound in haemophilia. J Bone Joint Surg Br 1987; 69(1): 103-7.
[PMID: 3546324]

[16] Hermann G, Gilbert MS, Abdelwahab IF. Hemophilia: evaluation of musculoskeletal involvement with CT, sonography, and MR imaging. AJR Am J Roentgenol 1992; 158(1): 119-23.
[http://dx.doi.org/10.2214/ajr.158.1.1727336] [PMID: 1727336]

[17] Acharya SS, Schloss R, Dyke JP, *et al*. Power Doppler sonography in the diagnosis of hemophilic synovitisa promising tool. J Thromb Haemost 2008; 6(12): 2055-61.
[http://dx.doi.org/10.1111/j.1538-7836.2008.03160.x] [PMID: 18823337]

[18] Park JS, Ryu KN. Hemophilic pseudotumor involving the musculoskeletal system: spectrum of radiologic findings. AJR Am J Roentgenol 2004; 183(1): 55-61.
[http://dx.doi.org/10.2214/ajr.183.1.1830055] [PMID: 15208110]

[19] Ng WH, Chu WC, Shing MK, *et al*. Role of imaging in management of hemophilic patients. AJR Am J Roentgenol 2005; 184(5): 1619-23.
[http://dx.doi.org/10.2214/ajr.184.5.01841619] [PMID: 15855127]

[20] Pettersson H, Ahlberg A. Computed tomography in hemophilic pseudotumor. Acta Radiol Diagn (Stockh) 1982; 23(5): 453-7.
[PMID: 7158409]

[21] Ribbens C, Hustinx R. Nuclear (Scintigraphic) methods and FDG-PET in rheumatoid arthritis and osteoarthritis. In: Bruno MA, Mosher TJ, Gold GE, Eds. Arthritis in Color, Advanced Imaging of Arthritis. Philadelphia, PA: Saunders, Elsevier 2009; pp. 138-49.
[http://dx.doi.org/10.1016/B978-1-4160-4722-3.00007-0]

[22] Bruno MA, Mosher TJ, Gold GE, Eds. Arthritis in Color, Advanced Imaging of Arthritis. Philadelphia, PA: Saunders, Elsevier 2009; pp. 153-70.

[23] Cross S, Vaidya S, Fotiadis N. Hemophilic arthropathy: a review of imaging and staging. Semin Ultrasound CT MR 2013; 34(6): 516-24.
[http://dx.doi.org/10.1053/j.sult.2013.05.007] [PMID: 24332203]

[24] Goddard NJ, Mann H. Diagnosis of haemophilic synovitis. Haemophilia 2007; 13 (Suppl. 3): 14-9.
[http://dx.doi.org/10.1111/j.1365-2516.2007.01535.x] [PMID: 17822516]

[25] Nuss R, Kilcoyne RF, Rivard GE, Murphy J. Late clinical, plain X-ray and magnetic resonance imaging findings in haemophilic joints treated with radiosynoviorthesis. Haemophilia 2000; 6(6): 658-63.
[http://dx.doi.org/10.1046/j.1365-2516.2000.00433.x] [PMID: 11122392]

[26] Yu W, Lin Q, Guermazi A, *et al*. Comparison of radiography, CT and MR imaging in detection of arthropathies in patients with haemophilia. Haemophilia 2009; 15(5): 1090-6.
[http://dx.doi.org/10.1111/j.1365-2516.2009.02044.x] [PMID: 19515027]

[27] Soler R, López-Fernández F, Rodríguez E, Marini M. Hemophilic arthropathy. A scoring system for magnetic resonance imaging. Eur Radiol 2002; 12(4): 836-43.
[http://dx.doi.org/10.1007/s003300101078] [PMID: 11960235]

[28] Lundin B, Pettersson H, Ljung R. A new magnetic resonance imaging scoring method for assessment of haemophilic arthropathy. Haemophilia 2004; 10(4): 383-9.
[http://dx.doi.org/10.1111/j.1365-2516.2004.00902.x] [PMID: 15230954]

[29] Doria AS, Babyn PS, Lundin B, *et al.* Reliability and construct validity of the compatible MRI scoring system for evaluation of haemophilic knees and ankles of haemophilic children. Expert MRI working group of the international prophylaxis study group. Haemophilia 2006; 12(5): 503-13.
[http://dx.doi.org/10.1111/j.1365-2516.2006.01310.x] [PMID: 16919081]

[30] Lundin B, Babyn P, Doria AS, *et al.* Compatible scales for progressive and additive MRI assessments of haemophilic arthropathy. Haemophilia 2005; 11(2): 109-15.
[http://dx.doi.org/10.1111/j.1365-2516.2005.01049.x] [PMID: 15810912]

[31] Feldman BM, Funk S, Lundin B, Doria AS, Ljung R, Blanchette V. Musculoskeletal measurement tools from the International Prophylaxis Study Group (IPSG). Haemophilia 2008; 14 (Suppl. 3): 162-9.
[http://dx.doi.org/10.1111/j.1365-2516.2008.01750.x] [PMID: 18510537]

[32] Lundin B, Manco-Johnson ML, Ignas DM, *et al.* An MRI scale for assessment of haemophilic arthropathy from the International Prophylaxis Study Group. Haemophilia 2012; 18(6): 962-70.
[http://dx.doi.org/10.1111/j.1365-2516.2012.02883.x] [PMID: 22765835]

[33] Foppen W, van der Schaaf IC, Witkamp TD, Fischer K. Is joint effusion on MRI specific for haemophilia? Haemophilia 2014; 20(4): 582-6.
[http://dx.doi.org/10.1111/hae.12338] [PMID: 24373059]

[34] Hassan TH, Badr MA, El-Gerby KM. Correlation between musculoskeletal function and radiological joint scores in haemophilia A adolescents. Haemophilia 2011; 17(6): 920-5.
[http://dx.doi.org/10.1111/j.1365-2516.2011.02496.x] [PMID: 21371193]

[35] Nägele M, Kunze V, Hamann M, *et al.* [Hemophiliac arthropathy of the knee joint. Gd-DTP--enhanced MRI; clinical and roentgenological correlation]. Rofo 1994; 160(2): 154-8.
[PMID: 8312513]

[36] Clunie GP, Wilkinson ID, Lui D, *et al.* Changes in articular synovial lining volume measured by magnetic resonance in a randomized, double-blind, controlled trial of intra-articular samarium-153 particulate hydroxyapatite for chronic knee synovitis. Rheumatology (Oxford) 1999; 38(2): 113-7.
[http://dx.doi.org/10.1093/rheumatology/38.2.113] [PMID: 10342622]

[37] Lundin B, Berntorp E, Pettersson H, *et al.* Gadolinium contrast agent is of limited value for magnetic resonance imaging assessment of synovial hypertrophy in hemophiliacs. Acta Radiol 2007; 48(5): 520-30.
[http://dx.doi.org/10.1080/02841850701280775] [PMID: 17520428]

[38] Rand T, Trattnig S, Male C, *et al.* Magnetic resonance imaging in hemophilic children: value of gradient echo and contrast-enhanced imaging. Magn Reson Imaging 1999; 17(2): 199-205.
[http://dx.doi.org/10.1016/S0730-725X(98)00148-9] [PMID: 10215474]

[39] Dardzinski BJ, Mosher TJ, Li S, Van Slyke MA, Smith MB. Spatial variation of T2 in human articular cartilage. Radiology 1997; 205(2): 546-50.
[http://dx.doi.org/10.1148/radiology.205.2.9356643] [PMID: 9356643]

[40] Hargreaves BA, Gold GE, Lang PK, *et al.* MR imaging of articular cartilage using driven equilibrium. Magn Reson Med 1999; 42(4): 695-703.
[http://dx.doi.org/10.1002/(SICI)1522-2594(199910)42:4<695::AID-MRM11>3.0.CO;2-Z] [PMID: 10502758]

[41] Glaser C. New techniques for cartilage imaging: T2 relaxation time and diffusion-weighted MR imaging. Radiol Clin North Am 2005; 43(4): 641-653, vii.
[http://dx.doi.org/10.1016/j.rcl.2005.02.007] [PMID: 15893528]

[42] Eckstein F, Hudelmaier M, Wirth W, *et al.* Double echo steady state magnetic resonance imaging of knee articular cartilage at 3 Tesla: a pilot study for the Osteoarthritis Initiative. Ann Rheum Dis 2006; 65(4): 433-41.
[http://dx.doi.org/10.1136/ard.2005.039370] [PMID: 16126797]

[43] Nieminen MT, Rieppo J, Silvennoinen J, *et al.* Spatial assessment of articular cartilage proteoglycans with Gd-DTPA-enhanced T1 imaging. Magn Reson Med 2002; 48(4): 640-8.
[http://dx.doi.org/10.1002/mrm.10273] [PMID: 12353281]

[44] Foppen W, Sluiter D, Witkamp TD, Mali WP, Fischer K. Haemophilic magnetic resonance imaging score in healthy controls playing sports. Haemophilia 2013; 19(6): 939-43.
[http://dx.doi.org/10.1111/hae.12191] [PMID: 23710616]

[45] McQueen F, Lassere M, Østergaard M. Magnetic resonance imaging in psoriatic arthritis: a review of the literature. Arthritis Res Ther 2006; 8(2): 207-14.
[http://dx.doi.org/10.1186/ar1934] [PMID: 16569257]

[46] Olivieri M, Kurnik K, Pfluger T, Bidlingmaier C. Identification and long-term observation of early joint damage by magnetic resonance imaging in clinically asymptomatic joints in patients with haemophilia A or B despite prophylaxis. Haemophilia 2012; 18(3): 369-74.
[http://dx.doi.org/10.1111/j.1365-2516.2011.02682.x] [PMID: 22032268]

[47] Den Uijl IE, De Schepper AM, Camerlinck M, Grobbee DE, Fischer K. Magnetic resonance imaging in teenagers and young adults with limited haemophilic arthropathy: baseline results from a prospective study. Haemophilia 2011; 17(6): 926-30.
[http://dx.doi.org/10.1111/j.1365-2516.2011.02513.x] [PMID: 21435115]

[48] Pergantou H, Platokouki H, Matsinos G, *et al.* Assessment of the progression of haemophilic arthropathy in children. Haemophilia 2010; 16(1): 124-9.
[http://dx.doi.org/10.1111/j.1365-2516.2009.02109.x] [PMID: 19744251]

[49] Mauser-Bunschoten EP, Jansen NW, Doria AS, Oldenburg J. New images in haemophilia. Haemophilia 2008; 14 (Suppl. 3): 147-52.
[http://dx.doi.org/10.1111/j.1365-2516.2008.01719.x] [PMID: 18510535]

[50] Rodriguez-Merchan EC. The haemophilic pseudotumour. Haemophilia 2002; 8(1): 12-6.
[http://dx.doi.org/10.1046/j.1365-2516.2002.00577.x] [PMID: 11886459]

[51] Jaovisidha S, Ryu KN, Hodler J, Schweitzer ME, Sartoris DJ, Resnick D. Hemophilic pseudotumor: spectrum of MR findings. Skeletal Radiol 1997; 26(8): 468-74.
[http://dx.doi.org/10.1007/s002560050268] [PMID: 9297751]

[52] Rodriguez-Merchan EC, Goddard NJ. Muscular bleeding, soft-tissue haematomas and pseudotumours in Musculoskeletal aspect of Haemophilia. Blackwell Science Ltd 2000.

[53] Stafford JM, James TT, Allen AM, Dixon LR. Hemophilic pseudotumor: radiologic-pathologic correlation. Radiographics 2003; 23(4): 852-6.
[http://dx.doi.org/10.1148/rg.234025154] [PMID: 12853660]

[54] Kerr R. Imaging of musculoskeletal complications of hemophilia. Semin Musculoskelet Radiol 2003; 7(2): 127-36.
[http://dx.doi.org/10.1055/s-2003-41346] [PMID: 12920650]

[55] Bush CH. The magnetic resonance imaging of musculoskeletal hemorrhage. Skeletal Radiol 2000; 29(1): 1-9.
[http://dx.doi.org/10.1007/s002560050001] [PMID: 10663582]

[56] Allen DJ, Goddard NJ, Mann HA, Rodriguez-Merchan EC. Primary malignancies mistaken for pseudotumours in haemophilic patients. Haemophilia 2007; 13(4): 383-6.
[http://dx.doi.org/10.1111/j.1365-2516.2007.01438.x] [PMID: 17610552]

[57] Traivaree C, Blanchette V, Armstrong D, Floros G, Stain AM, Carcao MD. Intracranial bleeding in haemophilia beyond the neonatal periodthe role of CT imaging in suspected intracranial bleeding. Haemophilia 2007; 13(5): 552-9.
[http://dx.doi.org/10.1111/j.1365-2516.2007.01545.x] [PMID: 17880443]

CHAPTER 7

Sonographic Findings and Scoring Method of Target Joints

Daniela Melchiorre* and Marco Matucci-Cerinic

Rheumatology Unit, University of Florence, Florence, Italy

Abstract: In haemophilic arthropathy (HA), a spontaneous joint bleeding may trigger and perpetuate synovitis, and cartilage damage may follow even after a single exposure to blood, leading to a progressive and permanent joint damage. Ultrasonography (US) may detect articular and periarticular structures, muscles, tendons, tendon-sheats and enthesys. While power Doppler (PDUS) detects synovial inflammation and local blood flow. The US is based on technique, concepts and method widely accepted. We describe a US protocol to study the typical target joint (elbows, knees, and ankles). Knees, elbows, and ankles can be systematically and easily evaluated by means of conventional US machines, including portable machines, with a linear probe 13-4 MHz. The presence of haemarthrosis and the evidence of a synovial neoangiogenesis is assessed by PDUS in longitudinal scan. In the last decade, some scoring methods were proposed. Our scoring system requires a practice of US technique without necessarily being expert sonographers and allow to study all joints in static and dynamic position through nine items. This scoring method is applied to each target joint with a range from 0 to 21 and with cut off ≤ 5 or >5 useful to define the early stage of arthropathy.

Keywords: Haemophilic arthropathy, Power doppler, Scoring method, Target joint, Uultrasonography.

INTRODUCTION

Spontaneous joint bleeding in haemophilia A and B may trigger and perpetuate synovitis, and cartilage damage may follow even after a single exposure to blood [1 - 3], leading to a progressive and permanent joint damage, *i.e.* haemophilic arthropathy (HA). This results in loss of joint function and muscle hypotrophy, especially involving the larger joints (target joint) [4, 5].

Synovitis with synovial changes, cartilage, and bone damages with resulting disability may occur even after few bleeding episodes.

---

* **Corresponding author Daniela Melchiorre:** Rheumatology Unit, University of Florence, Florence, Italy; Tel: +39 0552751688; Email: daniela.melchiorre@unifi.it

The ultrasonographic examination (US) has shown its validity for the diagnosis of musculoskeletal diseases. It is easily available at any facility, results as a non-invasive evaluation, and allows for a quick and recurrent study of joint status. This relatively recent technique has been employed in Haemophilia starting from the pioneering work proposed by Wilson in 1987 [6] who first made a specific reference to the significance of the diagnosis by US in Haemophilia, and the routine control of bleeding in soft tissues.

US is an imaging method detecting joint structures, muscles, tendons, sheats, and entheses [9]. It is helpful to detect bone and cartilage alterations and synovitis [10]. It is also well known that power Doppler US (PDUS) may identify the synovial blood flow [11, 12]. The early diagnosis and evaluation of an acute haemarthrosis by US may optimize the Haemophilia treatment fostering the achievement of a satisfactory health condition of patients [7 - 10]. US is fast and effective, safe and widely available; it is a dynamic, real-time, comparative study that can confirm the clinical examination in haemophilic patients. This type of imaging evidences the presence of bleeding, its extension, exact location, relationships with adjacent anatomic structures, its evolution, and finally possible complications.

PDUS may identify bleeding also in asymptomatic joints and is able to show different types of haemarthrosis [11, 12].

Sonographic Findings

The US is based on technique, concepts and method widely accepted and described elsewhere [9, 11 - 14]. Here, we describe a US protocol to study the typical target joint (elbows, knees, and ankles).

Knees, elbows, and ankles can be systematically and easily evaluated by means of conventional US machines, including portable machines, with a linear probe 13-4 MHz.

The presence of haemarthrosis and the evidence of a synovial neoangiogenesis is assessed by PDUS in longitudinal scan.

The positioning of the probe and relevant US images for target joints are shown in the Figs. (**1-9**).

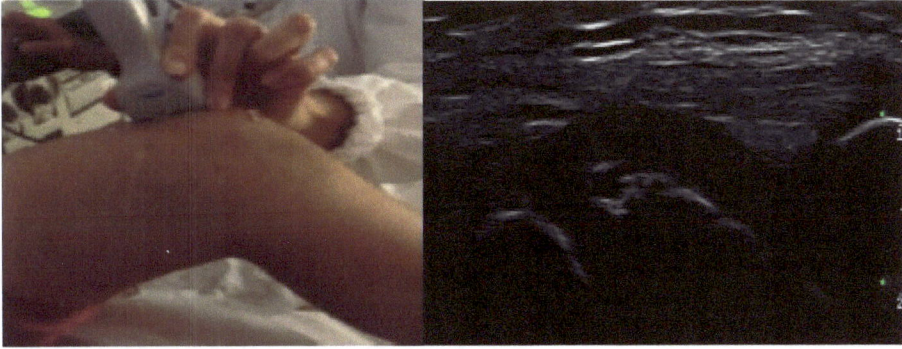

Fig. (1). Knee: the probe scans the joint in the longitudinal view in the supine position with the knee in full or moderate extension (30°-45°) to detect the superior (suprapatellar) recess and the presence of the joint effusion or haemarthrosis and thickening of synovial tissue.

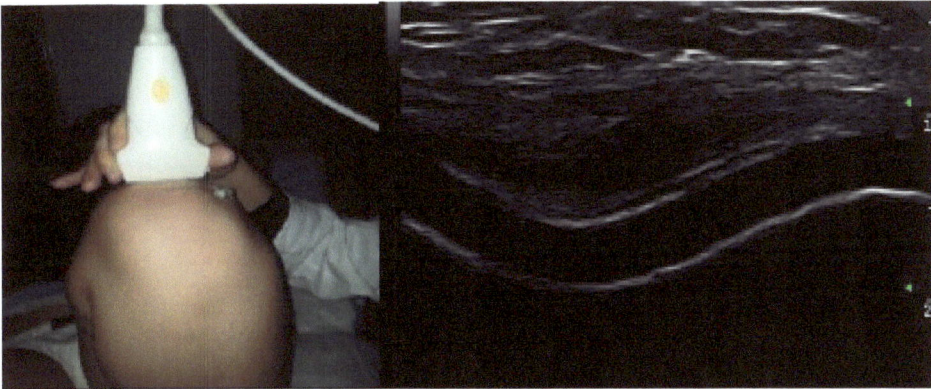

Fig. (2). Knee: the probe scans the joint in transverse view and supine position with maximal knee flexion to study the cartilage.

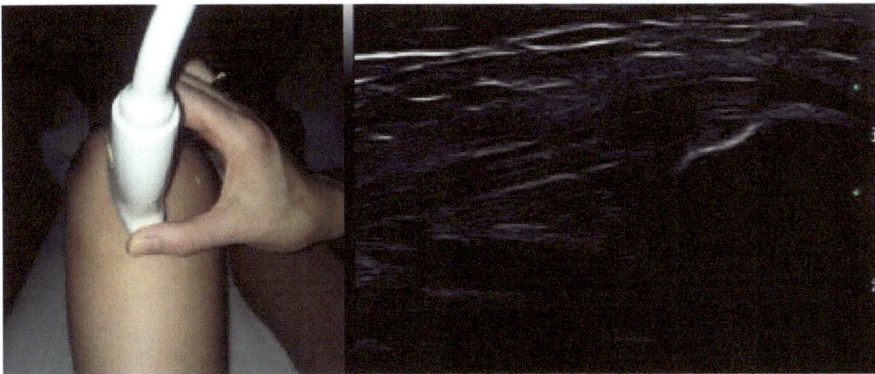

Fig. (3). Knee: in this view it is possible to detect the patellar tendon and Hoffa body.

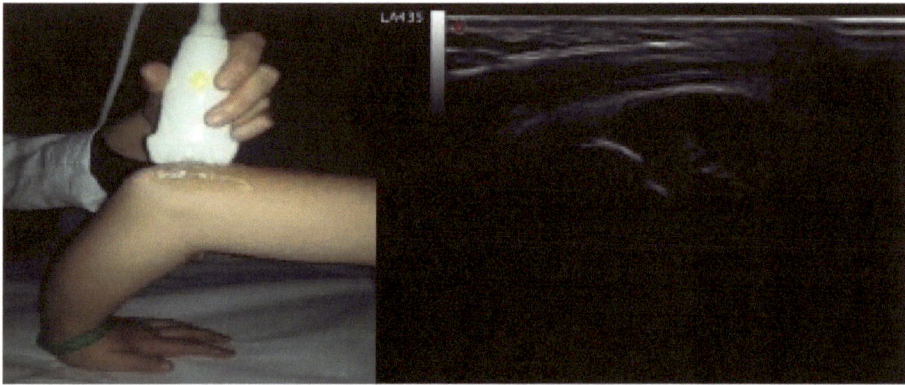

Fig. (4). Elbow: the probe is placed in the longitudinal scan with the elbow flexed 90° and with the palm posed on the bed to study the posterior (olecranon) recess.

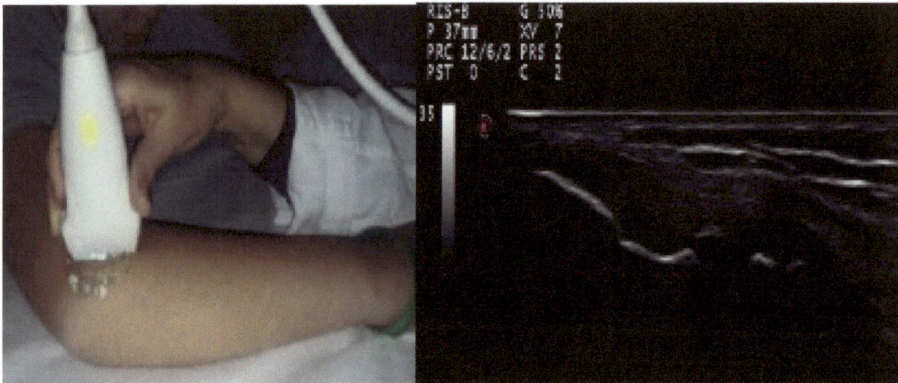

Fig. (5). Elbow: the probe is placed in the longitudinal scan with the elbow in moderate flexion (35°-40°) to study the joint line.

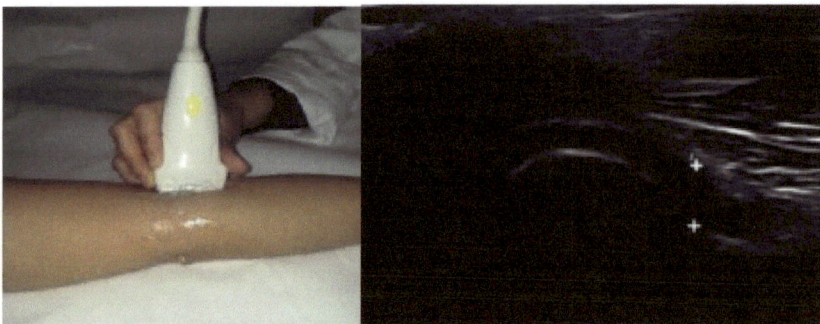

Fig. (6). Elbow: the probe is placed in the longitudinal scan with the elbow in maximal extension to study the coronoid recess and the presence of the joint effusion or haemarthrosis and thickening of synovial tissue.

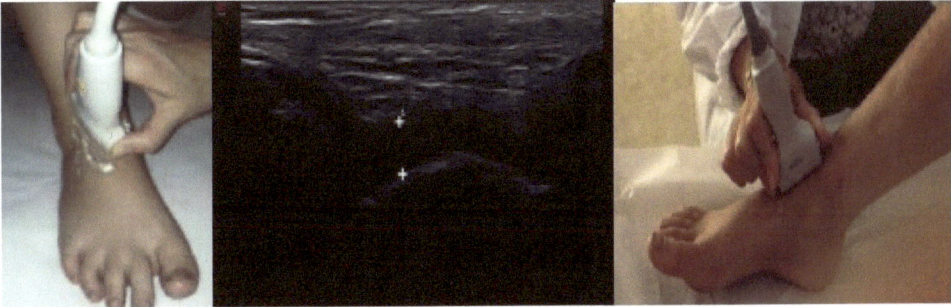

Fig. (7). Ankle: the ankle is studied with the foot on the bed. The probe scans the joint in longitudinal view to detect the anterior recess.

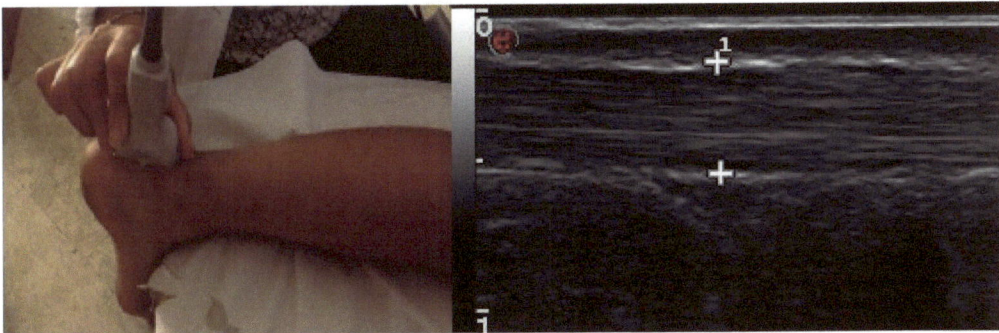

Fig. (8). Ankle: the probe scans the Achilles tendon in longitudinal view and in the supine position with maximal foot flexion.

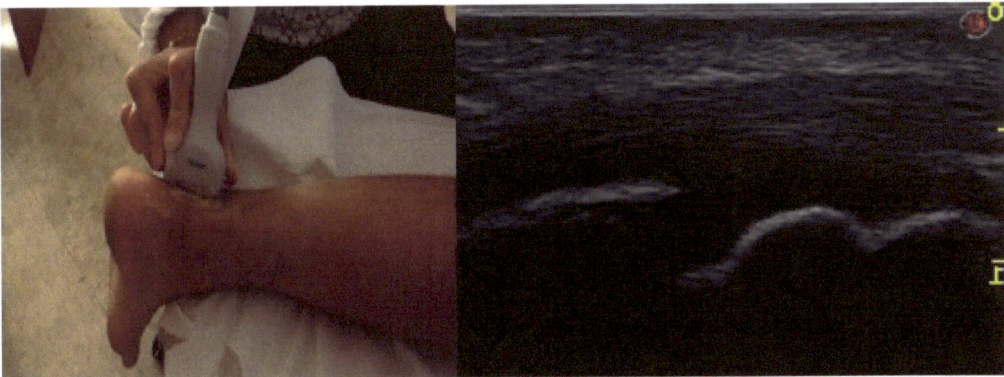

Fig. (9). Ankle: the probe is placed in the sagittal scan over supracalcanear portion of the Achilles tendon to examine the posterior recess.

POWER DOPPLER

The PDUS is performed to detect the synovial neoangiogenesis, which is defined as colour-flow signals in structures between the capsule and the bone surface [15,

16]. To maximize the sensitivity of PDUS, variables are adjusted to the lowest permissible pulse repetition frequency (PRF= 7,50 Hz). A flow is additionally demonstrated in two planes and confirmed by pulsed-wave Doppler spectrum [15 - 21]. Power Doppler settings are standardized with PRF of 750 Hertz and a power Doppler gain of 50/53 dB.

The intra-articular PDUS signal is scored on a semiquantitative scale from 0 to 2: 0= absence, no vessel signals; 1= vessel signals in the region of interest (ROI) <3 flags; 2= vessel signals in region of interest (ROI) >3 flags or in more than half of the intraarticular area (Fig. **10**).

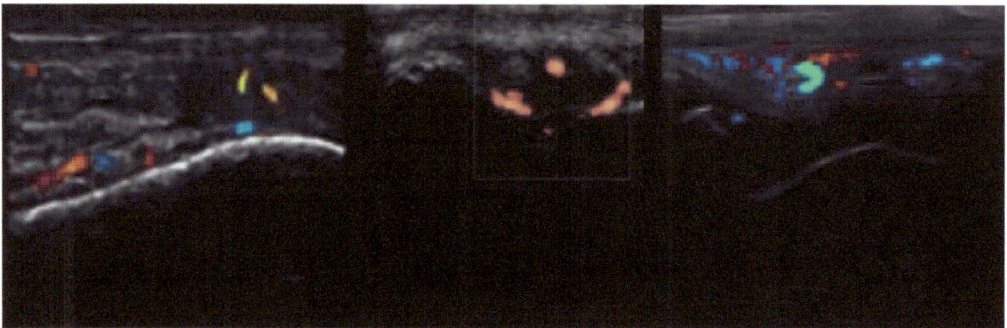

Fig. (10). Example of Power Doppler.

Scoring Method

In the last decade, some scoring methods were proposed [12, 14]. The HEAD-US method [14] was designed to allow an easier implementation of US score compared to what will be described subsequently, and it was supposed to be particularly useful for unexperienced sonographers. The HEAD-US scanning protocol evaluates joints of patients with HA by including also a systematic evaluation of synovial recesses and selection of a single osteochondral surface for the damage analysis. This method scoring however does not include a PDUS evaluation.

Our scoring system (Table **1**) requires a practice of US technique without necessarily being expert sonographers [11]. By this means, both the severity (due to damage) and the activity (due to bleeding) of the disease may be evaluated. Moreover, the monitoring of the progression of HA is easily feasible. The US can be carried out in static and dynamic position in all joints and the following items are investigated:

1. Presence of joint effusion in the joint recesses
2. Joint bleeding with a diffuse hyperechoic signal with or without flags on PDUS
3. Synovial hypertrophy measured in mm
4. Fibrous septa
5. Haemosiderin deposition, which appears as a diffuse hyperechoic signal
6. Presence of bone irregularity as incongruence between joint surface (remodelling)
7. Osteophytes, as enlargement of epiphysis and marginal hypertrophic bone formation
8. Erosions, as cortical "break" or defect with irregular shape seen in the longitudinal or in the coronal plane
9. Cartilage alterations.

This scoring method is applied to each target joint with a range from 0 to 21 and with cut off $\leq$ 5 or >5 useful to define the early stage of arthropathy [11].

Table 1. Personal scoring system for haemophilic arthropathy.

Item	Concept	Evaluation	Score
1	Effusion: hydrarthrosis or haemarthrosis	Absent = 0; small = 1; moderate = 2; Absent = 0; small = 1; moderate = 2;	
2	Fibrotic septa	Absent = 0; present = 1	
3	Synovial hyperthrophy with flags on PDUS	1 = <3 flags; 2= >3 flags	
4	Synovial hyperthrophy without flags on PDUS	Thickness <1.5 mm = 1 Thickness 1.5-2.5 mm = 2 Thickness >2.5 mm = 3	
5	Haemosiderin deposition	Absent = 0; small = 1; moderate = 2; large = 3	
6	Bone erosion	Absent = 0; present = 1	
7	Osteophytes	Absent = 0; present = 1	
8	Bone remodelling	Absent = 0; present = 1	
9	Cartilage modifications	Hyperechogenicity = 1; irregular profile = 2; calcification = 3	

Scoring Method "Step by Step"

Furthermore, it is useful to differentiate the early and severe stages of the arthropathy in Haemophilia A and B, and the introduction of the cut off represents an important tool in the diagnosis. The daily use of US and the scoring method can be a valid support for the physician, in the clinical practice and in the management of therapy (see below).

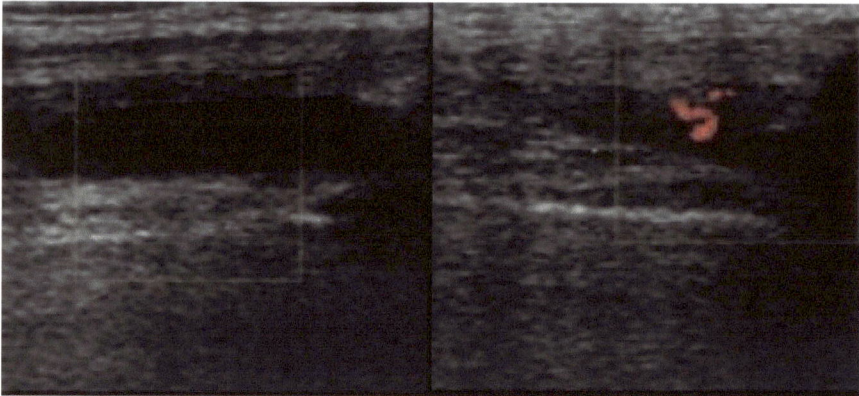

1	Effusion: hydrarthrosis or haemarthrosis	Absent = 0; small = 1; moderate = 2; Absent = 0; small = 1; moderate = 2;

Knee

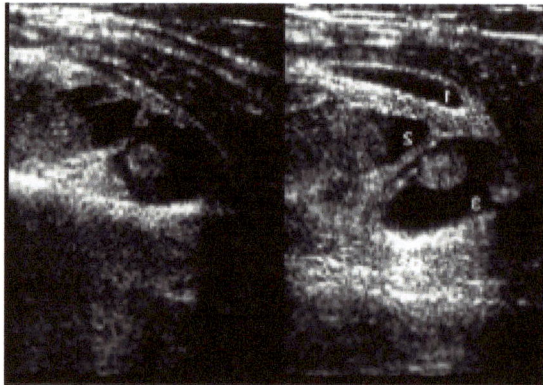

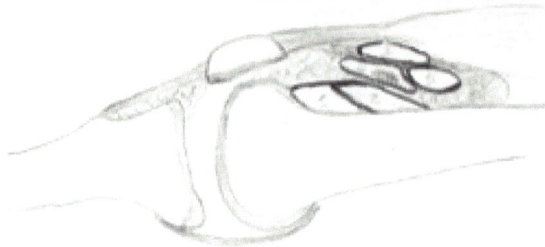

2	Fibrotic septa	Absent = 0; present = 1

Knee

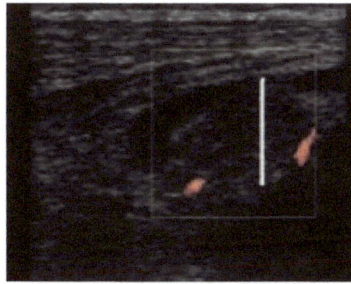

3	*Synovial hyperthrophy with flags on PDUS*	*1 = <3 flags; 2= >3 flags*

Knee

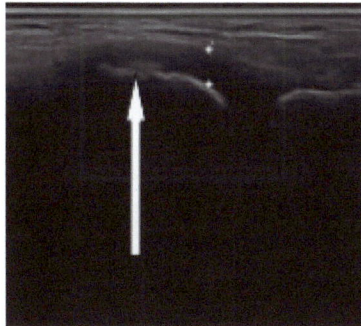

4	*Synovial hyperthrophy without flags on PDUS*	*Thickness <1.5 mm = 1* *Thickness 1.5-2.5 mm = 2* *Thickness >2.5 mm = 3*

Ankle

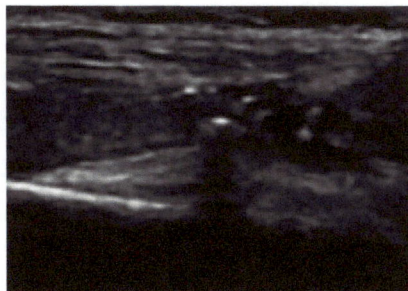

5	*Haemosiderin deposition*	*Absent = 0; small = 1; moderate = 2; large = 3*

Knee

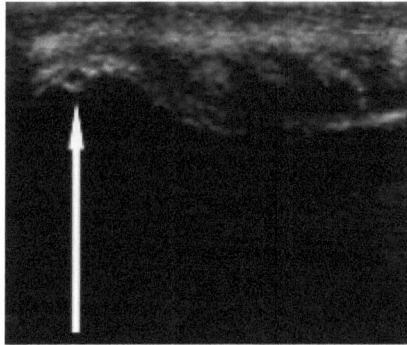

6	Bone erosion	Absent = 0; present = 1

Elbow

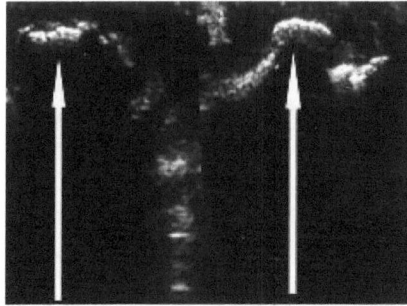

7	Osteophytes	Absent = 0; present = 1

Knee

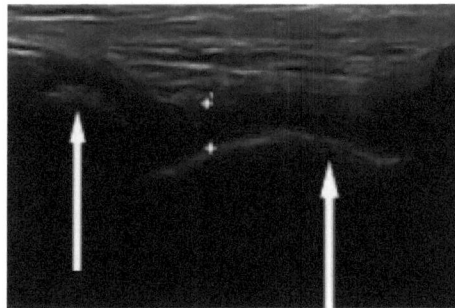

8	Bone remodelling	Absent = 0; present = 1

Ankle

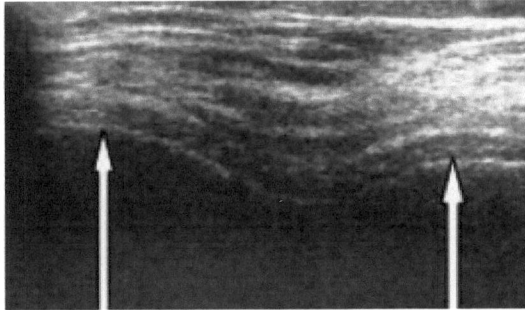

| 9 | *Cartilage modifications* | Hyperechogenicity = 1; irregular profile = 2; calcification = 3 |

Knee

CONFLICT OF INTEREST

The authors confirm that they have no conflict of interest to declare for this publication.

ACKNOWLEDGEMENTS

A special acknowledgment to Giancarlo Castaman, MD for his precious cooperation.

REFERENCES

[1]   Hakobyan N, Kazarian T, Jabbar AA, Jabbar KJ, Valentino LA. Pathobiology of hemophilic synovitis I: overexpression of mdm2 oncogene. Blood 2004; 104(7): 2060-4.
[http://dx.doi.org/10.1182/blood-2003-12-4231] [PMID: 15172967]

[2]   Wen FQ, Jabbar AA, Chen YX, Kazarian T, Patel DA, Valentino LA. c-myc proto-oncogene expression in hemophilic synovitis: *in vitro* studies of the effects of iron and ceramide. Blood 2002; 100(3): 912-6.
[http://dx.doi.org/10.1182/blood-2002-02-0390] [PMID: 12130502]

[3]   Jansen NW, Roosendaal G, Lafeber FP. Understanding haemophilic arthropathy: an exploration of current open issues. Br J Haematol 2008; 143(5): 632-40.
[http://dx.doi.org/10.1111/j.1365-2141.2008.07386.x] [PMID: 18950457]

[4]   Pettersson H, Ahlberg A, Nilsson IM. A radiologic classification of hemophilic arthropathy. Clin Orthop Relat Res 1980; 149(149): 153-9.
[PMID: 7408294]

[5]   Doria AS. State-of-the-art imaging techniques for the evaluation of haemophilic arthropathy: present and future. Haemophilia 2010; 16 (Suppl. 5): 107-14.
[http://dx.doi.org/10.1111/j.1365-2516.2010.02307.x] [PMID: 20590865]

[6]   Wilson DJ, McLardy-Smith PD, Woodham CH, MacLarnon JC. Diagnostic ultrasound in haemophilia. J Bone Joint Surg Br 1987; 69(1): 103-7.
[PMID: 3546324]

[7]   Keen HI, Brown AK, Wakefield RJ, Conaghan PG. MRI and musculoskeletal ultrasonography as diagnostic tools in early arthritis. Rheum Dis Clin North Am 2005; 31(4): 699-714.
[http://dx.doi.org/10.1016/j.rdc.2005.07.002] [PMID: 16287592]

[8]   Jelbert A, Vaidya S, Fotiadis N. Imaging and staging of haemophilic arthropathy. Clin Radiol 2009; 64(11): 1119-28.
[http://dx.doi.org/10.1016/j.crad.2009.07.005] [PMID: 19822246]

[9]   Querol F, Rodriguez-Merchan EC. The role of ultrasonography in the diagnosis of the musculo-skeletal problems of haemophilia. Haemophilia 2012; 18(3): e215-26. [Review].
[http://dx.doi.org/10.1111/j.1365-2516.2011.02680.x] [PMID: 22044728]

[10]   Rodriguez-Merchan EC. Cartilage damage in the haemophilic joints: pathophysiology, diagnosis and management. Blood Coagul Fibrinolysis 2012; 23(3): 179-83.
[http://dx.doi.org/10.1097/MBC.0b013e32835084dd] [PMID: 22261870]

[11]   Melchiorre D, Linari S, Innocenti M, *et al.* Ultrasound detects joint damage and bleeding in haemophilic arthropathy: a proposal of a score. Haemophilia 2011; 17(1): 112-7.
[http://dx.doi.org/10.1111/j.1365-2516.2010.02380.x] [PMID: 21070482]

[12]   Acharya SS, Schloss R, Dyke JP, *et al.* Power Doppler sonography in the diagnosis of hemophilic synovitisa promising tool. J Thromb Haemost 2008; 6(12): 2055-61.
[http://dx.doi.org/10.1111/j.1538-7836.2008.03160.x] [PMID: 18823337]

[13]   Zukotynski K, Jarrin J, Babyn PS, *et al.* Sonography for assessment of haemophilic arthropathy in children: a systematic protocol. Haemophilia 2007; 13(3): 293-304.
[http://dx.doi.org/10.1111/j.1365-2516.2006.01414.x] [PMID: 17498079]

[14]   Martinoli C, Della Casa Alberighi O, Di Minno G, *et al.* Development and definition of a simplified scanning procedure and scoring method for Haemophilia Early Arthropathy Detection with Ultrasound (HEAD-US). Thromb Haemost 2013; 109(6): 1170-9.
[http://dx.doi.org/10.1160/TH12-11-0874] [PMID: 23571706]

[15]   Lim GY, Im SA, Jung WS, Lee JM, Lee AW. Evaluation of joint effusion in rabbits by color Doppler, power Doppler, and contrast-enhanced power Doppler ultrasonography. J Clin Ultrasound 2005; 33(7): 333-8.
[http://dx.doi.org/10.1002/jcu.20160] [PMID: 16196009]

[16]   Kiris A, Ozgocmen S, Kocakoc E, Ardicoglu O. Power Doppler assessment of overall disease activity in patients with rheumatoid arthritis. J Clin Ultrasound 2006; 34(1): 5-11.
[http://dx.doi.org/10.1002/jcu.20175] [PMID: 16353227]

[17]   Schmidt WA, Völker L, Zacher J, Schläfke M, Ruhnke M, Gromnica-Ihle E. Colour Doppler ultrasonography to detect pannus in knee joint synovitis. Clin Exp Rheumatol 2000; 18(4): 439-44.
[PMID: 10949717]

[18]   Naredo E, Rodríguez M, Campos C, *et al.* Validity, reproducibility, and responsiveness of a twelve-joint simplified power doppler ultrasonographic assessment of joint inflammation in rheumatoid arthritis. Arthritis Rheum 2008; 59(4): 515-22.
[http://dx.doi.org/10.1002/art.23529] [PMID: 18383408]

[19]   Klauser A, Demharter J, De Marchi A, *et al.* Contrast enhanced gray-scale sonography in assessment of joint vascularity in rheumatoid arthritis: results from the IACUS study group. Eur Radiol 2005; 15(12): 2404-10.
[http://dx.doi.org/10.1007/s00330-005-2884-9] [PMID: 16132921]

[20]   DiMichele DM. The potential role of power Doppler ultrasound in the diagnosis of haemophilic arthropathy. Haemophilia 2010; 16: 67-8.
[http://dx.doi.org/10.1111/j.1365-2516.2010.02263.x] [PMID: 20590859]

[21]   Keshava S, Gibikote S, Mohanta A, Doria AS. Refinement of a sonographic protocol for assessment of haemophilic arthropathy. Haemophilia 2009; 15(5): 1168-71.
[http://dx.doi.org/10.1111/j.1365-2516.2009.02016.x] [PMID: 19493019]

CHAPTER 8

The Conservative Management of the Haemophilic Arthropathy

Christian Carulli[*], **Caterina Martini** and **Irene Felici**

Orthopaedic Clinic, University of Florence, Florence, Italy

Abstract: The combination of bleeding control strategies associated with lifestyle modifications, gentle physical activity, and the eventual use of ortheses are the basic principles to prevent the haemophilic arthropathy in its severe stages that represent the most common clinical manifestation of Haemophilia. Several conservative treatments may be also useful. Intraarticular injections of hyaluronic acid (viscosupplementation), Rifampicine (chemical synoviorthesis), and radioactive colloids (radiosynoviorthesis) with their different indications have been associated with good results. Other approaches as platelet-rich-plasma injections or synovial endovascular embolization have still to be validated and understood to ensure their safety or effectiveness.

Keywords: Chemical synoviorthesis, Endovascular embolization, Haemophilia, Haemophilic arthropathy, Hyaluronic acid, Platetet rich plasma, Physical synoviorthesis rifampicine Radiocolloids, Viscosupplementation.

INTRODUCTION

Modern bleeding-preventing drugs and tailored haematologic protocols have represented the milestones for the prevention of the complications of Haemophilia from the middle '90s in developed countries [1, 2]. To date, the musculoskeletal alterations represent the most common affection of haemophilic patients. The combination of the primary haematologic prophylaxis associated with medical therapy, lifestyle modifications, gentle physical activity, and the eventual use of ortheses have to be considered the historical basic principles to prevent the arthropathy or to limit its progression in case of early alterations. In cases of subjects not treated by a primary prophylaxis (patients >30years and middle aged), patients with poor bleeding control (particularly those with inhibitors), and in mild to advanced joint diseases such approaches may be associated to poor outcomes. In this population, the purposes of the treatment are the temporary

---

[*] **Corresponding author Christian Carulli:** Orthopaedic Clinic, University of Florence, Florence, Italy; Tel: 0039 055 794 8200; Email: christian.carulli@unifi.it

Christian Carulli (Ed.)

modulation of symptoms or the delay of a surgical procedure [3]. On the other hand, surgery is mandatory to obtain adequate clinical results in cases of persistent symptoms or bleedings.

In the last years, new conservative or non-surgical therapies as injections of drugs with effect on synovial tissue and cartilage have been proposed. Recently, other minimally invasive treatments as Platelet-rich-plasma (PRP) and endovascular embolization have arised interest on the haemophilic population. These treatments, to be considered "modern" conservative strategies, have specific indications in Haemophilia: symptomatic early stages of arthropathy, acute or recurrent synovitis, and late stages of arthropathy in subjects with contrain-dications to surgery, waiting or just delaying a surgical procedure [3, 4].

The following is an overview of the historical and modern conservative orthopaedic treatments.

Viscosupplementation

Viscosupplementation is the intraarticular administration of hyaluronic acid (HA), and has been considered the treatment of choice of early knee Osteoarthritis with clinical results equal to or better than placebo and corticosteroids [5, 6]. Over the years, it has been hypothesized its efficacy in other arthritic joints even not reaching a full evidence but with good clinical outcomes, and an advantageous cost/benefit ratio [7, 8]. Moreover, given the substantially absence of complications, HA injections have been proposed also in other types of arthropathy as Rheumatoid Arthritis and Haemophilic Arthropathy with encouraging results in several target joints [3, 4, 9].

HA is a complex polysaccharide containing glucosamine and glucuronic acid produced by synovial cells, and highly represented in synovial fluid. It is involved in several biological mechanisms, such as joint lubrication, shock absorption, and viscoelasticity of synovial fluid. Theoretic effects of HA on inhibition of tissue nociceptors, stimulation of endogenous hyaluronan, direct anti-inflammatory effects, and inhibition of matrix metalloproteinase activity, have been demonstrated *in vitro* and *in vivo* over the years [6]. Degenerative joint diseases are related to modifications of HA concentration causing a reduced viscoelasticity of the synovial fluid. By inducing metabolic changes, intraarticular HA showed a certain efficacy principally related to the induction of effects as *disease modifying* more than *symptoms modifying drug*.

As widely known, haemophilic arthropathy is characterized by destructured joints, bone deformities, almost complete closure of intra-articular spaces, and significant malalignment. In most cases, typically in younger patients, radiological aspects do not necessarily correspond to the clinical situation, thus involved joints are modestly painful, with little limitation in ROM, and fair flexion contractures. In these cases, surgery is usually not recommended. However, symptoms may be not tolerated, or poorly controlled with drugs and/or physical therapy, so further treatments are needed. Viscosupplementation may be considered one of the most indicated approaches given the ascertained improvements on pain reduction and functional abilities. Moreover, as mentioned before, it seems that this approach may ensure a delay for more invasive procedures even maintaining unmodified the joint from an anatomical and radiographic point of view [3, 4].

Fernandez-Palazzi *et al.* were the first authors to hypothesize the effectiveness and safety of HA in Haemophilia. In their latest report 25 subjects underwent viscosupplementation with a mean follow-up of about 2 years. The majority of patients reported satisfactory and persistent improvements, with only 10% requesting further treatments [10]. Wallny *et al.* reported their experience of viscosupplementation in knees of 20 haemophilic patients with good clinical results in 14 subjects and no complications at 2-years follow-up [11]. Athanassiou-Metaxa *et al.* reported only partial results in a population of eight children affected by haemophilic arthropathy treated with injections of HA and Rifampicine. In both groups, the authors noted several withdrawals related to low compliance, and complications not tolerated by too young patients particularly after rifampicine injections [12].

Carulli *et al.* reported the first prospective series of 46 haemophilic patients affected by arthropathy in elbows, knees, and ankles undergoing viscosupplementation and evaluated at a long-term follow-up [3]. More than 60% of them was in secondary prophylaxis and affected by severe stages of arthropathy (Petterson score>9). Administration protocols consisted in 3 to 5 injections of low molecular weight HA in sterile setting with 1–4 weeks intervals. All subjects were evaluated by the Visual Analogue Scale (VAS), the World Federation of Haemophilia score (WFH), and the Short Form-36 (SF-36). All patients completed at least two cycles of HA injections, 6 patients received three cycles. At a mean follow-up time of 6.3 years no adverse effect was recorded and almost all the patients reported significant improvements in pain control, joint function, and quality of life at 6 months follow-up. The best effects were achieved after the first HA cycle with respect to the others. At the long-term evaluation, 6 of the 24 patients with knee arthropathy needed surgery for persistent pain and functional impairment that injections temporarily limited in a period from 2 to 4 years after the first HA cycle (3 TKAs, 2 arthroscopies, 1 high tibial osteotomy). One patient among 22 affected by ankle arthropathy referred no effects requiring an ankle replacement, while the remainders reported satisfactory outcomes. All patients with elbow arthropathy showed significant improvements. Of noting that the reported outcomes were not correlated to the type or severity of Haemophilia, to the associated infectious diseases, and to the type of recombinant factor used for the prophylaxis.

A brand new indication of viscosupplementation may be also the hip arthropathy, even it is one of the less involved target joint due to its scarce presence of synovial tissue. Such kind of injections have to be necessarily performed by an US-guide in order to prevent any complications (vascular or neurologic lesions).

Finally, further ongoing studies will ascertain the long-term effect of viscosupplementation combined with other strategies and also the potential differences between the type of HA nowadays available.

Synoviorthesis

Synoviorthesis is the intraarticular injection of chemical or radioactive substances able to produce fibrosis of the hypertrophic synovium. Two main types of synoviorthesis have been proposed in Haemophilia during the last decades: the chemical synoviorthesis by the introduction of low cost antibiotic substances (rifampicine, tetracycline), and the synoviorthesis with radiocolloids.

The indication for synoviorthesis is a chronic synovitis causing recurrent haemarthroses, unresponsive to the basic conservative treatment. Contraindications include: intolerance to radiocolloids or rifampicine, acute bleedings, and joint infections.

The efficacy of such procedures is reported with a range from 76% to 80%, and can be repeated up to three times with 3-month intervals if radiocolloids are used, or weekly up to 3-4 times if rifampicine is used [13]. A future perspective is the use of synoviorthesis for patients with inhibitors.

Chemical Synoviorthesis

Rifampicine is a cheap antibiotic used for long time in the treatment of soft tissues infections. Recently, it was used for the treatment of haemophilic patients, however using different protocols [13]. Caviglia *et al.* reported the use of rifampicin as more effective when used in small joints (elbows, ankles) with respect to knees [14]. Fernandez-Palazzi and colleagues presented a study on synoviorthesis with a different drug, reporting satisfactory results in terms of pain relief and functional recovery in elbows, ankles, knees, and shoulders. Seventy-seven patients out of 84 underwent a treatment with four weekly injections of oxytetracycline chlorhydrate, antibiotic belonging to the family of tetracyclines (active on the proteic synthesis with a bacteriostatic effect) without significant complications [15]. Athanassiou-Metaxa *et al.* reported their preliminary experience with rifampicine and HA injections in a population of eight haemophilic children. However, they recorded a low compliance to the treatment and complications (intolerance, transient swelling, and occasional pain) in these very young patients particularly after rifampicine injections [12]. Same results and limitations were reported by Molho and colleagues [16].

Radiosynoviorthesis

Radiosynoviorthesis consists in the intraarticular injection of beta-emittents drugs, which can be used in a colloidal or particulate form. After contact with the synovium, local phagocytic cells absorb the drug allowing the transmission of the radiant dose to the synovium itself.

Historically, radiosynoviorthesis was used for the first time in 1952 by Fellinger for the local treatment of rheumatologic diseases [17]. For the first time it was proposed as a treatment of haemophilic synovitis in 1971 by Ahlberg *et al* [18]. The rationale was that radiations would cause a reduction of the synovial vasculature, consequently preventing the progression of the arthropathy.

The "ideal" radionuclide which resumes the best pharmacological and physical characteristics should have some features. It should be a pure beta-emittent nuclide, or minimal gamma-emitting; it should have a tissue penetration between 5 and 10mm, and a short half-life; it should have a high chemical purity, and it should not be toxic; finally, it should have a low cost.

In the first experimentations, the radionuclide used was gold. Then, a lot of drugs were used: the more commonly used were Yttrium 90 and Rhenium 186, because of their nearness to the "perfect" radionuclide. Classically, Yttrium was used adopted in larger joints (knees), while Rhenium was used in smaller joints (elbows, ankles) [18, 19]. More recently, new drugs have been introduced: Erbium 169 and Samarium 153. Er169 has a lesser beta-energy, and it suites best small joints. Sm153 is more widely used to treat haemophilic knees, especially at higher doses [20]. The drug is transported towards the synovium by a particular carrier, which exist in several forms: as a colloid (*i.e.* Y90 citrate or silicate, Re186 colloidal sulfur, Er169 citrate), albumine microspheres, hydroxyapatite crystals, or polylactic acid particles. In all these forms, radioactive drugs are transported inside the joint to dispatch their action. Radiocolloids are then phagocytized by synovial cells, as mentioned acting in a double manner: early and later effect. The early effect is the reduction on the thickness of the synovium, the thrombotic occlusion of capillaries, and the increase in deposition of fibrin. The later effect includes an interstitial fibrosis, a further reduction of thickness of the synovium, a reduction of the number of vessels, and the consequential reduction of the bleedings.

Radioactive synoviorthesis has showed a 75% to 80% satisfactory outcomes at a long-term evaluation, evaluable by the decrease in the number of haemorragic episodes [21, 22].

Platelet-Rich-Plasma Injections

Platelet-rich therapies have been recently introduced and increasingly used in the treatment of several musculoskeletal pathologies, as main approach or associated to surgery [23]. Particularly, Platelet-rich-plasma (PRP) is produced by the centrifugation of an amount of the patient's own blood and extraction of the active fraction. Platelets have the ability to produce several growth factors, so these therapies should theoretically enhance various tissue healing processes. However, even the great resonance and enthusiasm arisen during last years, there is not currently a sufficient evidence to support the use of PRP in the treatment of musculoskeletal diseases. Moreover, it is to date difficult to reach a standard-isation of PRP preparation methods [24]. Thus, indications in haemophilic arthropathy are reasonably debated and would surely need a deep analysis of long-term effects and cost/benefit ratio [25].

Endovascular Embolization

Endovascular embolization is a form of minimally invasive surgery based on the rationale of limiting hemorrhages or stopping the blood supply of specific regions by intravascular devices positioned by peripheral accesses. Generally indicated in vascular and oncologic surgery, it has been proposed in haemophiliacs for the treatment of pseudotumours [26] and pseudoaneurisms [27, 28], for the control of severe bleedings not responding to other therapies [29 - 33], and recently for the management of haemoartrosis related to chronic synovitis [34]. By the embolization of specific arteries in knees and elbows, it has been hypothesized that synovial blood supply may be reduced up to 80%, thus inducing a necrosis of synovial tissue and preventing further bleedings [35]. Results have been encouraging even the very few indications: recalcitrant synovitis in knees and elbows without any improvement after standard treatments, and before a surgical treatment not accepted by patients [34, 35]. We believe that this kind of approach may be considered only after a close evaluation by patients and multidisciplinary team, given the potential complications. Individual anatomic variability of the local vascular network, prolonged radiologic exposition, limited accessibility of the patients to equipped facilities on a side, and infections in the surgical access site, vascular lesions, and ischemic sequelae (particularly in ankles, where the procedure is contraindicated) are the main limitations of this technique.

CONCLUDING REMARKS

Conservative orthopaedic treatments are useful in association with adequate bleeding strategies, medical therapy, and lifestyle modifications in the management of early to moderate stages of joint disease. Actually, such approaches may be used to reduce pain and functional impairment, improving the bleeding control by the use of intraarticular injections of hyaluronic acid, radioactive substances, or rifampicine. Such injections have been associated to short- and mid-term satisfactory outcomes and no complications also in very young patients. Non-surgical options may also be considered to delay surgery in case of mild to severe arthropathy. The future perspective is to prevent the arthropathy in haemophilic patients by medical or gene therapies, and to adopt conservative strategies only for the pain control or improvement of the functional ability.

CONFLICT OF INTEREST

The authors confirm that they have no conflict of interest to declare for this publication.

ACKNOWLEDGEMENTS

Declared none.

REFERENCES

[1] Houghton GR, Duthie RB. Orthopedic problems in hemophilia. Clin Orthop Relat Res 1979; (138): 197-216.
[PMID: 445900]

[2] Roosendaal G, Van Der Berg HM, Lafeber FP, Bijilsma JW. Blood induced joint damage: an overview of musculoskeletal research in Haemophilia. In: Rodriguez-Merchan EC, Goddard NJ, Lee CA, Eds. Muscoloskeletal Aspects of Haemophilia. Cambridge: Blackwell Science Ltd 2000; pp. 18-26.

[3] Carulli C, Civinini R, Martini C, et al. Viscosupplementation in haemophilic arthropathy: a long-term follow-up study. Haemophilia 2012; 18(3): e210-4.
[http://dx.doi.org/10.1111/j.1365-2516.2011.02654.x] [PMID: 21951693]

[4] Carulli C, Matassi F, Civinini R, Morfini M, Tani M, Innocenti M. Intra-articular injections of hyaluronic acid induce positive clinical effects in knees of patients affected by haemophilic arthropathy. Knee 2013; 20(1): 36-9.
[http://dx.doi.org/10.1016/j.knee.2012.05.006] [PMID: 22704969]

[5] Evanich JD, Evanich CJ, Wright MB, Rydlewicz JA. Efficacy of intraarticular hyaluronic acid injections in knee osteoarthritis. Clin Orthop Relat Res 2001; (390): 173-81.
[http://dx.doi.org/10.1097/00003086-200109000-00020] [PMID: 11550864]

[6] Bellamy N, Campbell J, Robinson V, Gee T, Bourne R, Wells G. Viscosupplementation for the treatment of osteoarthritis of the knee. Cochrane Database Syst Rev 2006; 2(2): CD005321.
[PMID: 16625635]

[7]   Migliore A, Giovannangeli F, Bizzi E, *et al.* Viscosupplementation in the management of ankle osteoarthritis: a review. Arch Orthop Trauma Surg 2011; 131(1): 139-47.
      [http://dx.doi.org/10.1007/s00402-010-1165-5] [PMID: 20697901]

[8]   Migliore A, Massafra U, Bizzi E, *et al.* Comparative, double-blind, controlled study of intra-articular hyaluronic acid (Hyalubrix) injections *versus* local anesthetic in osteoarthritis of the hip. Arthritis Res Ther 2009; 11(6): R183.
      [http://dx.doi.org/10.1186/ar2875] [PMID: 20003205]

[9]   Saito S, Momohara S, Taniguchi A, Yamanaka H. The intra-articular efficacy of hyaluronate injections in the treatment of rheumatoid arthritis. Mod Rheumatol 2009; 19(6): 643-51.
      [http://dx.doi.org/10.3109/s10165-009-0207-8] [PMID: 19649562]

[10] Fernández-Palazzi F, Viso R, Boadas A, Ruiz-Sáez A, Caviglia H, De Bosch NB. Intra-articular hyaluronic acid in the treatment of haemophilic chronic arthropathy. Haemophilia 2002; 8(3): 375-81.
      [http://dx.doi.org/10.1046/j.1365-2516.2002.00627.x] [PMID: 12010437]

[11] Wallny T, Brackmann HH, Semper H, *et al.* Intra-articular hyaluronic acid in the treatment of haemophilic arthropathy of the knee. Clinical, radiological and sonographical assessment. Haemophilia 2000; 6(5): 566-70.
      [http://dx.doi.org/10.1046/j.1365-2516.2000.00413.x] [PMID: 11012703]

[12] Athanassiou-Metaxa M, Koussi A, Economou M, *et al.* Chemical synoviorthesis with rifampicine and hyaluronic acid in haemophilic children. Haemophilia 2002; 8(6): 815-6.
      [http://dx.doi.org/10.1046/j.1365-2516.2002.00696.x] [PMID: 12410653]

[13] Rodriguez-Merchan EC, Wiedel JD. General principles and indications of synoviorthesis (medical synovectomy) in haemophilia. Haemophilia 2001; 7 (Suppl. 2): 6-10.
      [http://dx.doi.org/10.1046/j.1365-2516.2001.00102.x] [PMID: 11564137]

[14] Caviglia HA, Fernandez-Palazzi F, Galatro G, Perez-Bianco R. Chemical synoviorthesis with rifampicin in haemophilia. Haemophilia 2001; 7 (Suppl. 2): 26-30.
      [http://dx.doi.org/10.1046/j.1365-2516.2001.00105.x] [PMID: 11564141]

[15] Fernández-Palazzi F, Cedeño M, Maldonado JC, *et al.* Chemical synoviorthesis with oxytetracycline clorhydrate (Emicine) in recurrent haemarthrosis. Haemophilia 2008; 14(1): 21-4.
      [PMID: 18005152]

[16] Molho P, Verrier P, Stieltjes N, *et al.* A retrospective study on chemical and radioactive synovectomy in severe haemophilia patients with recurrent haemarthrosis. Haemophilia 1999; 5(2): 115-23.
      [http://dx.doi.org/10.1046/j.1365-2516.1999.00287.x] [PMID: 10215960]

[17] Fellinger K, Schmid J. [Local therapy of rheumatic diseases]. Wien Z Inn Med 1952; 33(9): 351-63.
      [PMID: 13006334]

[18] Fernandez-Palazzi F, Caviglia H. On the safety of synoviorthesis in haemophilia. Haemophilia 2001; 7 (Suppl. 2): 50-3.
      [http://dx.doi.org/10.1046/j.1365-2516.2001.00110.x] [PMID: 11564146]

[19] Rodriguez-Merchan EC. Aspects of current management: orthopaedic surgery in haemophilia. Haemophilia 2012; 18(1): 8-16.
      [http://dx.doi.org/10.1111/j.1365-2516.2011.02544.x] [PMID: 21535324]

[20] Calegaro JU, Machado J, Furtado RG, *et al.* The use of 185 Mbq and 740 MBq of 153-samarium and oxyapatite for knee synovectomy in hemophilia. Hemophilia 2014; 20: 421-5.

[21] Rodriguez-Merchan EC, Quintana M, De la Corte-Rodriguez H, Coya J. Radioactive synoviorthesis for the treatment of haemophilic synovitis. Haemophilia 2007; 13 (Suppl. 3): 32-7.
      [http://dx.doi.org/10.1111/j.1365-2516.2007.01538.x] [PMID: 17822519]

[22] Eraghi AS, Kaseb MH, Espandar R, Mardookhpour S. The long-term effects of radioactive phosphorous synoviorthesis on hemophilic arthropathy. Blood Cells Mol Dis 2015; 55(1): 68-70.
[http://dx.doi.org/10.1016/j.bcmd.2015.03.011] [PMID: 25976470]

[23] Moraes VY, Lenza M, Tamaoki MJ, Faloppa F, Belloti JC. Platelet-rich therapies for musculoskeletal soft tissue injuries. Cochrane Database Syst Rev 2013; 12(12): CD010071.
[PMID: 24363098]

[24] Moraes VY, Lenza M, Tamaoki MJ, Faloppa F, Belloti JC. Platelet-rich therapies for musculoskeletal soft tissue injuries. Cochrane Database Syst Rev 2014; 4(4): CD010071.
[PMID: 24782334]

[25] Silva M. 14th International Musculoskeletal Congress of World Federation of Haemophilia; Belfast (North Ireland). 2015.7-10 May;

[26] Lim MY, Nielsen B, Ma A, Key NS. Clinical features and management of haemophilic pseudotumours: a single US centre experience over a 30-year period. Haemophilia 2014; 20(1): e58-62.
[http://dx.doi.org/10.1111/hae.12295] [PMID: 24354486]

[27] Saris DB, van Rinsum AC, Dhert WJ, Roosendaal G, Mali WP. Periarticular aneurysm formation in haemophilia. Lancet 1997; 349(9054): 766-8.
[http://dx.doi.org/10.1016/S0140-6736(96)09177-5] [PMID: 9074576]

[28] Rodriguez-Merchan EC. Pseudoaneurysms in haemophilia. Blood Coagul Fibrinolysis 2013; 24(5): 461-4.
[http://dx.doi.org/10.1097/MBC.0b013e32835e42aa] [PMID: 23337709]

[29] Rodriguez-Merchan EC, Jimenez-Yuste V, Gomez-Cardero P, Rodriguez T. Severe postoperative haemarthrosis following a total knee replacement in a haemophiliac patient caused by a pseudoaneurysm: early treatment with arterial embolization. Haemophilia 2014; 20(1): e86-9.
[http://dx.doi.org/10.1111/hae.12286] [PMID: 24165398]

[30] Park JJ, Slover JD, Stuchin SA. Recurrent hemarthrosis in a hemophilic patient after revision total knee arthroplasty. Orthopedics 2010; 33(10): 771.
[PMID: 20954656]

[31] Espandar R, Heidari P, Rodriguez-Merchan EC. Management of haemophilic pseudotumours with special emphasis on radiotherapy and arterial embolization. Haemophilia 2009; 15(2): 448-57.
[http://dx.doi.org/10.1111/j.1365-2516.2008.01942.x] [PMID: 19175421]

[32] Klamroth R, Gottstein S, Essers E, Landgraf H, Wilaschek M, Oldenburg J. Successful angiographic embolization of recurrent elbow and knee joint bleeds in seven patients with severe haemophilia. Haemophilia 2009; 15(1): 247-52.
[http://dx.doi.org/10.1111/j.1365-2516.2008.01842.x] [PMID: 18691374]

[33] Mauser-Bunschoten EP, Zijl JA, Mali W, van Rinsum AC, van den Berg HM, Roosendaal G. Successful treatment of severe bleeding in hemophilic target joints by selective angiographic embolization. Blood 2005; 105(7): 2654-7.
[http://dx.doi.org/10.1182/blood-2004-06-2063] [PMID: 15613551]

[34] Galli E, Baques A, Moretti N, Candela M, Caviglia H. Hemophilic chronic synovitis: therapy of hemarthrosis using endovascular embolization of knee and elbow arteries. Cardiovasc Intervent Radiol 2013; 36(4): 964-9.
[http://dx.doi.org/10.1007/s00270-012-0480-3] [PMID: 23150120]

[35] Caviglia H. 14th International Musculoskeletal Congress of World Federation of Haemophilia.; Belfast (North Ireland). 2015.7-10 May;

CHAPTER 9

Lifestyle Strategies and Physical Therapy

Francesco Demartis[1,*] and **Massimiliano Tani**[2]

[1] *Center for Bleeding Disorders, Department of Heart and Vessels, Azienda Ospedaliero-Universitaria Careggi, Florence, Italy*

[2] *Orthopaedic Clinic, University of Florence, Florence, Italy*

Abstract: Haemophilia is a condition that has to be kept under full control. A "3 M's" approach aiming to the patient's Mindfulness, Muscles and physical activity Maintenance is nowadays suggested. In association, an appropriate program of physical therapy with strategies fitting all needs and abilities of patients is mandatory and reasonable, particularly when acute or chronic musculoskeletal affections occur.

Keywords: Haemophilia, lifestyle strategies, Physical therapy.

LIFESTYLE STRATEGIES

In affective neuroscience it is common to quote an African proverb that says: "it only takes one woman to give birth to a child, but it takes a whole village to bring up that child". This same proverb can apply to hemophiliac children, who have the same need of friendship, emotions, incitements and childhood experiences than any other child in the world. Their only specific characteristic is their tendency to bleed. They will still grow, learn and have the same culture such as any other child, and they will become totally grown up adults only if they will have the opportunity to interact with their own environment just like any other child [1].

At some time in the '70s, for a month per year, the Olympic fields close to a Comprehensive Care Haemophilia Center, in Pisa, Italy, were opened to young Italian and European haemophiliacs. These teenagers had the opportunity to run, jump and test themselves in the most competitive sports in order to strengthen their body along with their self-esteem. This experience lasted almost one decade and allowed us to understand that Haemophilia requires understanding, adequate therapies, and commitment, but that it also allows a remarkable muscular

---

* **Corresponding author Francesco Demartis:** Center for Bleeding Disorders , AOU Careggi, University of Florence, Florence, Italy; Email: drfrancescodemartis@gmail.com

Christian Carulli (Ed.)

development together with an outstanding social integration. Most of those teenagers, today, are active and graduated adults, many of which have become head of a family [2, 3].

So, which are the steps to take once the diagnosis of Haemophilia has been achieved? We suggest the 3 M's Approach to Haemophilia, as follows.

Mindfulness: "fully control the Haemophilia instead of letting it control you";

Muscles: "a harmonious physical development decreases the risk of haemorrhagic events whilst it increases self-esteem and socialization";

Maintenance: "an adequate physical activity needs to be pursued and maintained for the whole lifespan in order to enhance patients' lives and joints".

Mindfulness

In order to reach the first target of our program, it is important to deepen the knowledge of Haemophilia itself by speaking with the Reference Center doctors. This is due to be informed and have questions answered to, as well as obtaining a precise diagnosis (A or B, severe, moderate or mild Haemophilia). It is important to be aware that with the same level of factor, clinically milder forms exist, and these are detectable by careful observation of the child, the only person who will show us the clinical phenotype. It is also important to read about Haemophilia, bearing in mind that scientific literature is normally revised by many doctors and scientists who filter the many enthusiasms and take into consideration only demonstrated facts. On the other hand, the information found inside the web can be diffused by anybody, so it is important to read only official scientific organizations or patients associations websites in order to avoid unreliable sources [4, 5].

After obtaining appropriate medical information from the Haemophilia Center's health care staff members, the second - and sometimes amazing - step is understanding that you are not alone but that there is an international network ready to support you and provide you with very important information. The WFH (World Federation of Haemophilia) in Canada is committed to provide data, information, therapeutic guidelines or directions of Comprehensive Haemophilia Center of your own area or Nation. This makes possible to meet families of haemophilic children in order to obtain direct reports on the quality of life of their family, as well as to participate to a large number of social events such as summer camps, periodical meetings and even winter holidays! Nowadays haemophilic people rightfully belong to an international community [6 - 8].

Furthermore, it is important to consider that among congenital blood disorders Haemophilia has achieved a high standard of efficacious and safe treatments. As a consequence, also quality of life is definitely better compared to other inherited blood disorders. Over the recent years safer drugs for haemophiliacs have been developed and today long-acting recombinant drugs (rFVIII and rFIX) are available. So, now more than ever before, it is important to maintain a positive attitude towards this pathology and to understand that, with social and therapeutic efforts, it is possible to live a normal life. Comprehensive Care is a team aimed to approach the care and treatment of Haemophilia. The main target of this approach is to give the child the most normal life as possible [9, 10].

During the pre-scholar period we suggest to:

1. Build a solid relationship between the parents in order to take care, in the best possible way, of the characteristic of the child during the most delicate moment of his life, the early childhood;
2. Obtain an accurate and updated knowledge about Haemophilia, as previously said, referring to a Comprehensive Care Center, its members and to families;
3. Be aware that during this period (from the diagnosis to the beginning of primary school) three main difficulties will have to be dealt with:
   a. Avoiding the child's overprotection, in order to not interfere with his normal activities and to not limit his interaction with other children (for example, avoiding to take him to the nursery for fear of injuries or uncontrollable bleedings). Considering that we are next to commercialize second-generation long-lasting drugs, probably with non-intravenous injections, and we should certainly avoid provoking more damages with a wrong parents-child relationship than the pathology itself. It is then important to refer to Haemophilia experienced doctors in order to not fall in a harmful iatrogenic overprotection. Having a very clear idea of the family's function is really important during this age: that is, to support a person who is blossoming in order to have, one day, an autonomous individual who has his own family. Do not keep your child in the shade [11]!
   b. Learning how to distinguish intensity and location of traumas in order to decide if the child has to be infused or not. Remember that healthy children are full of energy and have often little accidents that cause bruises. When they start crawling they may hit their head against the coffee table or against its legs, they may get bruises on their bottoms when they fall down whilst trying to stand up. The most dangerous body parts are the inextensible ones, such as the spine and cranium. When the kinetic energy of the bump is strong enough to cause a bruise it is important to infuse the child and bring him immediately to the Hospital or to the Haemophilic

Center for an evaluation. The same applies in case of car accidents as a pedestrian or as a passenger, or other sorts of injuries that may involve spine, cranium or throat [12, 13]. It is impossible to avoid the randomness, but we can always reduce the frequency of these events, for example improving the area where the child plays by covering the furniture edges and covering the floor with soft pads in order to soften the contact between knees and the floor when crawling or in case of falls. For especially lively children it is advisable to sew small foam rubber pads on the baby's rompers in order to protect knees and elbows, while bottoms are usually well protected in the early years by diapers.

c. Learning how to inject your child: many Centers have learning classes where parents can learn how to inject their children, as well teenager self-injection learning classes, fundamental in order to reach the independence of the patient. Keep handy everything needed in order to inject FVIII and FIX, and be informed exactly on which structure to rely on in case of need in any moment of the day or the night [14].

4. Have an adequate nutrition. A suitable diet is important for the development of every child, but whereas haemophilic children have excellent intellectual and muscular resources as any other, their joints are more fragile than others. This is because, despite the prophylaxis, there may be spontaneous or posttraumatic bleedings provoking different patterns of arthropathy [15]. Lower limb joints must sustain the weight of the body through very small contact surfaces, with a quite impressive load per square centimeter and jumping or standing on a single leg increases the load. In our experience, young severe haemophiliacs treated by appropriate prophylaxis, following fitness courses will obtain strong and flexible bodies, as long as they (and their family) avoid obesity. Obesity, particularly if pathological, becomes a vicious cycle that limits extensively our patients, increasing the number of haemarthrosis and resulting in the loss of days of school or play, and risking to socially isolate the teenager [16]. Anybody can get an idea of what it means to be overweight by 10 kg by using a 5 kg soft weight belt per leg and walking for three miles. The result would be sore ankles and aching legs, and 10 kg overweight is not much nowadays if we consider the amount of junk food commercials tormenting our children daily while watching television. It is therefore important to have a varied diet avoiding excesses, and to be aware that industrial products and sweetened drinks, as well as high in fat food such as French fries, butter and lard, are not the best that you can give to a child. On the other hand, fruit smoothies or sugarless fresh-squeezed juice are perfect to provide fibers and vitamins. Obviously excesses must always be avoided. We believe that the Mediterranean diet is advisable thanks to the high assumption of fruits, cereals and vegetables, and its reduced consumption of fats, but always bear in mind

that the total calories intake should be related to age, physical activity, and body surface. The Mediterranean diet is well balanced itself, but quantities should be individualized [17]. Please consider that a normal daily diet can include components such as ginseng, gingko, high quantities of garlic or green tea, that facilitates blood circulation in normal people, but that can even cause haemorrhages to those who have coagulation defects. Similarly, an excessive assumption of Omega three or Docosahexaenoic acid (DHA) present in the diet or added in the form of supplement pills, as well as high amounts of blue fish, especially if associated to excessive amounts of olive oil, can create bleeding complications. The target is to obtain a balanced diet with all the fundamental nutritional components, from vitamins to carbohydrates, from mineral salts to protein, to consume in a varied manner and with no caloric overload [18].

Muscles

Sports are a great tool for socializing and for reaching an adequate muscular development; as for any other activity, it is important to choose it in complete accordance with the child so as to support his choices, but it is also important to discuss it with the Haemophilia Comprehensive Center members. Developing a strong musculature helps protecting joints and induces to a lower incidence of spontaneous bleedings. Furthermore, the muscular strength, especially in central bearing muscles, helps avoiding strong impacts on the joints, as for example, toned and strong quadriceps helps avoiding heavy impacts on knees [19, 20].

We suggest approaching sports during the pre-scholar age, possibly under the guidance of an instructor in order to learn how to properly warm-up. Also an appropriate proprioceptive training is necessary for children, in order to enhance the awareness of their own bodies within the surrounding space and to have a greater promptness to retrieve adequate balanced positions. Many sports use these techniques for their professional athletes or as basic techniques (e.g. Tai Chi or Judo). For children aged 4 to 6 years, sports as volleyball-game, tennis-game or swimming-game are preferable, just because it is important to play encouraging the children as much as possible by using their own language, which stands truly far away from rules and discipline. This is the basis that will allow today's children to become tomorrow's athletes, when they will have the feeling that their choice has been respected and they will then be able to maintain sport activities as a part of their life. Some physical and extreme sports should be avoided, and in Table 1 we provide a list of the most suitable sports thanks to their limited possibilities of trauma. It is also important to remember that in order to have an adequate protection the level of coagulative factor of the blood is normally supposed to be over 5%, whereas during physical activities it should reach at least 15%. However, there are many roles inside the sport community such as the coach, the physiotherapist, the masseur, the referee, who are an active part of this amazing world but who also have a lesser risk of traumas and, therefore, have more enduring careers [21, 22].

Table 1. Sports recommended or discouraged in haemophilic patients.

Recommended Sports	The Least Favoured Sports
Swimming	Boxing
Table tennis	Rugby / football
Tai chi	American football
Fishing	Karate
Dance	Wrestling
Badminton	Motorcycling
Sailing	Judo
Golf	Hockey
Bowls	
Cycling	

Maintenance

Keeping a haemophilic patient healthy needs physical activity being maintained for the whole lifespan. We can reach this goal elaborating strategies together with the patient and by counseling approaches, listening to the personal anamnesis and evaluating his physical scores (i.e. Haemophilia Joint Health Score, HJHS) [23]. The main outcome of a lifelong training is a psychological well-being feeling that can overcome the time necessary to go to the gym. Because of this, we usually ask the patients which physical activities are common in their areas, if they are married or not, if they can take classes with their partner indoor or if they prefer to commit themselves in outdoor activities. Often, if we are dealing with over 50 years-old patients, we have to elaborate again their own feeling towards free time and towards prophylaxis, and quite often we have to suggest a step by step increase of prophylaxis (i.e. by bypassing agents) in order to increase their own self confidence. When they can keep their body free from bleedings and haemarthroses then they can collaborate much more with your efforts, and the joy of the physical activity itself can booster your medical advices much more than any scientific conference. Physical activity may increase endorphins synthesis, endogenous neuropeptides reducing pain and increasing the well-being feeling. On the other hand, exercising itself increases the production of synovial fluid that keep the joints lubricated, reduce stiffness, and bring nutrients into joints [24].

Group therapy is the top we can aim to, because of a mutual positive feedback. Tai Chi, Nordic walking, dancing classes, golf, and water aerobics all share the same social and physical advantages and patients who exercise regularly can improve overall fitness.

Home workout can also be a convenient way to exercise for very motivated patients and today it is quite common to see fitness machines such as treadmills, exercise bikes, rowing machines in private homes. They are much easier to use today compared to few years ago. They can be connected via web and patients can compete with their friends and also keep positive feedbacks at any time, following their own schedules. A daily warm-up routine, squat jumps, pushups, abs, plank hold, stretching, and bicycle exercises can complete a single machine equipment, keeping the patient in good physical health. In few words, exercising is a gift for your health!

PHYSICAL THERAPY

Some patients present muscular and articular impairments secondary to haemorrhagic events despite the substitutive therapy. Many reasons, such as the insufficient compliance with the prophylaxis, the functional overload, or the development of inhibitors, may explain these problems. In other cases, young patients present a mild Haemophilia phenotype, hard to be diagnosed until a severe posttraumatic haemorrhage occurs [25].

Each child has his own development pace but normally they all pass through the same steps, and with the same order. During the first year of life every child is attracted by everything accessible, they roll on their belly in order to change from the prone to the supine position, and they struggle in order to crawl. During this stage haemophilic babies can get bruises while rolling on toys within the cradle or while crawling. Within the first and second year babies will start standing without a support and walking always more actively moved by the curiosity towards everything that surrounds them. Together with the first intents they will start falling, increasing the possibility of bruises to arms, knees, and head. Two to three years-old babies keep exploring the surrounding environment, learning to coordinate their movements, and increasing their speed. Obviously, during this period of time they fall even more frequently due to the increased speed of their movements and their inexperience in quickly dodging obstacles. Normally, three to five years-old children can use staircases, ride a tricycle, jump, and kick or throw a ball. As they keep growing also increases the chance to get in posttraumatic or spontaneous joint bleedings, especially on load-bearing joints such as ankles and knees [26, 27].

Once they start attending school they also start participating to recreational-motoric activities and sports. During this stage, such activities were proved to be fundamental for the prevention of haematomas, even if bleeding and functional overloads increase [28]. As previously described, the Comprehensive Center doctors and physiotherapists would provide their patients with adequate information and help them pondering over the cost/benefits ratio of their physical activities [29].

Physiotherapists' first goal in Haemophilia, particularly in children is to prevent and treat musculoskeletal problems [30]. Physical therapy must be adapted focusing on the cognitive and motoric abilities of haemophilic patients, in relation to their age. Adults can perform sessions of exercises divided by series and repetitions of therapeutic movements, whereas children need to be engaged with recreational strategies, having short "working sessions" repeated often during the day. Adults need to properly warm-up before physical activity and inject themselves in case of high-intensity activities.

This chapter aims to provide physical therapists, health professionals in general, patients, and their families with directions and informations about the strategies that best may suit needs and abilities of the patient in case of musculoskeletal problems, both in acute and chronic phases [31].

Diagnosis

In order to evaluate all functional limitations caused by Haemophilia and the best therapeutic strategies, the therapist must have knowledge of the exact anatomical site and the causes of the injury. Does it involve a muscle, an articulation or both? Which are the causes of the injury: spontaneous bleeding, arthropathy, trauma, overload, postsurgical setting, or unknown cause? Which is the diagnosis? In order to assess it, the use of diagnostic tools such as a standard radiographic examination [32], ultrasounds [33], and MRI [34] may be useful. In addition to these instrumental examinations, specific questionnaires such as HJHS, Haemophilia Activity List [35] or Haemophilia-Specific Quality of Life Index (HRQL) [36 - 39] may help the therapist in order to test the functional capacity of the musculoskeletal system in relationship to the patients' daily activities. The final goal of the physiotherapy is to restore and improve the functional ability, to reduce pain and symptoms, to treat the consequences of each bleeding evaluating and adapting the individual needs of each patient. Finally, further targets are the proposal of a lifestyle centered on the best health condition possible [40].

Treatment

Several therapeutic strategies are available for haemophiliacs but unfortunately there is a little consensus about length, intensity, and kind of treatment. Many authors agree with the need to follow specific treatments for pain management, muscular strength, elasticity, and proprioceptive enhancement [41 - 44]. For this purpose physical therapy, muscular increasing exercises, hydrotherapy, and several other forms of physical exercises can be used [45 - 47]. Nonetheless, there is no evidence about which should the most effective treatment protocol. The physical therapy should pursue the therapeutic goals without resulting aggressive, in order not to be harmful. The early recognition of bleeding and the administration of the missing clotting factor are the keys to the success of all the approach to Haemophilia, and also for the physiotherapic treatment.

Infants and children are unable to communicate their parents if they have bleedings, but by a careful observation it is possible to assess if they are not using properly a limb, or if they may have symptoms of an inflammatory state. The earlier a bleeding is detected the faster is the beginning of an adequate treatment. Haemarthrosis or haematomas not promptly treated can cause functional limitations which may result in chronical arthropathy [48, 49].

In order of frequency, the most affected joints and muscles are reported in Table 2.

Table 2. Target joints and related involved muscles.

Joints	Muscles
Ankles	Quadriceps
Knees	Calves
Elbows	Forearm flectors

• How can we recognize a haemarthrosis?

Haemarthrosis is characterized by swollen, warm, redden, and painful joints with functional impairments. Recurrent haemarthrosis leads to haemophilic arthropathy with consequent severe disability. The most common joint abnormalities are valgus knees with tibial extrarotation, varus knees with tibial intrarotation, and valgus elbows.

• How can we recognize a haematoma?

Haematomas cause swollen and stiff muscles, showing the typical signs of an inflammatory state. They favor analgesic compensations in relation to the affected muscle, such as the hip flexion when iliopsoas muscle is involved. Also, injuries to the calf muscle can lead to the retraction of the Achilles tendon with consequent difficulties for the gait ability. Furthermore, when the anterior forearm musculature is affected, it often causes flexion deformities of wrists and fingers, and sensory and motoric limitations.

The following represent examples of treatment of haematoma and haemarthrosis, according to acute and subacute phase. Moreover, the management of chronic arthropathy will be discussed.

Acute Phase

The physiotherapic approach during the inflammatory phase of haemarthrosis and haematoma is based upon the "P.R.I.C.E." protocol:

• Protection
• Rest
• Ice
• Compression
• Elevation

A proper intervention should aim at stopping effusions and reducing pain and swelling. The affected area needs to be immobilized in order to ensure protection, and the patient should rest in a comfortable position for at least 48 hours. For the immobilization it is possible to use a thermoformable splint. The local application of ice for 15 minutes every two hours should be repeated for at least 5-6 times per day. During this phase it is useful to use a compression bandage, and the limb affected by bleeding should be kept in elevation. When ankles or knees are involved, the use of crutches can favor, according to the age, the mobility of the patient during the healing period. Adults, children, and patients' relatives should know the P.R.I.C.E. protocol in order to be able to use it whenever needed [48, 49].

Subacute Phase

Subacute phases start when muscular or articular bleedings have been stopped. The aim of the treatment in this phase is to improve the range of movement (ROM) and the muscular strength. Joint integrity depends on muscles tone supporting them; if muscles are not strengthened over the time, the functional overload increases together with the risk of repetitive effusions. During this phase is important to start the mobilization, which should be passive or assisted, together with the isometric strengthen of muscles in combination with ice applications. A therapeutic exercise program to do at home ensuring its proper execution is important especially for children. In order to do so it is desirable to share efforts with parents and relatives during home-treatment. Exercises should be as more enjoyable as possible, introducing, if possible, swimming sessions or hydrotherapy, which are useful ways to increase strength and mobility. It is advisable to start exercising at an early age and repeat the exercises several times a day after the period of immobilization without forcing the joints. Later, a progressive increasing of the intensity of the exercise especially in children is suggested [29].

The musculoskeletal system of children should not work under excessive loads, but keeping movements under control, and avoiding ballistic movements. In case of further bleedings, an increase of the prophylactic factor dosing may be sufficient; however, some children may also develop synovitis. The treatment of chronic synovitis consists in an adequate prophylaxis with substitutive therapy, together with physiotherapy intensive classes. Once reduced the synovial thickening the child will need physical and moral support in order to complete the program which can last up to 18 months [29].

Chronic Arthropathy

Chronic arthropathy is characterized by the contraction of soft tissues, articular destruction, and deformities. Nowadays less and less children suffer for chronic arthropathy thanks to the introduction of the prophylaxis and home-treatment programs. However, a single haemarthrosis is enough to begin chronic and progressive articular damage (see chapter 1). For this reason, it is important to prevent the haemarthrosis as much as possible, or to treat it as early as possible. After noting the first signs of an arthropathy it is important to control pain, maintaining ROM and muscular strength, as keeping an appropriate articular function. If not treated adequately, haemophilic patients may develop a bilateral arthropathy over the time, with further impairments and loss of a physiological gait [50]. Parents should be trained to early recognize and treat such clinical settings.

Inhibitors

Patients with severe A or B Haemophilia may develop inhibitors to FVIII or FIX [51]. The development of inhibitors is a serious complication for hemophiliacs, predisposing patients to more frequent and prolonged episodes of bleeding (see chapter 19). Physiotherapy for patients with inhibitors is rather complex. Any therapeutic intervention must be carefully monitored and tailored, and should be performed with delayed times and no hurry. In case of acute haemarthrosis the P.R.I.C.E. protocol should be used. Physiotherapy has no contraindications for patients with inhibitions as long as the patient is carefully monitored and evaluated by a multidisciplinary Haemophilia team [29]. Because of the extreme fragility of these patients it is important to be sure that the bleeding has stopped before starting any rehabilitative activity.

Functional Taping

Functional taping is effective in both subacute and acute phases because it supports and protects the damaged tissues thanks to the use of rigid, semi-rigid, and elastic materials. Bandages protect the affected joints and segments, reducing the mechanical stress while allowing minimal but physiological movements. Studies on severe injuries of ligaments of the ankle on non-hemophilic patients show that the use of bandages with semi-rigid materials allow a faster return to work than those with rigid materials The use of different types of materials associated with bandages does not show significant improvements in relation to pain relief, reduction of the oedema, and of the residual joint instability [52 - 54].

Massotherapy

Therapeutic massages are used in order to improve soft tissues healing, to obtain pain relief, to reduce the mechanical stress caused by the compression or traction of connective tissues [55], to enhance the lymphatic drainage, and to prevent adhesions [56]. The massage favors vasodilatation among muscles and skin, improving their cellular metabolism [57]. Once the acute phase has been limited, massages can be introduced as a therapeutic tool. The association of the massage to eccentric contraction can increase the analgesic effect on muscles [58].

TENS (transcutaneous Electrical Nerve Stimulation)

The transcutaneous electrical nerve stimulation can have two types of application: a local and immediate effect, and a systemic and delayed effect. By local applications the analgesic effect should occur within few minutes, otherwise it is possible that the electrodes have not been placed on the favorable zone. The effect of TENS is based upon the gate-control theory postulated by Melzack and Wall [59 - 61]. Its effectiveness has been proved on knee arthritis [62, 63], low back pain [60], and tension cephalea [61]. The frequency commonly used is between 100 and 150Hz, associated by a 150 a 250µs pulse width. This analgesic therapy can be accompanied by ice applications during acute phases or with massages in the subacute stage, in order to reduce muscular contractures.

The systematic analgesia favors the endogenous production of endorphinic substances increasing the threshold of perception of pain, which can be useful in painful phases, tiredness, or as a sedative. This effect can be obtained by electrical parameters with frequency between 2 and 5Hz and stimulus width around 350µs. The intensity can be increased in order to obtain a significant muscular contraction and maintained for 30 minutes. The application of the electrodes should be carried out in any area of the body, even if the interscapular area is particularly recommended [64].

Ultrasounds

Ultrasounds are a type of physical therapy which penetrates tissues through unionizing radiation in the form of acoustic energy, while producing heat.

Working parameters are generally used between 1.0 and 3.0MHz, which allows acting up to 5cm deep under the cutaneous surface. Ultrasounds as any other diathermic physical therapies can be administered in continuous or pulsed mode in order to achieve a thermal or athermal effect. The goal of thermal therapies is to increase the pain threshold, improve the local blood circulation, the cellular metabolism and cellular permeability, as well as to enhance the nerve conduction. On the other hand, athermal therapies, using the mechanical component of the acoustic energy, increase the cellular activity and proteic synthesis, finally originating cavitation and reducing the oedema [65]. However, excessive thermal or mechanical effects could induce some form of damage to tissues [66, 67].

Nevertheless, ultrasounds application shows as non-thermal effects prevail over thermal ones [68]. High intensities ($2W/cm^2$) are recommended in order to stimulate a fibrinolytic effect (protein denaturalization) in case of adherences and fibrosis typical of capsulate haematomas. Low intensities (1W/cm2) are recommended in order to treat fibroblasts proliferation as well as to stimulate the restoration of damaged tissues. Eccentric physical activity can be combined with low intensity ultrasounds applications in order to stimulate the collagen synthesis and improve its tensile property.

Deep Thermotherapy, Hyperthermia, Radiofrequency

Hyperthermia is a form of deep thermotherapy applied through a device that may, or may not, be in contact with patients' skin. Temperatures can be reached thanks to substantial energy frequencies. The thermal profundity of the treatment depends on the patient's fat tissue width and the modality of use of the device. Main effects of the deep heat are the increase of the cellular metabolism [69], vasodilatation, and lymphatic drainage [70, 71]. The increase of the temperature on the deep tissue, combined with stretching exercises, can favor the reabsorption together with the extension of tissues. However, therapeutic heating on deep structures has to be used extremely carefully because of the vasodilatative effect. In fact, during the acute phase, the increase of the blood circulation caused by the produced vasodilatation may worsen the bleeding tendency. For this reason, the therapy should not be started until a stable haemostasis is achieved.

Therapeutic Exercises

Each modality of physiotherapy (active, passive, and counterforce) represents the fundamental basis for the recovery after any injury. The current literature on the experimental treatment of severe injuries of soft tissues conveys the preference of early mobilization over the complete immobilization, in order to obtain an optimal recovery. The early mobilization of damaged tissues should be carefully performed, and only after an efficient haemostasis is ensured [72].

The therapeutic exercise aims to improve muscular strength, cardiovascular and muscular endurance, and to increase ROM. The most frequently used exercises are those aimed at muscles strengthening and hypertrophy through isometric, concentric and eccentric contractions, electrical muscular stimulations (EMS), stretching, and proprioceptive and postural assessment.

Several studies have shown that any musculoskeletal injury causes a loss of strength which should be avoided considering that in only a week it can reach extremely high levels. Exercises can be done in closed and open kinetic chain. The first offers greater joint stability and simulates the daily joint activity: however, there is a greater load transmission to joints, and it is not recommended for altered joints. In such cases the open kinetic chain exercise is preferable. Working parameters are typically 2 or 3 sets of 10-15 repetitions per muscular groups with three sessions per week. The intensity of the load has to be adapted to the physical condition of patients and should stimulate a muscle strain without causing overloads and consequent damages of already affected muscles and joints [73].

CONCLUDING REMARKS

Haemophilia is a life-long disease. It needs a positive cultural attitude and training aimed to a continuous personal improvement. Each developmental step needs an accurate knowledge of the disease and family commitment in order to cope appropriately with all associated physical and psychological aspects. Maintenance of a good balance between physical activity and musculoskeletal strength and flexibility is the gold standard that each hemophilic patient should reach.

CONFLICT OF INTEREST

The authors confirm that they have no conflict of interest to declare for this publication.

ACKNOWLEDGEMENTS

Declared none.

REFERENCES

[1]   Panksepp J. Affective Neuroscience: The Foundations of Human and Animal Emotions. Oxford University Press 1998; p. 403.

[2]   Panicucci F, Sabbatini AM, Testi A, Bastianini C. Holidays and Sports for Haemophiliacs in Italy. Haemostasis 1981; 10: 244.

[3]   Panicucci F, Sagripanti A, Conte B, Sabbatini AM, Bastianini C, Testi A. Prevention of Haemophilia risks through comprehensive care haemostasis 1981; 10: 173.

[4]   Silberg WM, Lundberg GD, Musacchio RA. Assessing, controlling, and assuring the quality of medical information on the Internet: Caveant lector et vieworLet the reader and viewer beware. JAMA 1997; 277(15): 1244-5.
        [http://dx.doi.org/10.1001/jama.1997.03540390074039] [PMID: 9103351]

[5]   Winker MA, Flanagin A, Chi-Lum B, *et al.* American Medical Association. Guidelines for medical and health information sites on the internet: principles governing AMA web sites. JAMA 2000; 283(12): 1600-6.
        [http://dx.doi.org/10.1001/jama.283.12.1600] [PMID: 10735398]

[6]   Beeton K, Neal D, Lee C. An exploration of health-related quality of life in adults with haemophiliaa qualitative perspective. Haemophilia 2005; 11(2): 123-32.
        [http://dx.doi.org/10.1111/j.1365-2516.2005.01077.x] [PMID: 15810914]

[7]   VON Mackensen S. Quality of life and sports activities in patients with haemophilia. Haemophilia 2007; 13 (Suppl. 2): 38-43.
        [http://dx.doi.org/10.1111/j.1365-2516.2007.01505.x] [PMID: 17685923]

[8]   Oladapo AO, Epstein JD, Williams E, Ito D, Gringeri A, Valentino LA. Health-related quality of life assessment in haemophilia patients on prophylaxis therapy: a systematic review of results from prospective clinical trials. Haemophilia 2015; 21(5): e344-58.
        [http://dx.doi.org/10.1111/hae.12759] [PMID: 26390060]

[9]   Plug I, Peters M, Mauser-Bunschoten EP, *et al.* Social participation of patients with hemophilia in the Netherlands. Blood 2008; 111(4): 1811-5.
        [http://dx.doi.org/10.1182/blood-2007-07-102202] [PMID: 17986664]

[10]   Mahdi AJ, Obaji SG, Collins PW. Role of enhanced half-life factor VIII and IX in the treatment of haemophilia. Br J Haematol 2015; 169(6): 768-76.
        [http://dx.doi.org/10.1111/bjh.13360] [PMID: 25754016]

[11]   Laffan M. New products for the treatment of haemophilia. Br J Haematol 2015. [ahead of press].
        [PMID: 26456702]

[12]   Witmer CM. Low mortality from intracranial haemorrhage in paediatric patients with haemophilia. Haemophilia 2015; 21(5): e359-63.
        [http://dx.doi.org/10.1111/hae.12716] [PMID: 26010533]

[13]   Witmer CM, Manno CS, Butler RB, Raffini LJ. The clinical management of hemophilia and head trauma: a survey of current clinical practice among pediatric hematology/oncology physicians. Pediatr Blood Cancer 2009; 53(3): 406-10.
        [http://dx.doi.org/10.1002/pbc.22126] [PMID: 19489052]

[14]   Rosendaal FR, Smit C, Briët E. Hemophilia treatment in historical perspective: a review of medical and social developments. Ann Hematol 1991; 62(1): 5-15.
        [http://dx.doi.org/10.1007/BF01714977] [PMID: 1903310]

[15]   Manco-Johnson MJ, Abshire TC, Shapiro AD, *et al.* Prophylaxis versus episodic treatment to prevent joint disease in boys with severe hemophilia. N Engl J Med 2007; 357(6): 535-44.
        [http://dx.doi.org/10.1056/NEJMoa067659] [PMID: 17687129]

[16]   Wong TE, Majumdar S, Adams E, *et al.* Healthy Weight Working Group. Overweight and obesity in hemophilia: a systematic review of the literature. Am J Prev Med 2011; 41(6) (Suppl. 4): S369-75.
        [http://dx.doi.org/10.1016/j.amepre.2011.09.008] [PMID: 22099360]

[17]   Schröder H, Marrugat J, Vila J, Covas MI, Elosua R. Adherence to the traditional Mediterranean diet is inversely associated with body mass index and obesity in a spanish population. J Nutr 2004; 134(12): 3355-61.
        [PMID: 15570037]

[18] Schröder H. Protective mechanisms of the Mediterranean diet in obesity and type 2 diabetes. J Nutr Biochem 2007; 18(3): 149-60.
[http://dx.doi.org/10.1016/j.jnutbio.2006.05.006] [PMID: 16963247]

[19] VON Mackensen S. Quality of life and sports activities in patients with haemophilia. Haemophilia 2007; 13 (Suppl. 2): 38-43.
[http://dx.doi.org/10.1111/j.1365-2516.2007.01505.x] [PMID: 17685923]

[20] Heijnen L. The role of rehabilitation and sports in haemophilia patients with inhibitors. Haemophilia 2008; 14 (Suppl. 6): 45-51.
[http://dx.doi.org/10.1111/j.1365-2516.2008.01889.x] [PMID: 19134033]

[21] Petrini P, Seuser A. Haemophilia care in adolescents compliance and lifestyle issues. Haemophilia 2009; 15 (Suppl. 1): 15-9.
[http://dx.doi.org/10.1111/j.1365-2516.2008.01948.x] [PMID: 19125936]

[22] Seuser A, Boehm P, Kurme A, Schumpe G, Kurnik K. Orthopaedic issues in sports for persons with haemophilia. Haemophilia 2007; 13 (Suppl. 2): 47-52.
[http://dx.doi.org/10.1111/j.1365-2516.2007.01507.x] [PMID: 17685925]

[23] Feldman BM, Funk SM, Bergstrom BM, *et al.* Validation of a new pediatric joint scoring system from the International Hemophilia Prophylaxis Study Group: validity of the hemophilia joint health score. Arthritis Care Res (Hoboken) 2011; 63(2): 223-30.
[http://dx.doi.org/10.1002/acr.20353] [PMID: 20862683]

[24] Wittmeier K, Mulder K. Enhancing lifestyle for individuals with haemophilia through physical activity and exercise: the role of physiotherapy. Haemophilia 2007; 13 (Suppl. 2): 31-7.
[http://dx.doi.org/10.1111/j.1365-2516.2007.01504.x] [PMID: 17685922]

[25] Kasper CK. Mild haemophilia is less of a burden than severe haemophilia. Isn't it? Or is it? Haemophilia World 1996; 3: 3.

[26] Buzzard BM, Heim M. A study to evaluate the effectiveness of Air-Stirrup splints as a means of reducing the frequency of ankle haemarthroses in children with haemophilia A and B. Haemophilia 1995; 1(2): 131-6.
[http://dx.doi.org/10.1111/j.1365-2516.1995.tb00054.x] [PMID: 27214323]

[27] Boone DC. Management of musculoskeletal problems of hemophilia. Phys Ther 1974; 54(2): 122-7.
[PMID: 4460014]

[28] Buzzard BM, Saeed C. The physiotherapy management of sports injuries in haemophilia. In: Heijnen L, Ed. Recent Advances in Rehabilitation in Haemophilia. Hove, East Sussex: Medical Education Network 1995; pp. 73-7.

[29] Rodríguez-Merchan EC, Goddard NJ, Lee CA. Musculoskeletal Aspects of Haemophilia. Physiotherapy management of haemophilia in children. Oxford: Blackwell 2000; pp. 169-76.

[30] Heijnen L, de Klein P. Recent Advances in Rehabilitation in Haemophilia Hove: Medical Education Network. 1995; pp. 66-72.

[31] Mulder K. Exercise for People with Hemophilia. Montreal, Canada: World Federation of Hemophilia 2006.

[32] Pettersson H, Ahlberg A, Nilsson IM. A radiologic classification of hemophilic arthropathy. Clin Orthop Relat Res 1980; (149): 153-9.
[PMID: 7408294]

[33] Zukotynski K, Jarrin J, Babyn PS, *et al.* Sonography for assessment of haemophilic arthropathy in children: a systematic protocol. Haemophilia 2007; 13(3): 293-304.
[http://dx.doi.org/10.1111/j.1365-2516.2006.01414.x] [PMID: 17498079]

[34]   Doria AS, Lundin B, Miller S, *et al.* Expert Imaging Working Group of The International Prophylaxis Study Group. Reliability and construct validity of the compatible MRI scoring system for evaluation of elbows in haemophilic children. Haemophilia 2008; 14(2): 303-14.
[http://dx.doi.org/10.1111/j.1365-2516.2007.01602.x] [PMID: 18179575]

[35]   Groen WG, van der Net J, Helders PJ, Fischer K. Development and preliminary testing of a Paediatric Version of the Haemophilia Activities List (pedhal). Haemophilia 2010; 16(2): 281-9.
[http://dx.doi.org/10.1111/j.1365-2516.2009.02136.x] [PMID: 19906160]

[36]   Bradley CS, Bullinger M, McCusker PJ, Wakefield CD, Blanchette VS, Young NL. Comparing two measures of quality of life for children with haemophilia: the CHO-KLAT and the Haemo-QoL. Haemophilia 2006; 12(6): 643-53.
[http://dx.doi.org/10.1111/j.1365-2516.2006.01346.x] [PMID: 17083516]

[37]   Bullinger M, von Mackensen S. Quality of life assessment in haemophilia. Haemophilia 2004; 10 (Suppl. 1): 9-16.
[http://dx.doi.org/10.1111/j.1355-0691.2004.00874.x] [PMID: 14987244]

[38]   Bullinger M, von Mackensen S, Fischer K, *et al.* Pilot testing of the Haemo-QoL quality of life questionnaire for haemophiliac children in six European countries. Haemophilia 2002; 8 (Suppl. 2): 47-54.
[http://dx.doi.org/10.1046/j.1351-8216.2001.114.doc.x] [PMID: 11966854]

[39]   Gringeri A, Mantovani L, Mackensen SV. Quality of life assessment in clinical practice in haemophilia treatment. Haemophilia 2006; 12 (Suppl. 3): 22-9.
[http://dx.doi.org/10.1111/j.1365-2516.2006.01257.x] [PMID: 16683993]

[40]   Cuesta-Barriuso R, Gómez-Conesa A, López-Pina JA. Physiotherapy treatment in patients with hemophilia and chronic ankle arthropathy: a systematic review. Rehabil Res Pract 2013; 2013: 305249.
[http://dx.doi.org/10.1155/2013/305249] [PMID: 23997955]

[41]   Heijnen L, de Kleijn P. Physiotherapy for the treatment of articular contractures in haemophilia. Haemophilia 1999; 5 (Suppl. 1): 16-9.
[http://dx.doi.org/10.1046/j.1365-2516.1999.0050s1016.x] [PMID: 10365295]

[42]   Gurcay E, Eksioglu E, Ezer U, Cakir B, Cakci A. A prospective series of musculoskeletal system rehabilitation of arthropathic joints in young male hemophilic patients. Rheumatol Int 2008; 28(6): 541-5.
[http://dx.doi.org/10.1007/s00296-007-0474-7] [PMID: 17943258]

[43]   Hilberg T, Herbsleb M, Puta C, Gabriel HH, Schramm W. Physical training increases isometric muscular strength and proprioceptive performance in haemophilic subjects. Haemophilia 2003; 9(1): 86-93.
[http://dx.doi.org/10.1046/j.1365-2516.2003.00679.x] [PMID: 12558784]

[44]   Garcia MK, Capusso A, Montans D, Massad E, Battistella LR. Variations of the articular mobility of elbows, knees and ankles in patients with severe haemophilia submitted to free active movimentation in a pool with warm water. Haemophilia 2009; 15(1): 386-9.
[http://dx.doi.org/10.1111/j.1365-2516.2008.01871.x] [PMID: 18771424]

[45]   Hill K, Fearn M, Williams S, *et al.* Effectiveness of a balance training home exercise programme for adults with haemophilia: a pilot study. Haemophilia 2010; 16(1): 162-9.
[http://dx.doi.org/10.1111/j.1365-2516.2009.02110.x] [PMID: 19804383]

[46]   Czepa D, von Mackensen S, Hilberg T. Haemophilia & Exercise Project (HEP): the impact of 1-year sports therapy programme on physical performance in adult haemophilia patients. Haemophilia 2013; 19(2): 194-9.
[http://dx.doi.org/10.1111/hae.12031] [PMID: 23039074]

[47]   Rodríguez-Merchan EC, Goddard NJ, Lee CA. Musculoskeletal Aspects of Haemophilia. Physiotherapy for adult patients with haemophilia. Oxford: Blackwell 2000; pp. 177-86.

[48]   Buzzard B, Beeton K. Physiotherapy Management of Haemophilia. Muscle Imbalance in Haemophilia. Blackwell Sciences 2000; pp. 51-63.

[49]   Buzzard BM. Physiotherapy for prevention and treatment of chronic hemophilic synovitis. Clin Orthop Relat Res 1997; (343): 42-6.
[PMID: 9345204]

[50]   Rodriguez-Merchan EC, Jimenez-Yuste V, Aznar JA, *et al.* Joint protection in haemophilia. Haemophilia 2011; 17 (Suppl. 2): 1-23.
[http://dx.doi.org/10.1111/j.1365-2516.2011.02615.x] [PMID: 21819491]

[51]   Brettler DB. Inhibitors of factor VIII and IX. Haemophilia 1995; 1 (Suppl. 1): 35-9.
[http://dx.doi.org/10.1111/j.1365-2516.1995.tb00108.x] [PMID: 27214738]

[52]   White R, Schuren J, Konn DR. Semi-rigid vs rigid glass fibre casting: a biomechanical assessment. Clin Biomech (Bristol, Avon) 2003; 18(1): 19-27.
[http://dx.doi.org/10.1016/S0268-0033(02)00167-5] [PMID: 12527243]

[53]   Avci S, Sayli U. Comparison of the results of short-term rigid and semi-rigid cast immobilization for the treatment of grade 3 inversion injuries of the ankle. Injury 1998; 29(8): 581-4.
[http://dx.doi.org/10.1016/S0020-1383(98)00129-6] [PMID: 10209587]

[54]   Kerkhoffs GM, Rowe BH, Assendelft WJ, Kelly K, Struijs PA, van Dijk CN. Immobilisation and functional treatment for acute lateral ankle ligament injuries in adults. Cochrane Database Syst Rev 2002; 3(3): CD003762.
[PMID: 12137710]

[55]   Stecco L, Stecco A. Manipolazione fasciale. Piccin Nuova Libraria 2010.

[56]   Casley-Smith JR, Boris M, Weindorf S, Lasinski B. Treatment for lymphedema of the arm the Casley-Smith method: a noninvasive method produces continued reduction. Cancer 1998; 83(12) (Suppl American): 2843-60.
[http://dx.doi.org/10.1002/(SICI)1097-0142(19981215)83:12B+<2843::AID-CNCR38>3.0.CO;2-U] [PMID: 9874410]

[57]   Gregory MA, Mars M. Compressed air massage causes capillary dilation in untraumatised skeletal muscle: a morphometric and ultrastructural study. Physiotherapy 2005; 91: 131-7.
[http://dx.doi.org/10.1016/j.physio.2004.11.007]

[58]   Zainuddin Z, Newton M, Sacco P, Nosaka K. Effects of massage on delayed-onset muscle soreness, swelling, and recovery of muscle function. J Athl Train 2005; 40(3): 174-80.
[PMID: 16284637]

[59]   Melzack R, Wall PD. Pain mechanisms: a new theory. Science 1965; 150(3699): 971-9.
[http://dx.doi.org/10.1126/science.150.3699.971] [PMID: 5320816]

[60]   Gadsby JG, Flowerdew M. Transcutaneous electrical nerve stimulation and acupuncture-like transcutaneous electrical nerve stimulation for chronic low back pain. Cochrane Database Syst Rev 2006; 1: CD000210.

[61]   Vernon H, McDermaid CS, Hagino C. Systematic review of randomized clinical trials of complementary/alternative therapies in the treatment of tension-type and cervicogenic headache. Complement Ther Med 1999; 7(3): 142-55.
[http://dx.doi.org/10.1016/S0965-2299(99)80122-8] [PMID: 10581824]

[62]   Rutjes AW, Nüesch E, Sterchi R, *et al.* Transcutaneous electrostimulation for osteoarthritis of the knee. Cochrane Database Syst Rev 2009; 4(4): CD002823.
[PMID: 19821296]

[63]   Puett DW, Griffin MR. Published trials of nonmedicinal and noninvasive therapies for hip and knee osteoarthritis. Ann Intern Med 1994; 121(2): 133-40.
       [http://dx.doi.org/10.7326/0003-4819-121-2-199407150-00010] [PMID: 8017727]

[64]   Wojtys EM, Carpenter JE, Ott GA. Electrical stimulation of soft tissues. Instr Course Lect 1993; 42: 443-52.
       [PMID: 8463694]

[65]   Webster DF, Harvey W, Dyson M, Pond JB. The role of ultrasound-induced cavitation in the in vitro stimulation of collagen synthesis in human fibroblasts. Ultrasonics 1980; 18(1): 33-7.
       [http://dx.doi.org/10.1016/0041-624X(80)90050-5] [PMID: 7350723]

[66]   Dyson M, Suckling J. Stimulation of tissue repair by ultrasound: a survey of the mechanisms involved. Physiotherapy 1978; 64(4): 105-8.
       [PMID: 349580]

[67]   Baker KG, Robertson VJ, Duck FA. A review of therapeutic ultrasound: biophysical effects. Phys Ther 2001; 81(7): 1351-8.
       [PMID: 11444998]

[68]   Prentice WE. Therapeutic modalities in sports medicine. 3rd ed., St Louis: Mosby 1994.

[69]   Horsman MR. Tissue physiology and the response to heat. Int J Hyperthermia 2006; 22(3): 197-203.
       [http://dx.doi.org/10.1080/02656730600689066] [PMID: 16754339]

[70]   Akyürekli D, Gerig LH, Raaphorst GP. Changes in muscle blood flow distribution during hyperthermia. Int J Hyperthermia 1997; 13(5): 481-96.
       [http://dx.doi.org/10.3109/02656739709023547] [PMID: 9354933]

[71]   Nah BS, Choi IB, Oh WY, Osborn JL, Song CW. Vascular thermal adaptation in tumors and normal tissue in rats. Int J Radiat Oncol Biol Phys 1996; 35(1): 95-101.
       [http://dx.doi.org/10.1016/S0360-3016(96)85016-4] [PMID: 8641932]

[72]   Woo SL, Hildebrand KA. Healing of ligament injuries: from basic science to clinical practice. Clin Orthop Relat Res 1997; (2): 63-79.

[73]   Kannus P, Jozsa L, Renström P, *et al.* The effects of training, immobilization and remobilization on musculoskeletal tissue. 2: remobilization and prevention of immobilization atrophy. Scand J Med Sci Sports 1992; 2: 164-76.
       [http://dx.doi.org/10.1111/j.1600-0838.1992.tb00340.x]

Frontiers in Arthritis, 2017, *Vol. 2*, 138-146

CHAPTER 10

Arthroscopy

Christian Carulli* and **Massimo Innocenti**

Orthopaedic Clinic, University of Florence, Florence, Italy

Abstract: Arthroscopy in haemophilic subjects is nowadays considered a procedure associated with good clinical outcomes and a low rate of complications. Once addressed as the minimally invasive way to obtain a synovectomy, to date it is performed for several other procedures, as loose bodies removal and joint debridement. It is also useful as assistance for a mini-open ankle fusion. The modern aim of an arthroscopy in a target joint is to delay a more aggressive surgical approach. Thus, critical are the indications: early to moderate or mild arthropathies, in adult or young subjects after failure of conservative treatments. Knees and ankles are the most arthroscopically treated joints, followed by elbows and shoulders.

Keywords: Arthroscopy, Ankle, Arthrolysis, Debridement, Elbow, Haemophilia, Knee, Loose bodies removal, Paediatric patients, Shoulder, Synovectomy.

INTRODUCTION

Arthroscopy is a minimally invasive procedure nowadays successfully performed in almost all joints, and associated with good outcomes and a very low rate of complications [1 - 5]. A-part from traumatic intraarticular lesions and sport-related injuries, in which arthroscopy is currently considered the gold standard of treatment, this procedure is also indicated in cases of degenerative joint alterations as Osteoarthritis to delay a more aggressive surgical treatment. In such cases, the arthroscopic treatment showed however variable short- to mid-term results [6 - 10]. Arthroscopy has been similarly advocated for the initial treatment of inflammatory diseases as Rheumatoid arthritis, mainly for synovial tissue removal and to provide a transitory relief from symptoms [11 - 14].

In haemophilic patients, over the decades, arthroscopy was used as a primary minimally invasive approach in order to delay a further aggressive surgery, specifically for the knee arthropathy [15 - 25]. It has been later indicated for ankles, and recently for shoulders and elbows, with satisfactory outcomes

* **Corresponding author Christian Carulli:** Orthopaedic Clinic, University of Florence, Florence, Italy; Tel: 0039 055 794 8200; Email: christian.carulli@unifi.it

[26 - 36]. It is now debated if there is indication for a joint debridement in hips and wrists that on the other side represent very uncommon sites of haemophilic arthropathy.

The following is an overview of the indications, techniques, and complications of arthroscopic procedures in the main target joints affecting patients with Haemophilia.

INDICATIONS & CLINICAL SETTINGS

The most frequent indications are: joint debridement, synovectomy, removal of loose bodies (osteochondral or meniscal fragments), meniscal alterations, treatment of chondral lesions (Figs. **1** and **2**).

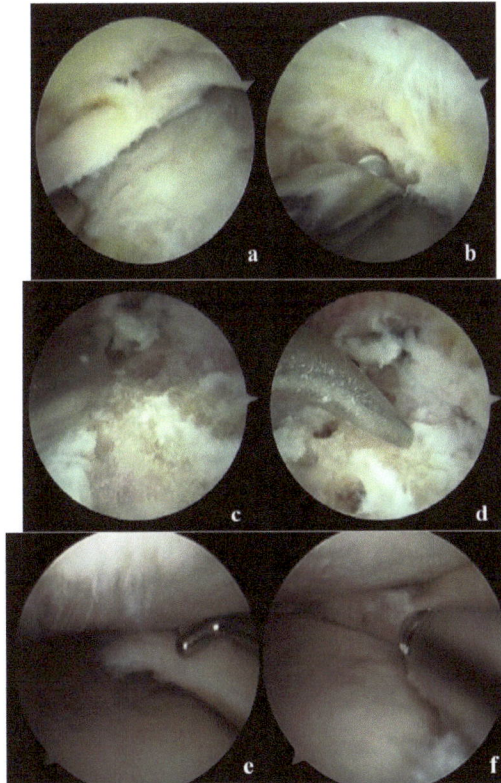

Fig. (1). Unstable ostechondral fragment of the anterior lip of the tibial side of an ankle of a 28-years old haemophilic patient with inhibitors (a) and its removal by a burr (b). Chondral lesion of a talar dome in an ankle of a 31-years old haemophilic subject affected by Haemophilia B (c) treated by shaving and microfractures (d). Global alterations in a knee of a severe Haemophilia A patient (e) managed by debridement (f).

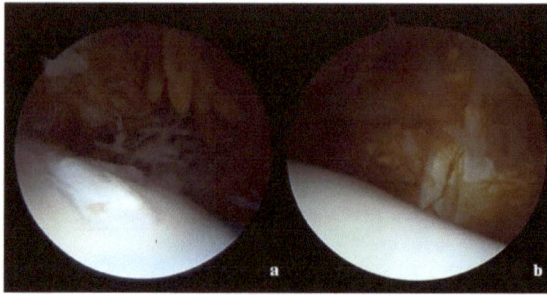

Fig. (2). Chronic hypertrophic synovitis in the lateral aspect of the ankle of a 20-years old patient affected by Haemophilia A (a). Synovectomy by shaver and radiofrequencies (b).

In ankles, arthroscopy is very useful to assist a mini-open joint fusion that represented a step forward in this surgical technique (See Chapter 13) [31, 33]. Moreover, also tendon release or repair, arthrolysis for flexion contractures after recurrent bleedings or related to previous fractures are in selected cases indicated [35, 37]. Paediatric patients with severe arthropathy or recalcitrant bleedings may be successfully treated by arthroscopic procedures associated with a very low psychological and physical impact [27, 28]. Finally, arthroscopy may find a role in the treatment of specific sequelae after joint replacements as stiff joints (typically after knee or ankle replacements), and for the management of its intraarticular complications as arteriovenous fistulae or portals haematoma [38, 39].

SURGICAL TECHNIQUE

As for other types of surgery in Haemophilia, the preparation of an arthroscopy requires a multidisciplinary planning, and specifically a tailored haematological prophylaxis. Perioperative doses of clotting factors are generally similar to other more aggressive procedures, as the high risk of bleeding associates particularly for synovectomy [35, 37]. General anaesthesia and standard antibiotic prophylaxis are required. Tourniquet is generally used to allow a better and clear visualization of the joint.

An arthroscopy with two (ankle, elbow) or three (shoulder, knee) portals is generally accepted as the standard approach to ensure a global visualization of joint space. However, accessory portals are required in case of loose bodies removal and synovectomy [35, 40 - 43].

Standard knee portals are the superomedial, anterolateral, and anteromedial. Posterolateral and posteromedial (transseptal) portals have been performed in haemophiliacs to ensure a full synovectomy [35, 40, 41]. The use of drainages are suggested but not always applied [35]. In the ankle the anteromedial and anterolateral portals are used, even if additional posterior portals are useful in case of synovectomy or loose bodies removal [26, 28, 35].

Shoulders and elbows are usually approached by standard portals. Shoulders may be approached by anterior and posterior (soft spot) portals. Further portals are made in case of necessity. In elbows, anteromedial, anterolateral, and posterior (soft spot) portals are generally created [35]. Posteromedial and posterolateral accesses are useful to ensure a complete synovectomy or a full release for flexion contractures. A supplemental regional nerve block may be performed after general anaesthesia for postoperative pain control. An arthroscopic radial head resection in end-stage arthropathies of the radiohumeral joint has been reported [35].

A single experience of three knee arthroscopic synovectomies by Holmium: Yag laser in two haemophilic patients with inhibitors has been reported [44]. Laser has showed a potential efficacy in bleeding control and precise cutting properties in water medium. However, despite good clinical outcomes, very high related costs (4 or 5 times superior to standard procedures) represent an undoubtful limit of such technique.

Independently by the operated joint, continuous passive mobilization has been addressed as the most important postoperative prescription. In association, compressive dressings and protected weight bearing are useful in the first two to three weeks after surgery [19, 35, 42].

RESULTS

Since its introduction and the release of the first related papers [16 - 20], arthroscopy showed a superiority with respect to open surgery: similar outcomes associated to a lower morbidity and inferior costs. These aspects were related to a single indication and a very little number of patients (mostly less than 10 subjects): the chronic synovitis of the knee. Later such features were demonstrated also for other indications, other target joints, and increased numbers of subjects (up to 44 haemophiliacs) [26 - 31, 33 - 35, 40]. Comparative studies showed also faster times of recovery, shorter hospital stays and days of haematological prophylaxis [22, 27]. Improvements on ROM and functional ability were almost always present after arthroscopy whereas remained unchanged or poorly modified in high percentages of cases after open surgery. All joints showed similar outcomes, particularly in children. No significant differences were reported in cases of Haemophilia A or B. Such results were persistent over time, as reported in long-term follow-up series (up to 25 years postoperatively) [25, 41 - 43]. Recurrence of synovitis and worsening of arthropathy were generally related to stage of arthropathy at the time of arthroscopy, patients' aging, persistent tendency to bleedings, and presence of inhibitors. Different types of scoring systems were used to evaluate arthroscopic outcomes (WFH, IKDC, KSS, HSS, DASH, Constant-Murley, WOMAC, SF-36): as reported for other procedures, it was and still is difficult to assess a specific and precise score for haemophilic arthropathy.

COMPLICATIONS

Even if arthroscopy represents the ideal model of minimally invasive surgery, it is not free from complications. Rates of complications in standard sport-related or arthritic settings are very low (<2%). In haemophilic subjects, unfortunately the incidence of problems or sequelae are higher, mainly related to bleedings [26 - 37]. Such percentages lead multidisciplinary Haemophilia teams to accurate haematological approaches to haemophilic patients, particularly in those with inhibitors. Tailored protocols and close postoperative monitoring have significantly reduced the rate of such complications. However, some authors reported specific complications after knee arthroscopy. A single case of an arterovenous fistula 19 months after an arthroscopic synovectomy was reported with a mixed open/arthroscopic approach and ligation of the communicating vessels. Such structure was found after an angiography in a HIV haemophilic patient referring persistent haemoartrosis in his target joint [38]. Expanding haematomas were reported in arthroscopic portals in two patients after knee synovectomies [39]. Mini-open approaches have been performed in both cases to remove large organized masses causing a recurrent clicking during flexion/extension activity of the subject's months after the index procedure, indicated for debridement and synovectomy.

CONCLUDING REMARKS

Arthroscopy in Haemophilia is a key procedure associated with good clinical outcomes and a low rate of complications. Arthroscopic treatment is nowadays not intended for synovectomy alone, but considered a procedure with several aims in any target joints. Thus, critical are the indications, usually early to moderate or mild arthropathies both for adult or underage subjects. The most important targets in such cases are synovectomy to reduce the bleedings, loose bodies removal, and joint debridement to delay a more aggressive surgical approach.

CONFLICT OF INTEREST

The authors confirm that they have no conflict of interest to declare for this publication.

ACKNOWLEDGEMENTS

Declared none.

REFERENCES

[1]   Chalmers PN, Mall NA, Moric M, *et al.* Does ACL reconstruction alter natural history?: A systematic literature review of long-term outcomes. J Bone Joint Surg Am 2014; 96(4): 292-300.
[http://dx.doi.org/10.2106/JBJS.L.01713] [PMID: 24553885]

[2]   Henry P, Wasserstein D, Park S, *et al.* Arthroscopic Repair for Chronic Massive Rotator Cuff Tears: A Systematic Review. Arthroscopy 2015; 31(12): 2472-80. Epub ahead of print
[http://dx.doi.org/10.1016/j.arthro.2015.06.038] [PMID: 26364549]

[3]   Adams JE, King GJ, Steinmann SP, Cohen MS. Elbow arthroscopy: indications, techniques, outcomes, and complications. Instr Course Lect 2015; 64: 215-24.
[PMID: 25745907]

[4]   MacDonald AE, Bedi A, Horner NS, *et al.* Indications and Outcomes for Microfracture as an Adjunct to Hip Arthroscopy for Treatment of Chondral Defects in Patients With Femoroacetabular Impingement: A Systematic Review. Arthroscopy 2015. Epub ahead of print
[PMID: 26385287]

[5]   Epstein DM, Black BS, Sherman SL. Anterior ankle arthroscopy: indications, pitfalls, and complications. Foot Ankle Clin 2015; 20(1): 41-57.
[http://dx.doi.org/10.1016/j.fcl.2014.10.001] [PMID: 25726482]

[6]   Hsu AR, Gross CE, Lee S, Carreira DS. Extended indications for foot and ankle arthroscopy. J Am Acad Orthop Surg 2014; 22(1): 10-9.
[http://dx.doi.org/10.5435/JAAOS-22-01-10] [PMID: 24382875]

[7]   Sayegh ET, Mascarenhas R, Chalmers PN, Cole BJ, Romeo AA, Verma NN. Surgical Treatment Options for Glenohumeral Arthritis in Young Patients: A Systematic Review and Meta-analysis. Arthroscopy 2015; 31(6): 1156-1166.e8.
[http://dx.doi.org/10.1016/j.arthro.2014.11.012] [PMID: 25543246]

[8]   Adams JE, King GJ, Steinmann SP, Cohen MS. Elbow arthroscopy: indications, techniques, outcomes, and complications. Instr Course Lect 2015; 64: 215-24.
[PMID: 25745907]

[9]   Domb BG, Gui C, Lodhia P. How much arthritis is too much for hip arthroscopy: a systematic review. Arthroscopy 2015; 31(3): 520-9.
[http://dx.doi.org/10.1016/j.arthro.2014.11.008] [PMID: 25543247]

[10]   Thorlund JB, Juhl CB, Roos EM, Lohmander LS. Arthroscopic surgery for degenerative knee: systematic review and meta-analysis of benefits and harms. Br J Sports Med 2015; 49(19): 1229-35.
[http://dx.doi.org/10.1136/bjsports-2015-h2747rep] [PMID: 26383759]

[11]   Gibbons CE, Gosal HS, Bartlett J. Long-term results of arthroscopic synovectomy for seropositive rheumatoid arthritis: 616 year review. Int Orthop 2002; 26(2): 98-100.
[http://dx.doi.org/10.1007/s00264-001-0309-1] [PMID: 12078886]

[12]   Kim SJ, Jung KA. Arthroscopic synovectomy in rheumatoid arthritis of wrist. Clin Med Res 2007; 5(4): 244-50.
[http://dx.doi.org/10.3121/cmr.2007.768] [PMID: 18086905]

[13]   Chalmers PN, Sherman SL, Raphael BS, Su EP. Rheumatoid synovectomy: does the surgical approach matter? Clin Orthop Relat Res 2011; 469(7): 2062-71.
[http://dx.doi.org/10.1007/s11999-010-1744-3] [PMID: 21213089]

[14]   Yeoh KM, King GJ, Faber KJ, Glazebrook MA, Athwal GS. Evidence-based indications for elbow arthroscopy. Arthroscopy 2012; 28(2): 272-82.
[http://dx.doi.org/10.1016/j.arthro.2011.10.007] [PMID: 22244102]

[15]   Wiedel JD. Arthroscopic synovectomy in hemophilic arthropathy of the knee. Scand J Haematol Suppl 1984; 40: 263-70.
[PMID: 6591393]

[16]   Kim HC, Klein K, Hirsch S, Seibold JR, Eisele J, Saidi P. Arthroscopic synovectomy in the treatment of hemophilic synovitis. Scand J Haematol Suppl 1984; 40: 271-9.
[PMID: 6591394]

[17]   Sim FH. Synovial proliferative disorders: role of synovectomy. Arthroscopy 1985; 1(3): 198-204.
[http://dx.doi.org/10.1016/S0749-8063(85)80012-8] [PMID: 4096771]

[18]   Wiedel JD. Arthroscopic synovectomy for chronic hemophilic synovitis of the knee. Arthroscopy 1985; 1(3): 205-9.
[http://dx.doi.org/10.1016/S0749-8063(85)80013-X] [PMID: 4096772]

[19]   Limbird TJ, Dennis SC. Synovectomy and continuous passive motion (CPM) in hemophiliac patients. Arthroscopy 1987; 3(2): 74-9.
[http://dx.doi.org/10.1016/S0749-8063(87)80019-1] [PMID: 3606769]

[20]   Klein KS, Aland CM, Kim HC, Eisele J, Saidi P. Long term follow-up of arthroscopic synovectomy for chronic hemophilic synovitis. Arthroscopy 1987; 3(4): 231-6.
[http://dx.doi.org/10.1016/S0749-8063(87)80116-0] [PMID: 3689521]

[21]   Servodio Iammarrone C, Lotito FM, Angrisani P, Bonocore C. [A case of hemophilic arthropathy of the knee: diagnostic and therapeutic considerations]. Chir Organi Mov 1988; 73(4): 405-11.
[PMID: 3251716]

[22]   Triantafyllou SJ, Hanks GA, Handal JA, Greer RB III. Open and arthroscopic synovectomy in hemophilic arthropathy of the knee. Clin Orthop Relat Res 1992; (283): 196-204.
[PMID: 1395245]

[23]   Zheng GZ. [Evaluation of synovectomy in hemophilic arthropathy follow-up of 26 cases]. Zhonghua Wai Ke Za Zhi 1993; 31(10): 585-7.
[PMID: 8033667]

[24]   Rodriquez Merchan EC, Galindo E, Ladreda JM, Pardo JA. Surgical synovectomy in haemophilic arthropathy of the knee. Int Orthop 1994; 18(1): 38-41.
[PMID: 8021067]

[25]   Eickhoff HH, Koch W, Raderschadt G, Brackmann HH. Arthroscopy for chronic hemophilic synovitis of the knee. Clin Orthop Relat Res 1997; (343): 58-62.
[PMID: 9345207]

[26]   Gilbert MS, Radomisli TE. Therapeutic options in the management of hemophilic synovitis. Clin Orthop Relat Res 1997; (343): 88-92.
[PMID: 9345212]

[27]   Tamurian RM, Spencer EE, Wojtys EM. The role of arthroscopic synovectomy in the management of hemarthrosis in hemophilia patients: financial perspectives. Arthroscopy 2002; 18(7): 789-94.
[http://dx.doi.org/10.1053/jars.2002.32621] [PMID: 12209438]

[28]   Dunn AL, Busch MT, Wyly JB, Sullivan KM, Abshire TC. Arthroscopic synovectomy for hemophilic joint disease in a pediatric population. J Pediatr Orthop 2004; 24(4): 414-26.
[http://dx.doi.org/10.1097/01241398-200407000-00013] [PMID: 15205625]

[29]   Strauss AC, Goldmann G, Ezziddin S, *et al.* Treatment options for haemophilic arthropathy of the elbow after failed conservative therapy. A single centre experience. Hamostaseologie 2014; 34 (Suppl. 1): S17-22.
[http://dx.doi.org/10.5482/HAMO-14-01-0009] [PMID: 25382765]

[30]   Pandya NK, Namdari S. Shoulder arthroscopy in children and adolescents. J Am Acad Orthop Surg 2013; 21(7): 389-97.
[PMID: 23818026]

[31]   Rodriguez-Merchan EC. Ankle surgery in haemophilia with special emphasis on arthroscopic debridement. Haemophilia 2008; 14(5): 913-9.
[http://dx.doi.org/10.1111/j.1365-2516.2008.01820.x] [PMID: 18637842]

[32]   Thomas JM, Tuddenham EG, Ahrens PM. Therapeutic shoulder arthroscopy in patients with clotting disorders. Haemophilia 2008; 14(4): 859-61.
[http://dx.doi.org/10.1111/j.1365-2516.2008.01683.x] [PMID: 18422609]

[33]   Bonnin M, Carret JP. [Arthrodesis of the ankle under arthroscopy. Apropos of 10 cases reviewed after a year]. Rev Chir Orthop Repar Appar Mot 1995; 81(2): 128-35.
[PMID: 7569187]

[34]   Hovy L. [Joint preserving operations and endoprosthetic joint substitutions in hemophiliacs. Indications and long term results]. Orthopade 1999; 28(4): 356-65.
[PMID: 10335530]

[35]   Verma N, Valentino LA, Chawla A. Arthroscopic synovectomy in haemophilia: indications, technique and results. Haemophilia 2007; 13 (Suppl. 3): 38-44.
[http://dx.doi.org/10.1111/j.1365-2516.2007.01539.x] [PMID: 17822520]

[36]   Rodríguez-Merchán EC, Magallón M, Galindo E, López-Cabarcos C. Hemophilic synovitis of the knee and the elbow. Clin Orthop Relat Res 1997; (343): 47-53.
[PMID: 9345205]

[37]   Rodriguez-Merchan EC. Aspects of current management: orthopaedic surgery in haemophilia. Haemophilia 2012; 18(1): 8-16.
[http://dx.doi.org/10.1111/j.1365-2516.2011.02544.x] [PMID: 21535324]

[38]   Cohen B, Griffiths L, Dandy DJ. Arteriovenous fistula after arthroscopic synovectomy in a patient with haemophilia. Arthroscopy 1992; 8(3): 373-4.
[http://dx.doi.org/10.1016/0749-8063(92)90072-J] [PMID: 1418213]

[39]   Heim M, Israeli A, Varon D, Chechic A, Engelberg S, Martinowitz U. Expanding portal haematomata as a complication of knee arthroscopies in persons with haemophilia. Haemophilia 1999; 5(3): 213-5.
[http://dx.doi.org/10.1046/j.1365-2516.1999.00315.x] [PMID: 10444291]

[40]   Dale TM, Saucedo JM, Rodríguez-Merchán EC. Hemophilic arthropathy of the elbow: prophylaxis, imaging, and the role of invasive management. J Shoulder Elbow Surg 2015; 24(10): 1669-78.
[http://dx.doi.org/10.1016/j.jse.2015.06.018] [PMID: 26385390]

[41]   Wiedel JD. Arthroscopic synovectomy of the knee in hemophilia: 10-to-15 year followup. Clin Orthop Relat Res 1996; (328): 46-53.
[http://dx.doi.org/10.1097/00003086-199607000-00010] [PMID: 8653977]

[42]   Yoon KH, Bae DK, Kim HS, Song SJ. Arthroscopic synovectomy in haemophilic arthropathy of the knee. Int Orthop 2005; 29(5): 296-300.
[http://dx.doi.org/10.1007/s00264-005-0666-2] [PMID: 16082543]

[43]   de Almeida AM, de Rezende MU, Cordeiro FG, *et al.* Arthroscopic partial anterior synovectomy of the knee on patients with haemophilia. Knee Surg Sports Traumatol Arthrosc 2015; 23(3): 785-91.
[http://dx.doi.org/10.1007/s00167-013-2706-6] [PMID: 25839071]

[44]   Ménart C, Lalain JJ, Lienhart A, Dechavanne M, Négrier C. Safety and efficacy of three arthroscopic procedures using Holmium: Yag laser in two high-responder haemophiliacs. Haemophilia 1999; 5(4): 278-81.
[http://dx.doi.org/10.1046/j.1365-2516.1999.00299.x] [PMID: 10469185]

CHAPTER 11

Total Knee Arthroplasty

Christian Carulli*, **Fabrizio Matassi** and **Massimo Innocenti**

Orthopaedic Clinic, University of Florence, Florence, Italy

Abstract: Total Knee Arthroplasty is one of the most performed procedures in the haemophilic population. Several series have been released over the last decades: despite good clinical outcomes, high rates of complications such as infection and loosening have been reported. Such complications have been mainly related to co-infected patients (HIV-positive) and subjects with inhibitors frequently affected by uncontrolled bleedings. Moreover, almost all arthroplasties have been performed using standard cemented Cobalt-Chrome knee implants and generally high constraints to ensure the stability of the prostheses. Recently new biomaterials with a better tribology and implants with less constraints have been used in haemophiliacs with encouraging results. The present mean survivorship is more than 90% at a mid-term follow-up while it was about 82.5% (range: 68%-96%) in the period '70-'90s. Dedicated multidisciplinary teams, appropriate bleeding management, and modern modular implants may ensure even better outcomes than the last decades with rates of success and complications very close to those of the non-haemophilic population.

Keywords: Haemophilia, Knee arthropathy, Oxidized zirconium, Total knee arthroplasty, Tribology.

INTRODUCTION

Total Knee Arthroplasty (TKA) is the most common surgical procedure performed in haemophilic patients. Since the very first releases focused on the surgical treatment of haemophilic patients published in the late '70s, TKA demonstrated good clinical results with dramatic improvements in the functional ability and daily life activities [1, 2]. However high rates of complications were reported. The clinical success of TKA in Haemophilia has been related to several facts: the functional recovery of a joint normally submitted to high forces and torques, in particular in patients affected by simultaneous arthropathy of elbows, hips, and ankles; the correction of the typical malalignment between femur and tibia affecting the gait ability of these subjects; the significant reduction of

---

* **Corresponding author Christian Carulli:** Orthopaedic Clinic, University of Florence, Florence, Italy; Tel: 0039 055 794 8200; Email: christian.carulli@unifi.it

bleedings of this target joint after the wide synovectomy usually performed during TKA [3, 4]. However, at a short follow-up, high percentages of complications and sequelae have been recorded [2, 3, 5 - 16]. Historically, the most common complications after primary TKA in Haemophilia have been represented by infections and aseptic loosening. Postoperative infections have been associated to co-infections, mainly to HIV, that was unfortunately very common after blood transfusions between '80s and '90s in haemophilic subjects [3, 10, 13]. On the other hand, aseptic loosening of TKAs have been frequently reported after postsurgical haemarthroses mostly related to difficult or uncontrolled bleeding management and the presence of inhibitors [3, 8, 10, 12, 13].

During last decades, modern bleeding management and perioperative prophylactic strategies in combination with multidisciplinary teams dedicated to coagulative disorders, and advanced surgical techniques and knee systems have significantly improved the clinical outcomes and reduced the postoperative complications. The last series reported with a mid- to long-term follow-up witness these substantial improvements [2, 4, 17 - 29].

CLINICAL SETTINGS AND INDICATIONS

Most of haemophilic patients suffer of a knee arthropathy given its large amount of synovial tissue representing the main target of bleedings [30]. The clinical features of a knee arthropathy are generally: pain, swelling, haemarthrosis; deformity, progressive malalignment; flexion contractures and loss of range of motion (ROM); loss of muscular masses; alterations of gait and limitation of the daily life activities. The more the number of bleedings, faster is the progression of arthropathy; in a similar manner, earlier haemarthroses are associated to a more severe arthropathy. However, different stages of arthropathy may be treated differently on the basis of the severity of the disease. Presently, early detection of the arthropathy and strategies of prevention of its worsening have reduced the incidence of severe patterns of diseases. Thus, surgery and particularly TKA are not considered the only options of the modern treatment of the haemophilic arthropathy (see Chapter 8) [4, 31]. During the decades several classifications have been proposed to evaluate the severity of arthropathy in order to associate the better orthopaedic management. The most used clinical scores are the Gilbert score [32] and the Haemophilia joint Health score [33]. From a radiologic point of view, the most used are the Arnold-Hilgartner classification [34] and the Petterson score [35]. Other well-known and widely diffused scores as Short Form 36, WOMAC, and Knee Society Score have seldom been used but are not validated for Haemophilia [36 - 38]. Radiographic-based classifications are particularly useful to plan any strategy of treatment. Rather similar, they have been equally used in several series released over the years in literature. TKA is usually indicated in advanced stages of disease corresponding to stages IV and V of the Arnold-Hilgartner classification, and with values from 9 to 13 of Petterson score [4]. Such stages usually correspond to the following clinical features: disabling pain unresponsive to medical treatments; severe deformity associated with flexion contractures (>15°), loss of ROM, and poor functional ability; tendency to bleedings even a close and tailored haematologic protocol; poor or unsatisfactory quality of life [3]. Actually, any of these features would represent a relative indication to TKA in a haemophilic patient; however, an association of various aspects may provide a strong basis to undergo a TKA. Nonetheless, it is mandatory to consider the very young age of patients affected by this arthropathy that may represent a reason to delay any invasive surgical procedure before an attempt of conservative approach [3, 4].

SURGICAL TECHNIQUE, CHOICE OF IMPLANTS, AND FIXATION

When approaching a case of haemophilic arthropathy of the knee, it is necessary to keep in mind that surgery is not a standard procedure. On the contrary, as for other specific diseases like rheumatoid arthritis, TKA in Haemophilia is a technically demanding surgery. Preoperative settings has to be carefully prepared by dedicated figures, as anaesthesiologists, haematologists, infective disease specialists, and skilled nurses. Haematologic protocols and storage of adequate quantities of recombinant or clotting factors have to be planned days before surgery. TKA should be scheduled in the morning and not in the afternoon. A central venous catheter is necessarily needed for the continuous infusion of FVII in patients with inhibitors. Prevision of blood bags for transfusion, urinary bladder catheter, and general anaesthesia are generally required. Furthermore, it is mandatory in our opinion for a modern management of such cases, a second-level antibiotic prophylaxis, strongly suggested both for the high risk of infections in Haemophilia and the high frequency of co-infections. Aminoglycosides and glycopeptides are efficient, wide spectrum, and diffused antibiotics useful to cover the extensive bacterial variety related to these cases [4]. Pneumatic ischemia of the leg is generally obtained after antibiotic administration. However, several series have been released reporting knee replacements conducted without tourniquet but with brilliant outcomes and rates of complications similar to other experiences [22, 26]. Both options have advantages and disadvantages, thus the use or not of the pneumatic tourniquet is a choice of the surgeon and his team depending on their experience.

Preoperative planning is usually difficult to be performed in haemophilic patients given the severe deformity and shape of bones, and the presence of adhesions and pseudocysts (Fig. **1**). The level of bone cuts, sizing of components, use of wedges, cones, offsets, and stems, and the level of constraint are generally intraoperative choices [4, 13, 19].

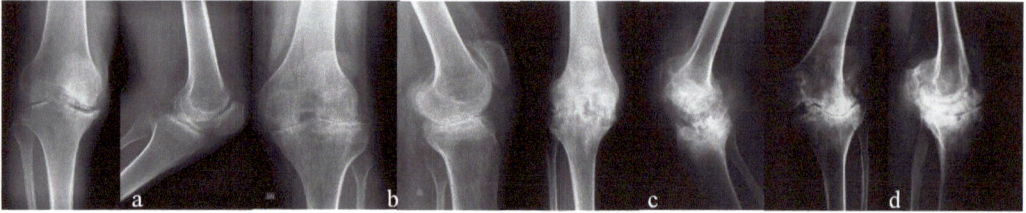

Fig. (1). Different stages of knee arthropathy in several haemophilic patients. To note the progression of the severity, well assessed by the Petterson score. Petterson score: 5 (a), 9 (b), 12 (c), and 13 (d). Preoperative planning may be seldom performed given the altered anatomy and *ligamenteous* setting.

The surgical approach in patients with no history of previous surgery should be the standard midline incision. When present, previous scars (generally related to previous open synovectomy) should be used following the classic rules of a knee revision [4, 39] (Fig. **2**).

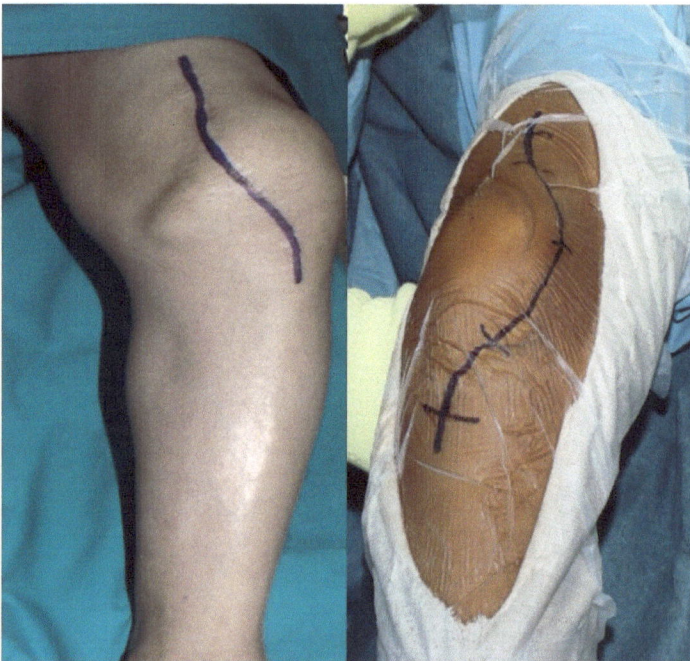

Fig. (2). Examples of previous surgical scars related to open synovectomy in haemophiliacs. These scars may be adequately used for the implant of a TKA.

Exposure in advanced stages of arthropathy is not easy, and frequently large quadriceps snips, V-Y tenotomy, and tibial tubercle osteotomies are often required [40] (Fig. **3**).

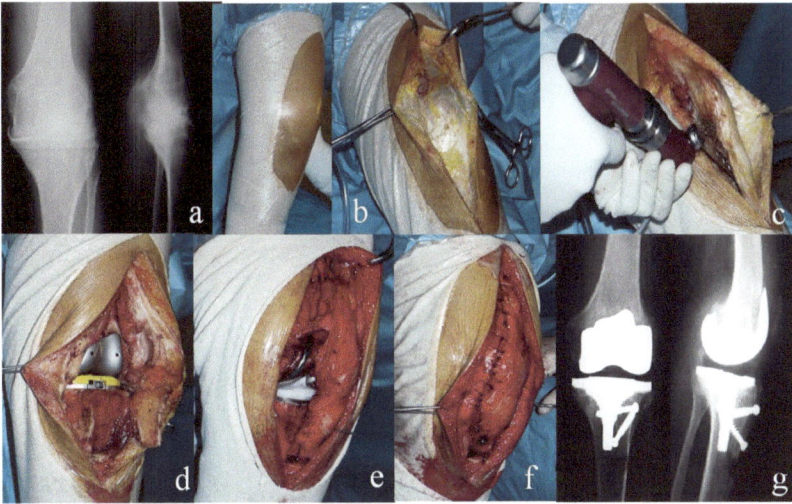

Fig. (3). Severe arthropathy of the left knee in a 38-years old haemophiliac (a). Large incision and wide approach (b), followed by a tibial tubercle osteotomy to allow the osteotomies of femoral and tibial bones (c). Trial components (d), final implant positioning (e), and tibial tubercle fixation by two screws (f). X-rays 3 years after surgery (g).

It is not uncommon in knees with severe stiffness to find an ankylosed patellofemoral joint: in such cases, an osteotomy (by saw or osteotome) should be performed trying to save as much bone possible from the patellar surface sacrificing the anterior femoral aspect (Fig. **4**).

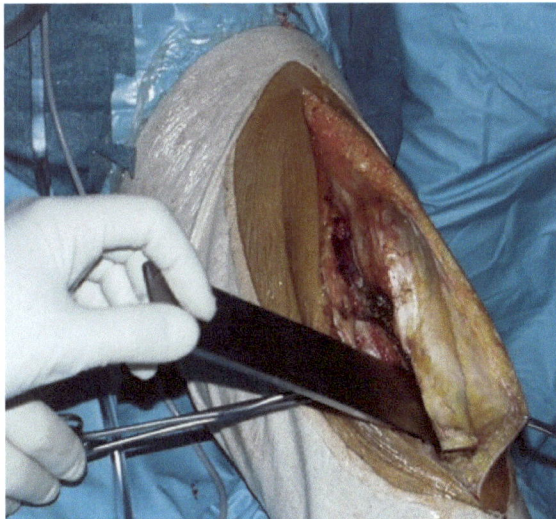

Fig. (4). Approach to an ankylosed patellofemoral joint in a haemophilic patient of 34-years old. An osteotome is gently beaten to divide the patella from the distorted trochlea without compromising the patellar bone stock.

A wide synovectomy and a following careful electrocautery should be performed, both to remove an important cause of postoperative bleeding, and to allow a better exposure of the intra-articular space (Fig. **5**).

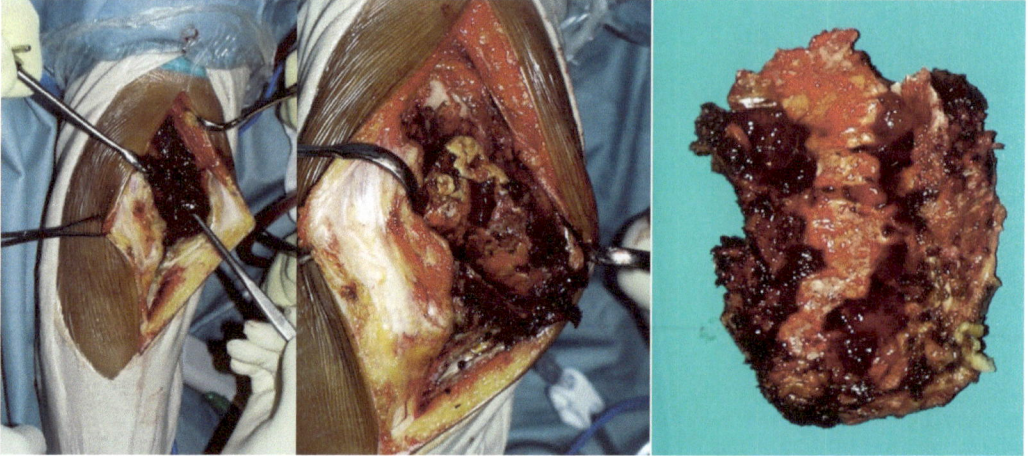

Fig. (5). Example of the standard synovectomy before performing a TKA: a large amount of chronic synovitis has been removed.

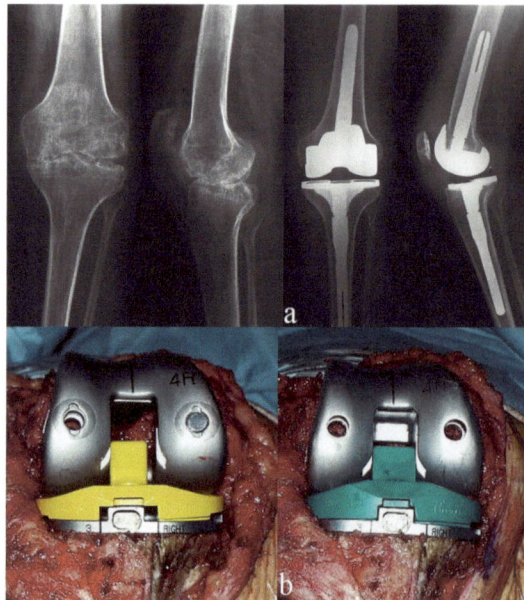

Fig. (6). The benefits related to the availability of a modern modular knee system in a haemophilic patient of 58-years old affected by Haemophilia A: cementless stems, offsets, wedges (a). Another advantage is the possibility to intraoperatively change the width and the level of constraint during the trial manoeuvre: flexion and extension gaps, and ligaments balancing may vary using a PS (yellow) or a constrained (green) tibial insert (b).

Cuts should be made as for personal experience starting either from tibial or femoral side. It is often necessary to perform very extensive cuts given the poor quality of tibial and/or femoral bones and the preoperative malalignment. For this reason, it is of paramount importance nowadays to have the availability of modular knee systems with tibial inserts, wedges, cones, offsets, and stems, different choices of constraint (cruciate retaining, posterior stabilized, constrained, hinged), and even bone grafts, in order to adapt the implant to the anatomy of the knee [41 - 43]. It is very common in primary TKA in Haemophilia for example to intraoperatively convert a CR into a PS implant, or a PS into a constrained TKA to achieve a better stability (Fig. **6**) [4]. This is far different from what done in the previous decades, when the only option was to adapt the operated knee to the available prostheses due to the limits of the first generation orthopaedic implants. Similarly, some authors reported their experience with "custom-made" implants with good clinical results [19].

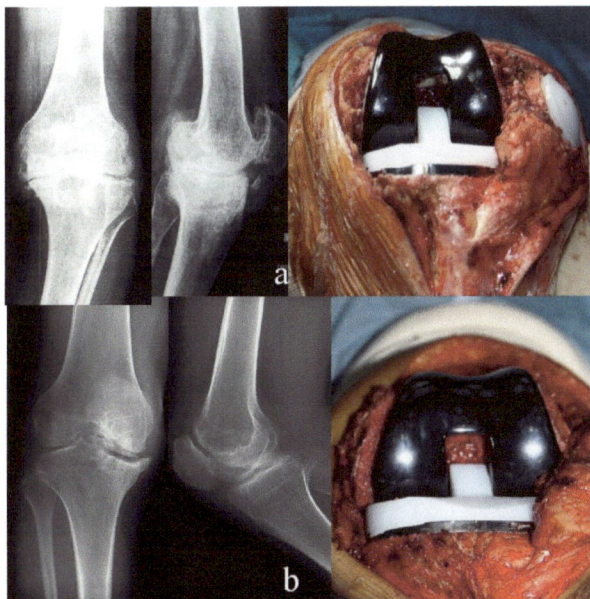

Fig. (7). Examples of TKA with patellar resurfacing in a 32-years old patient affected by severe Haemophilia A (a) and TKA without patellar resurfacing in a 39-years old affected by severe Haemophilia B (b). In both cases, an Oxidized zirconium femoral component and a posterior stabilized tibial insert was chosen.

Ligamentous and capsular releases have to be selectively made in a way to balance the gaps in extension and flexion, and to allow ROM as maximum as possible (full extension, flexion over 100°). Patellar resurfacing is generally performed with cemented domes, even if some series have been reported with selective resurfacing and brilliant outcomes also leaving the native patellae (Fig. 7) [4, 44]. Criteria not to resurface the patella are in our experience the following:

availability of a high tribologic properties material (for example, Oxidized Zirconium femoral components), good quality of the remaining articular cartilage, absence of eburnated bone, normal patellar shape, absence of inflammatory synovial tissue, adequate bone width of the residual patella, and congruent intraoperative patellar tracking [4, 44, 45].

One should believe that cemented fixation of components in patients affected by haemophilic arthropathy is undebatable: cemented tibial, femoral, and patellar components are reported in almost all series. However, some different experiences may be found. A raise of interest on the cementless fixation in young patients has been reported over the last years [46 - 48]. Given the very young mean age of haemophiliacs undergoing TKA this type of implants may be considered the best choice in order to facilitate any revision. However no specific series has been published, and the few cases managed by cementless fixation have obtained good results in terms of clinical outcomes and survivorship (Fig. **8**).

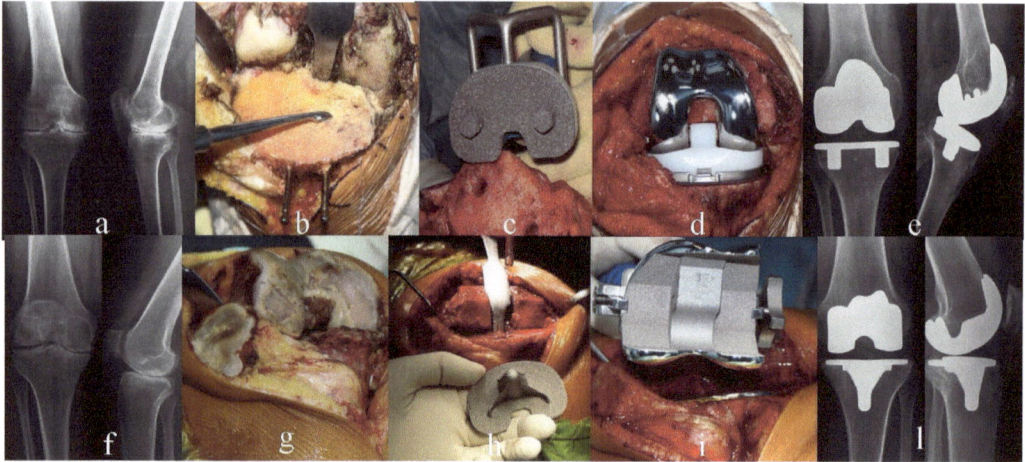

Fig. (8). Examples of cementless TKAs. A 23-years old haemophilic patient affected by Haemophilia A (a). Very good quality of tibial and femoral bone stock (b). Pictures of the trabecular metal tibial tray (c) and final implant (d). Follow-up after 4.5 years (e). A 25-years old haemophilic patient with inhibitors (f) undergone a cementless TKA. Intraoperative aspect of the knee after exposure (g). Aspect of the surface of tibial (h) and femoral (i) components before implanting. Follow-up at 4 years (l).

As mentioned, the not ideal quality of bone in such subjects should deserve a cemented TKA. There is no specific description of the actual type of cemented fixation in most of the published series, particularly referring to tibial components. In some papers the authors specify that tibial components are cemented both on the baseplate and keel [17 - 20]. In other series, tibial components have been cemented only in the baseplate leaving all keels pressfit (*hybrid fixation*) [4, 20, 44, 49]. There is still now debate on such type of fixation:

it may have advantages on the easier removal in case of failure or revision but may also have drawbacks related to relative micromovements with respect to all cemented components [47, 48]. On the other hand no significant differences have been reported over the years [4], and reported outcomes are similar to the standard fixation [45]. Before implanting the components, another session of electrocautery is recommended after deflation of tourniquet (if used). Drains are generally used and removed between 12 and 24 hours after TKA. Laboratory samplings of deficient factor are usually performed every day for the first days and after a week in case of actual necessity to progressively diminish the doses of the haematologic drugs. Postoperative rehabilitation is generally the same of standard TKA, even if dedicated and specifically trained therapists should follow the haemophilic patients. Moreover, an *in-patient* rehabilitative period should be considered in order to allow a close monitoring of the dedicated multidisciplinary team [50]. Specific bases of rehabilitation after TKA in haemophilic patients will be discussed in another section (see chapter 16). General principles of rehabilitation after a knee replacement in haemophiliacs are: tailored pain management over all the postoperative period; exercises sessions after the infusion of deficient factor; early rehabilitation by continuous passive mobilization (CPM) with immediate full extension and progressive flexion; isometrics exercises; gentle assisted active/resistive mobilization and passive flexion over 90° within 4-6 days; recovery of weight bearing and gait exercises with canes or crutches respecting the postoperative pain [51, 52].

COMPLICATIONS AND OUTCOMES

As mentioned, TKA in Haemophilia is a successful procedure in terms of reduction of pain and bleedings, recovery of joint function, and improvement of the quality of life. However, over the decades significant rates of complications and failures have been reported particularly in the first series: bleedings, mechanical problems, infections, and aseptic loosening were the main causes of failure mostly related to HIV-positive patients, presence of inhibitors, and limitations of the first generation knee implants [2 - 16]. Modern bleeding management, perioperative prophylactic strategies, dedicated multidisciplinary teams, advancements in the surgical technique, and high-tech orthopaedic implants have significantly reduced the complications after surgery and improved the clinical outcomes [17 - 29]. To date the mean survivorship is more than 90% at a mid-term follow-up with respect to a survival rate of 82.5% (range: 68%-96%) in the period between '70 and '90s [5 - 16, 24 - 29]. In our experience, the survivorship reaches up to 98.7 at 8.3 years after surgery [4]: this represents to date the only series without failures related to infection and mechanical loosening. Finally, from a clinical point of view it is expected that after a mean period of 5-6 years postoperatively a reduction of ROM (particularly in flexion) is usually reported by patients. However, they generally do not complaint this limitation as symptomatic or as a failure of TKA.

TKA in haemophilic patients has been associated with complications in the intraoperative and immediate postoperative period similar to standard TKA for other diseases as Osteoarthritis. However, given the peculiar pathogenesis and typical severity of the haemophilic arthropathy, some specific complication has been described. Skin necrosis, nerve palsies (mainly the peroneal nerve), and bleedings are examples of early complications often reported [3, 8, 10, 12, 13, 17, 20, 21]. Among the late postoperative complications we should make a distinction between biological and mechanical events. Regarding the former type, we should mention: recurrent bleedings, recurrence of synovitis, and infections [13, 17, 20]. Events as arthrofibrosis, stiffness and loss of extension (and less frequently flexion) are other peculiar events, related to the preoperative conditions but also to the surgical exposure [20 - 22]. It is well known that patients with stiff knees or severe flexion contractures will gain a wide ROM after surgery within the first 6-12 months after TKA. On the other hand, subjects with an extensive preoperative ROM (>90°) will suffer postoperatively for a small improvement particularly for the flexion [51, 52]. Patellar periprosthetic fracture is another relatively frequent event in haemophilic patients, particularly after resurfacing in case of an inadequate bone width of the residual patella [20]. This is the reason for not to resurface the patella if not necessary or in cases of small bone dimensions.

The classic mechanisms of failures (infection, aseptic loosening, instability) will be discussed in another section (see Chapter 15). Risk factors for all these complications and failures in Haemophilia are mostly related to the clinical conditions of patients. The most important are the type of deficient factor (deficiency of factor VIII is more at risk of complications than factor IX), associated infectious diseases (mainly HIV), and presence of inhibitors.

Regarding the type of deficiency, it has been demonstrated as Haemophilia A is associated with more sequelae and worse clinical outcomes with respect to Haemophilia B, that is a more relatively rare condition [15, 29, 30]. Co-infections induce patients undergoing TKA at higher risk of complications either at short- and long-term follow-up [53, 54]. HIV infection more than Hepatitis C has exposed subjects to a wide spectrum of complications, particularly in the late '80s and early '90s [10, 17, 18, 21]. Modern approaches to HIV-positive haemophilic patients have limited such high risks. The presence of inhibitors is still now a significant risk factor, and the improvements in these patients have been lesser consistent than for other conditions. Patients with inhibitors are more prone to develop postoperative bleedings and recurrence of haemarthrosis, presence of radiolucency lines at x-rays, pseudotumour, aseptic and septic loosening with respect to subjects without inhibitors [3, 12, 13, 21, 22].

CONCLUDING REMARKS

Knees represent the main target joints of Haemophilia and Total Knee Arthroplasty is the most performed major orthopaedic surgery in this population. A modern approach with an appropriate bleeding management, multidisciplinary teams, and the choice of new generation modular implants with high tribologic properties are the keys to ensure even better outcomes than last decades.

CONFLICT OF INTEREST

The authors confirm that they have no conflict of interest to declare for this publication.

ACKNOWLEDGEMENTS

Declared none.

REFERENCES

[1]   Marmor L. Total knee replacement in hemophilia. Clin Orthop Relat Res 1977; (125): 192-5.
        [PMID: 880765]

[2]   McCollough NC, Enis JE, Lovitt J, Lian EC, Niemann KC, Loughlin EC. Sinovectomy or total
        replacement of the knee in hemophilia. Clin Orthop Relat Res 1979; (61-A): 69-75.

[3]   Goddard NJ, Rodriguez-Merchan EC, Wiedel JD. Total knee replacement in haemophilia.
        Haemophilia 2002; 8(3): 382-6.
        [http://dx.doi.org/10.1046/j.1365-2516.2002.00604.x] [PMID: 12010438]

[4]   Innocenti M, Civinini R, Carulli C, Villano M, Linari S, Morfini M. A modular total knee arthroplasty
        in haemophilic arthropathy. Knee 2007; 14(4): 264-8.
        [http://dx.doi.org/10.1016/j.knee.2007.05.001] [PMID: 17601738]

[5]   Goldberg VM, Heiple KG, Ratnoff OD, Kurczynski E, Arvan G. Total knee arthroplasty in classic
        hemophilia. J Bone Joint Surg Am 1981; 63(5): 695-701.
        [http://dx.doi.org/10.2106/00004623-198163050-00002] [PMID: 7240292]

[6]   Small M, Steven MM, Freeman PA, *et al.* Total knee arthroplasty in haemophilic arthritis. J Bone
        Joint Surg Br 1983; 65(2): 163-5.
        [PMID: 6826622]

[7]   Lachiewicz PF, Inglis AE, Insall JN, Sculco TP, Hilgartner MW, Bussel JB. Total knee arthroplasty in
        hemophilia. J Bone Joint Surg Am 1985; 67(9): 1361-6.
        [http://dx.doi.org/10.2106/00004623-198567090-00009] [PMID: 3935651]

[8]   Rana NA, Shapiro GR, Green D. Long-term follow-up of prosthetic joint replacement in hemophilia.
        Am J Hematol 1986; 23(4): 329-37.
        [http://dx.doi.org/10.1002/ajh.2830230405] [PMID: 3788961]

[9]   Augerau B, Travers V, Le Balch T, Witvoet J. Les arthroplasties totals de hanche et de genou chez
        l'hemophile. A propos de 27 cas. Rev Chir Orthop Repar Appar Mot 1987; 73: 381-94.

[10]   Kjaersgaard-Andersen P, Christiansen SE, Ingerslev J, Sneppen O. Total knee arthroplasty in classic hemophilia. Clin Orthop Relat Res 1990; (256): 137-46.
[PMID: 2114246]

[11]   Karthaus RP, Novakova IR. Total knee replacement in haemophilic arthropathy. J Bone Joint Surg Br 1988; 70(3): 382-5.
[PMID: 3131346]

[12]   Figgie MP, Goldberg VM, Figgie HE III, Heiple KG, Sobel M. Total knee arthroplasty for the treatment of chronic hemophilic arthropathy. Clin Orthop Relat Res 1989; (248): 98-107.
[PMID: 2805504]

[13]   Unger AS, Kessler CM, Lewis RJ. Total knee arthroplasty in human immunodeficiency virus-infected hemophiliacs. J Arthroplasty 1995; 10(4): 448-52.
[http://dx.doi.org/10.1016/S0883-5403(05)80144-5] [PMID: 8523002]

[14]   Magone JB, Dennis DA, Weis LD. Total knee arthroplasty in chronic hemophilic arthropathy. Orthopedics 1986; 9(5): 653-7.
[PMID: 3714579]

[15]   Heeg M, Meyer K, Smid WM, Van Horn JR, Van der Meer J. Total knee and hip arthroplasty in haemophilic patients. Haemophilia 1998; 4(5): 747-51.
[http://dx.doi.org/10.1046/j.1365-2516.1998.00183.x] [PMID: 9873881]

[16]   Cohen I, Heim M, Martinowitz U, Chechick A. Orthopaedic outcome of total knee replacement in haemophilia A. Haemophilia 2000; 6(2): 104-9.
[http://dx.doi.org/10.1046/j.1365-2516.2000.00375.x] [PMID: 10781197]

[17]   Rodriguez-Merchan EC, Wiedel JD. Total knee arthroplasty in HIV-positive haemophilic patients. Haemophilia 2002; 8(3): 387-92.
[http://dx.doi.org/10.1046/j.1365-2516.2002.00610.x] [PMID: 12010439]

[18]   Norian JM, Ries MD, Karp S, Hambleton J. Total knee arthroplasty in hemophilic arthropathy. J Bone Joint Surg Am 2002; 84-A(7): 1138-41.
[http://dx.doi.org/10.2106/00004623-200207000-00007] [PMID: 12107312]

[19]   Legroux-Gerot I, Strouk G, Parquet A, Goodemand J, Gougeon F, Duquesnoy B. Total knee arthroplasty in hemophilic arthropathy. Joint Bone Spine 2003; 70: 22-32.
[http://dx.doi.org/10.1016/S1297-319X(02)00008-8]

[20]   Sheth DS, Oldfield D, Ambrose C, Clyburn T. Total knee arthroplasty in hemophilic arthropathy J Arthroplasty 2004; 19: 56-60.

[21]   Silva M, Luck JV jr. Long-term results of primary total knee replacement in patients with hemophilia. J Bone Joint Surg 2005; 87-A: 85-91.

[22]   Solimeno LP, Perfetto OS, Pasta G, Santagostino E. Total joint replacement in patients with inhibitors. Haemophilia 2006; 12 (Suppl.3): 113-6.
[http://dx.doi.org/10.1111/j.1365-2516.2006.01267.x]

[23]   Rodriguez-Merchan EC, Quintana M, Jimenez-Yuste V, Hernández-Navarro F. Orthopaedic surgery for inhibitor patients: a series of 27 procedures (25 patients). Haemophilia 2007; 13(5): 613-9.
[http://dx.doi.org/10.1111/j.1365-2516.2007.01520.x] [PMID: 17880452]

[24]   Rodriguez-Merchan EC. Total knee replacement in haemophilic arthropathy. J Bone Joint Surg Br 2007; 89(2): 186-8.
[http://dx.doi.org/10.1302/0301-620X.89B2.18682] [PMID: 17322432]

[25] Chiang CC, Chen PQ, Shen MC, Tsai W. Total knee arthroplasty for severe haemophilic arthropathy: long-term experience in Taiwan. Haemophilia 2008; 14(4): 828-34.
[http://dx.doi.org/10.1111/j.1365-2516.2008.01693.x] [PMID: 18510565]

[26] Solimeno LP, Mancuso ME, Pasta G, Santagostino E, Perfetto S, Mannucci PM. Factors influencing the long-term outcome of primary total knee replacement in haemophiliacs: a review of 116 procedures at a single institution. Br J Haematol 2009; 145(2): 227-34.
[http://dx.doi.org/10.1111/j.1365-2141.2009.07613.x] [PMID: 19236610]

[27] Sikkema T, Boerboom AL, Meijer K. A comparison between the complications and long-term outcome of hip and knee replacement therapy in patients with and without haemophilia; a controlled retrospective cohort study. Haemophilia 2011; 17(2): 300-3.
[http://dx.doi.org/10.1111/j.1365-2516.2010.02408.x] [PMID: 21070490]

[28] Zingg PO, Fucentese SF, Lutz W, Brand B, Mamisch N, Koch PP. Haemophilic knee arthropathy: long-term outcome after total knee replacement. Knee Surg Sports Traumatol Arthrosc 2012; 20(12): 2465-70. epub ahead of print
[http://dx.doi.org/10.1007/s00167-012-1896-7] [PMID: 22293897]

[29] Jenkins PJ, Ekrol I, Lawson GM. Total knee replacement in patients with haemophilia: the Scottish experience. Scott Med J 2013; 58(4): 223-7.
[http://dx.doi.org/10.1177/0036933013507870] [PMID: 24215041]

[30] Roosendaal G, Van Der Berg HM, Lafeber FP, Bijilsma JW. Blood induced joint damage: an overview of musculoskeletal research in Haemophilia. In: Rodriguez-Merchan EC, Goddard NJ, Lee CA, Eds. Muscoloskeletal Aspects of Haemophilia. Cambridge: Blackwell Science Ltd 2000; pp. 18-26.Chapter: 3

[31] Carulli C, Matassi F, Civinini R, Morfini M, Tani M, Innocenti M. Intra-articular injections of hyaluronic acid induce positive clinical effects in knees of patients affected by haemophilic arthropathy. Knee 2013; 20(1): 36-9.
[http://dx.doi.org/10.1016/j.knee.2012.05.006] [PMID: 22704969]

[32] Gilbert MS. Prophylaxis: musculoskeletal evaluation. Semin Hematol 1993; 30(3) (Suppl. 2): 3-6.
[PMID: 8367740]

[33] Hiliard P, Funk S, Zourikian N, *et al.* Haemophilia joint health score reliability study. Haemophilia 2006; 12: 518.

[34] Arnold WD, Hilgartner MW. Hemophilic arthropathy. Current concepts of pathogenesis and management. J Bone Joint Surg Am 1977; 59(3): 287-305.
[http://dx.doi.org/10.2106/00004623-197759030-00001] [PMID: 849938]

[35] Pettersson H, Ahlberg A, Nilsson IM. A radiologic classification of hemophilic arthropathy. Clin Orthop Relat Res 1980; (149): 153-9.
[PMID: 7408294]

[36] Ware JE Jr, Sherbourne CD. The MOS 36-item short-form health survey (SF-36). I. Conceptual framework and item selection. Med Care 1992; 30(6): 473-83.
[http://dx.doi.org/10.1097/00005650-199206000-00002] [PMID: 1593914]

[37] Bellamy N, Buchanan WW, Goldsmith CH, Campbell J, Stitt LW. Validation study of WOMAC: a health status instrument for measuring clinically important patient relevant outcomes to antirheumatic drug therapy in patients with osteoarthritis of the hip or knee. J Rheumatol 1988; 15(12): 1833-40.
[PMID: 3068365]

[38] Insall JN, Dorr LD, Scott RD, Scott WN. Rationale of the Knee Society clinical rating system. Clin Orthop Relat Res 1989; (248): 13-4.
[PMID: 2805470]

[39] Laskin RS. Ten steps to an easier revision total knee arthroplasty. J Arthroplasty 2002; 17(4) (Suppl. 1): 78-82.
[http://dx.doi.org/10.1054/arth.2002.32454] [PMID: 12068412]

[40] Whiteside LA, Ohl MD. Tibial tubercle osteotomy for exposure of the difficult total knee arthroplasty. Clin Orthop Relat Res 1990; (260): 6-9.
[PMID: 2225644]

[41] Innocenti M, Matassi F, Carulli C, Soderi S, Villano M, Civinini R. Joint line position in revision total knee arthroplasty: the role of posterior femoral off-set stems. Knee 2013; 20(6): 447-50.
[http://dx.doi.org/10.1016/j.knee.2013.05.012] [PMID: 23790671]

[42] Matassi F, Botti A, Sirleo L, Carulli C, Innocenti M. Porous metal for orthopedics implants. Clin Cases Miner Bone Metab 2013; 10(2): 111-5.
[PMID: 24133527]

[43] Carulli C, Matassi F, Civinini R, Innocenti M. Tissue engineering applications in the management of bone loss. Clin Cases Miner Bone Metab 2013; 10(1): 22-5.
[PMID: 23858306]

[44] Innocenti M, Civinini R, Carulli C, Matassi F, Villano M. The 5-year results of an oxidized zirconium femoral component for TKA. Clin Orthop Relat Res 2010; 468(5): 1258-63.
[http://dx.doi.org/10.1007/s11999-009-1109-y] [PMID: 19798541]

[45] Innocenti M, Matassi F, Carulli C, Nistri L, Civinini R. Oxidized zirconium femoral component for TKA: a follow-up note of a previous report at a minimum of 10 years. Knee 2014; 21(4): 858-61.
[http://dx.doi.org/10.1016/j.knee.2014.04.005] [PMID: 24835580]

[46] Carulli C, Matassi F, Nistri L, Civinini R, Innocenti M. Long-term survival of a flat-on-flat total condylar knee arthroplasty fixed with a hybrid cementing technique for tibial components. J Long Term Eff Med Implants 2012; 22(4): 305-12.
[http://dx.doi.org/10.1615/JLongTermEffMedImplants.2013007289] [PMID: 23662661]

[47] Mont MA, Pivec R, Issa K, Kapadia BH, Maheshwari A, Harwin SF. Long-term implant survivorship of cementless total knee arthroplasty: a systematic review of the literature and meta-analysis. J Knee Surg 2014; 27(5): 369-76.
[PMID: 24318196]

[48] Matassi F, Carulli C, Civinini R, Innocenti M. Cemented versus cementless fixation in total knee arthroplasty. Joints 2014; 8(1): 121-5.

[49] Kolisek FR, Mont MA, Seyler TM, et al. Total knee arthroplasty using cementless keels and cemented tibial trays: 10-year results. Int Orthop 2009; 33(1): 117-21.
[http://dx.doi.org/10.1007/s00264-007-0502-y] [PMID: 18185931]

[50] Viliani T, Zambelan G, Pandolfi C, et al. In-patient rehabilitation in haemophilic subjects with total knee arthroplasty. Haemophilia 2011; 17(5): e999-e1004.
[PMID: 21535326]

[51] Kamath AF, Horneff JG, Forsyth A, Nikci V, Nelson CL. Total knee arthroplasty in hemophiliacs: gains in range of motion realized beyond twelve months postoperatively. Clin Orthop Surg 2012; 4(2): 121-8.
[http://dx.doi.org/10.4055/cios.2012.4.2.121] [PMID: 22662297]

[52] Massin P, Petit A, Odri G, et al. Societè dorthopedie de louest (SOO). Total knee arthroplasty in patients with greater than 20 degresse flexion contracture. Orthop Traumatol Surg Res 2009; 95S: S7-S12.
[http://dx.doi.org/10.1016/j.otsr.2009.04.001] [PMID: 19442598]

[53]   Wilde JT. HIV and HCV coinfection in haemophilia. Haemophilia 2004; 10(1): 1-8.
        [http://dx.doi.org/10.1046/j.1351-8216.2003.00828.x] [PMID: 14962214]

[54]   Rodriguez-Merchan EC. HIV and HCV coinfected haemophilia patients: what are the best options of
        orthopaedic treatment? Haemophilia 2006; 12 (Suppl. 3): 90-101.
        [http://dx.doi.org/10.1111/j.1365-2516.2006.01264.x] [PMID: 16684002]

CHAPTER 12

Hip Arthroplasty

Christian Carulli*, **Roberto Civinini** and **Anna Rosa Rizzo**

Orthopaedic Clinic, University of Florence, Florence, Italy

Abstract: Hip arthropathy in patients with Haemophilia may be disabling. In early stages a conservative treatment may be useful, as in late stages a Total Hip Arthroplasty is indicated. During the '80s and '90s clinical outcomes after a hip arthroplasty were variable given the use of first generation cemented implants, and the significantly high rates of complications, as for other types of surgery. In the last decades modern cementless implants with high performing materials and less invasive surgical techniques have been introduced with expected improved results. Recently several series have been reported with very satisfactory outcomes, and longer survival rates of implants with respect to the past. A combination of multidisciplinary teams dedicated to haemophilic subjects, the use of modern cementless implants, and less invasive surgical approaches may represent the key to achieve good outcomes, fewer complications, and better prosthetic survivorship in such difficult patients.

Keywords: Ceramics, Ceramic on polyethylene coupling, Cementless arthroplasty, Total hip arthroplasty.

INTRODUCTION

Hips are not typical target joints of bleedings induced by Haemophilia, given the paucity of synovial tissue. However, the involvement of the hip induces a significant impairment in haemophilic subjects similarly to other joints affected by arthropathy. Several conservative approaches have been reported during recent years with high rates of clinical success before surgery (see chapter 8). Most of these approaches are indicated for the early stages of arthropathy of knees, elbows, and ankles: the main target of treatment in such joints is effectively the synovial tissue [1 - 3]. Unfortunately, these strategies have not shown similar effects in the hip, thus only a Total Hip Arthroplasty (THA) is considered useful, as reported by several series [4 - 6]. Historically, outcomes of hip surgery in haemophilic patients have shown acceptable rates of success, despite the high risk of complications related to comorbidities, mostly coinfections (HCV, HIV), liver

* **Corresponding author Christian Carulli:** Orthopaedic Clinic, University of Florence, Florence, Italy; Tel: 0039 055 794 8200; Email: christian.carulli@unifi.it

disease, and septic or aseptic loosening [7 - 10]. Such undefined results have been mostly related to the type of available implants (first-generation cemented implants), and to the difficult management of haemophilic patients before the introduction of the modern substitutive haematological therapy. Moreover, the lack of an actual multidisciplinary approach to such rare disease in those years implicated a further risk of failure.

In the recent years, several larger series of haemophiliacs undergoing THA with modern implants and followed by dedicated teams have been reported: excellent outcomes and transcurable rates of complications have underlined the crucial steps to achieve an ideal balance between clinical results and such demanding surgery in haemophilic patients.

INDICATIONS, CLINICAL SETTINGS, AND SURGICAL TECHNIQUE

As before mentioned, late stages of hip arthropathy in Haemophilia have to be treated by THA. A very little room is left to the conservative (medical) treatment: this has to be reserved to early stages [11]. THA may be addressed and planned as other major surgical procedures. General anaesthesia, antibiotic prophylaxis with appropriate antibiotics, tailored substitutive haematological prophylaxis, and close multidisciplinary perioperative evaluation are the basic procedures (see chapter 11).

Over the years, THA in haemophiliacs was performed by two main surgical approaches: lateral and posterolateral approach. As for hip Osteoarthritis, both have advantages and drawbacks, but the most important factor is surely the surgeon's experience. It is well known that the lateral approach is easier and safer for the lower risk of postoperative instability with respect to the posterolateral access. On the other side, the posterolateral approach is more conservative and no muscular impairment is left after surgery compared to the lateral access, where a limp due to abductor muscles deficiency may be present [12, 13].

The other key element is the choice of implant. For decades all THAs were cemented and with metal small-diameter heads, coupled with PolyEthylene (PE). Also in Haemophilia this represented for years the main option [4 - 10]. Later, few experiences with Metal-on-Metal (MOM) cementless THAs were reported with variable results [14]. Recently, series with cementless Metal-on-PE (MOP) or Ceramic-on-PE (COP) have been reported with consistent follow-up periods and satisfactory outcomes [15 - 19]. Given the young age of haemophilic patients (often <50years) it is nowadays reasonable to use cementless MOP or COP implants, for two main reasons: first of all, a young patient has higher functional requests, and an implant with a more favourable tribology and an expected low wear is desirable. Moreover, young subjects will surely undergo a revision for any reason in the future: a cementless THA will be easier to be removed with respect to cemented components [11].

Several series with modern short stems in Osteoarthritis have been reported, whereas no similar experience was presented in Haemophilia. A single series with such type of stems was successfully published at a medium-term follow-up with comparable results to standard femoral components [11].

Some technical aspects of THA in Haemophilia deserve a detailed analysis. Easy is to ensure an adequate limb length in modern THA: however, rarely a haemophilic patient shows an isolated hip arthropathy without any other involvement of target joints. Generally hard is to obtain such results when a multiple joints involvement is present. Flexion contractures of both knees, secondary scoliosis due to chronic postural changes, stiffness of ankles, and compensatory pelvis tilting are frequently present, creating an objective impossibility to realize an adequate length and an ideal hip centre restoration. Nevertheless, rarely a relative limb length discrepancy is source of pain or complaint by haemophiliacs [11].

Drains are generally used and removed between 12 and 24 hours after surgery. Laboratory samplings of deficient factor are usually performed every day for the first days and after a week in case of actual necessity to progressively diminish the doses of the haematologic drugs. Tailored rehabilitative protocols and dedicated physical therapy are mandatory to achieve an early recovery and muscular tone after THA. An *in-patient* rehabilitative period should be considered in order to allow a close monitoring by the dedicated multidisciplinary team. Specific principles of rehabilitation after THA in haemophilic patients will be discussed in another section (see chapter 16). As for TKA (see chapter 11), basic rehabilitation protocols after a hip replacement in haemophiliacs are: tailored pain management over all the postoperative period; exercises sessions after the infusion of deficient factor; early rehabilitation by passive mobilization without adduction and excessive intra and extrarotation of the hip; isometrics exercises; progressive recovery of weight bearing and gait exercises with canes or crutches respecting the postoperative pain.

Methods of objective evaluation of THAs in haemophiliacs do not differ from other type of patients. DeLee's and Charnley's criteria for cups positioning [20], Gruen's method for the analysis of radiolucency lines and osteolysis [21], and Brooker's classification for postoperative periarticular calcifications [22] are the main tools to evaluate the follow-up and the long-term survival of a hip replacement. The only subjective method applicable for haemophilic subjects is the Haemophilia Joint Health Score (HJHS) [23], that represents the most used scoring system specific for such patients, even if not accurate. On the other side, Harris Hip score, WOMAC, and SF-36 are not properly indicated given the poor clinical correspondence to this specific kind of patients.

Results and Complications

As for Osteoarthritis and Haemophilia, THA (with TKA) is one of the most successful surgical procedures of modern Orthopaedics. Specifically, even the multiple joint involvement of haemophilic subjects, such type of surgery usually produces a dramatic improvement in terms of pain relief and recovery of function ability. On the other hand, haemophiliacs are not easy patients. Intraoperative fractures mostly related to severe deformity than poor bone quality, infections in coinfected patients (mainly HIV-positive), tendency to postoperative bleedings, and early loosening due to wear, are the most common causes of failure in such this population [5 - 10].

Moreover, as for other type of surgery, small series of THA in Haemophilia have been reported because of the high risks of complications related to this rare disease [5, 8, 10].

The first consistent release was made by Luck *et al*, that reported their experience on 13 haemophilic patients treated by cemented components with almost 20 years of follow-up. They did not specify the actual survivorship of such implants, but reported some failures mainly related to infections and aseptic loosening [4].

Kelley *et al* conducted a retrospective study on 27 haemophiliacs (34 THAs) undergoing THA: 28 implants were cemented and only 6 cementless. The follow-up was about 8 years for the cemented THAs, with a survivorship of 65% for acetabular components and 44% for femoral stems; only 3 years for cementless implants [7].

Nelson *et al* reported a series of 39 patients undergoing THA with a survivorship of 70% at 8 years. The rate of complications was described as high: one patient deceased during surgery (cardiac arrest), one with a postoperative dislocation (managed by closed reduction), and five cases needing an early revision (two infections, three aseptic loosenings). Three additional cases showed a component migration with a scheduled revision [9].

Miles *et al* reported an experience with 30 haemophiliacs treated by 26 cemented and 4 uncemented implants with various couplings (Metal-on-PE, Ceramic-o--Ceramic) at 6.2 years. They recorded three deaths (not related to the procedure), three aseptic loosenings, and one deep infection, with a poor global survivorship [15].

Yoo *et al* presented a series of 27 THAs in 23 patients with a survival rate of 95.2% at 7.6 years. Better outcomes were found in patients undergoing a cementless THA, with only two failures related to aseptic loosening [16].

Sikkema *et al* reported a small series of 6 THAs in haemophilic patients at 7.6 years of follow-up: no failure was described, even if no information on the type of implants and couplings was specified [17].

Wang *et al* published their results in 18 THAs performed in 16 patients, with a mean follow-up of 8.5 years. Complications occurred in four hips, with two requiring revision arthroplasty. One case of transient sciatic nerve palsy, one case of intraoperative proximal femoral fracture, one case of aseptic acetabular component loosening at 7.5 years requiring revision, and one case of posttraumatic periprosthetic fracture (requiring revision) were reported. The overall survival rate was 89% at 8.5 years [18].

Panotopoulos *et al* recently published an interesting comparison between uncemented MOM *versus* COP THAs in a series of 12 haemophilic subjects, further compared to a control group of non-

haemophilic patients. Six were treated by a second-generation MOM (Metasul®) bearing, and six by a COP (alumina) coupling with a mean follow-up of 10.4 years. Their results were superior for the latter implants, while MOM THAs demonstrated substantially poor outcomes. The overall survival rate considering infection as cause of failure was 85.7% at 10 years. The authors finally suggested a cementless hard bearing coupling for THAs (other than MOM) in haemophiliacs [14].

Carulli *et al* reported about a series of 23 haemophilic patients undergoing a cementless THA with COP couplings at their multidisciplinar Haemophilia center [11]. In 14 subjects, a standard stem was used in 9 cases (Figs. **1** and **2**), while a modern short stem a was used Fig. (**3**).

No failures and no complications were recorded, with a survival rate of 100% at 8.1 years. Detailed descriptions of some features with respect to other experiences were reported. An adequate hip center restoration was achieved in 20 out of 23 cases, while a suboptimal hip center was reported in 3 subjects with severe involvement of other target joints. These patients did not complain of significant symptoms or functional impairment Fig. (**2**). No significant alterations of the periprosthetic space or radiolucencies were reported, whereas asymptomatic periarticular ossifications were found in some cases.

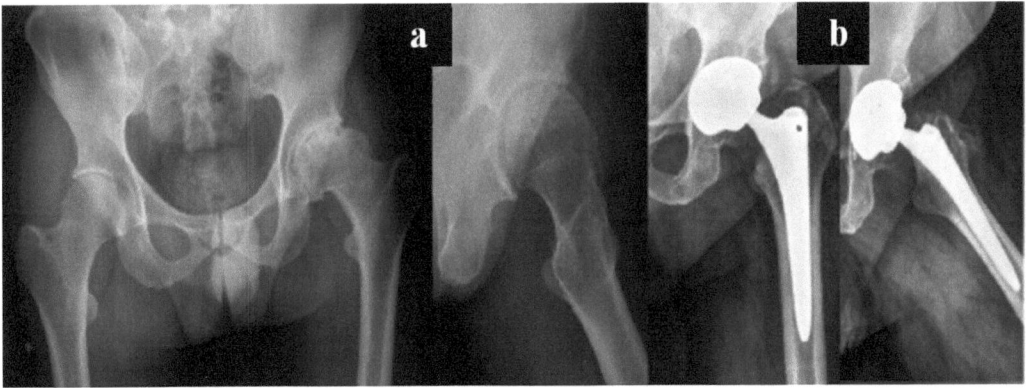

Fig. (1). Preoperative x-rays of the left hip of a 58 year-old patient with severe Haemophilia A. Petterson score: 12 (a). Radiographic aspect 6.5 years after surgery: COP coupling, standard tapered stem, restoration of the hip center, no residual limb length discrepancy, and asymptomatic ossifications Brooker stage 1. No progressive radiolucency lines or osteolysis were revealed (b).

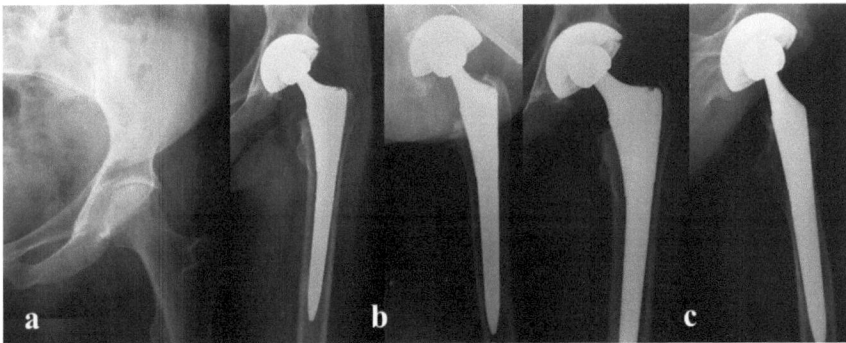

Fig. (2). Preoperative x-rays of the left hip of a 33 year-old patient with severe Haemophilia A. Petterson score: 11 (a). X-rays 2 years after surgery: standard stem and standard acetabular cup with COP coupling (b). No ossifications or significant radiolucency lines at 10 years after surgery (c).

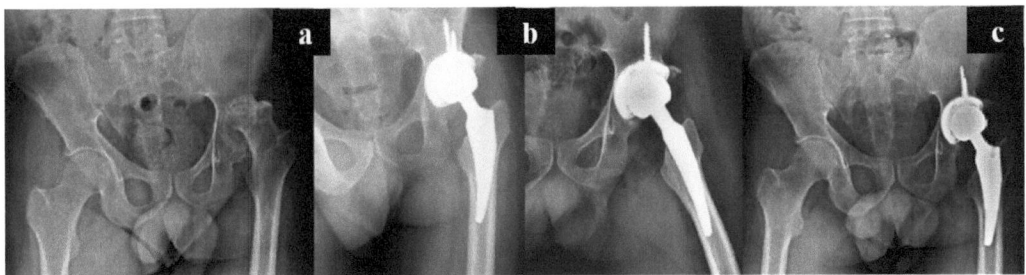

Fig. (3). Preoperative x-rays of the left hip of a 41 year-old patient with severe Haemophilia A. Petterson score: 13 (a). X-rays 6 months after surgery: of noting the modern short stem and COP coupling, the acetabular cup fixed by two screws, and no periarticular ossifications (b). Follow-up at 3 years after the index operation: no significant radiolucency, minimal length discrepancy but no complaints referred by the patient.

Lee *et al* evaluated their clinical and radiographic results of 21 cementless THAs in 17 Haemophilia patients at a mean follow-up of 134 months. According to revision rates and mortality, the 10-year survival rate was 95.2%. There were three cases requiring a revision. According to the authors' conclusions, the low revision rate in their series may be attributed to the adequate substitutive therapy, regular follow-up at the haemophilic center, and to the experienced surgical team [19].

CONCLUDING REMARKS

Hip arthropathy in haemophilic patients is less common than in other joints, but similarly disabling. Historically, THA in Haemophilia has demonstrated substantially good results with the use of first-generation cemented implants, but with rather high rates of complications. Recently, several series of modern and high-performance cementless THAs associated with a multidisciplinary approach to Haemophilia have been characterized by excellent results without complications. The survivorship of such implants has been reported as even higher than other pathologies. We strongly believe that the close cooperation between haematologists, orthopaedic surgeons, and rehabilitative physicians is the key to ensure brilliant outcomes. Moreover, it is mandatory to promote the use of uncemented implants in these young patients, also in order to facilitate further surgery.

CONFLICT OF INTEREST

The authors confirm that they have no conflict of interest to declare for this publication.

ACKNOWLEDGEMENTS

Declared none.

REFERENCES

[1]   Carulli C, Civinini R, Martini C, *et al.* Viscosupplementation in haemophilic arthropathy: a long-term follow-up study. Haemophilia 2012; 18(3): e210-4.
[http://dx.doi.org/10.1111/j.1365-2516.2011.02654.x] [PMID: 21951693]

[2]   Carulli C, Matassi F, Civinini R, Morfini M, Tani M, Innocenti M. Intra-articular injections of hyaluronic acid induce positive clinical effects in knees of patients affected by haemophilic arthropathy. Knee 2013; 20(1): 36-9.
[http://dx.doi.org/10.1016/j.knee.2012.05.006] [PMID: 22704969]

[3]   Fernández-Palazzi F, Cedeño M, Maldonado JC, *et al.* Chemical synoviorthesis with oxytetracycline clorhydrate (Emicine) in recurrent haemarthrosis. Haemophilia 2008; 14(1): 21-4.
[PMID: 18005152]

[4]   Luck JV Jr, Kasper CK. Surgical management of advanced hemophilic arthropathy. An overview of
        20 years experience. Clin Orthop Relat Res 1989; (242): 60-82.
        [PMID: 2650951]

[5]   Beeton K, Rodriguez-Merchan EC, Alltree J. Total joint arthroplasty in haemophilia. Haemophilia
        2000; 6(5): 474-81.
        [http://dx.doi.org/10.1046/j.1365-2516.2000.00443.x] [PMID: 11012688]

[6]   Mann HA, Choudhury MZ, Allen DJ, Lee CA, Goddard NJ. Current approaches in haemophilic
        arthropathy of the hip. Haemophilia 2009; 15(3): 659-64.
        [http://dx.doi.org/10.1111/j.1365-2516.2007.01563.x] [PMID: 19298385]

[7]   Kelley SS, Lachiewicz PF, Gilbert MS, Bolander ME, Jankiewicz JJ. Hip arthroplasty in hemophilic
        arthropathy. J Bone Joint Surg Am 1995; 77(6): 828-34.
        [http://dx.doi.org/10.2106/00004623-199506000-00003] [PMID: 7782355]

[8]   Löfqvist T, Sanzen L, Petersson C, Nilsson IM. Total hip replacement in patients with haemophilia.
        Acta Orthop Scand 1996; 67: 321.
        [http://dx.doi.org/10.3109/17453679609002323] [PMID: 8792731]

[9]   Nelson IW, Sivamurugan S, Latham PD, Matthews J, Bulstrode CJ. Total hip arthroplasty for
        hemophilic arthropathy. Clin Orthop Relat Res 1992; (276): 210-3.
        [PMID: 1537155]

[10]   Heeg M, Meyer K, Smid WM, Van Horn JR, Van der Meer J. Total knee and hip arthroplasty in
        haemophilic patients. Haemophilia 1998; 4(5): 747-51.
        [http://dx.doi.org/10.1046/j.1365-2516.1998.00183.x] [PMID: 9873881]

[11]   Carulli C, Felici I, Martini C, et al. Total hip arthroplasty in haemophilic patients with modern
        cementless implants. J Arthroplasty 2015; 30(10): 1757-60.
        [http://dx.doi.org/10.1016/j.arth.2015.04.035] [PMID: 25998131]

[12]   Masonis JL, Bourne RB. Surgical approach, abductor function, and total hip arthroplasty dislocation.
        Clin Orthop Relat Res 2002; (405): 46-53.
        [http://dx.doi.org/10.1097/00003086-200212000-00006] [PMID: 12461355]

[13]   Demos HA, Rorabeck CH, Bourne RB, MacDonald SJ, McCalden RW. Instability in primary total hip
        arthroplasty with the direct lateral approach. Clin Orthop Relat Res 2001; (393): 168-80.
        [http://dx.doi.org/10.1097/00003086-200112000-00020] [PMID: 11764347]

[14]   Panotopoulos J, Ay C, Schuh R, et al. Comparison of metal on metal *versus* polyethylene-ceramic
        bearing in uncemented total hip arthroplasty in patients with haemophilic arthropathy. Int Orthop
        2014; 38(7): 1369-73.
        [http://dx.doi.org/10.1007/s00264-014-2326-x] [PMID: 24728266]

[15]   Miles J, Rodríguez-Merchán EC, Goddard NJ. The impact of haemophilia on the success of total hip
        arthroplasty. Haemophilia 2008; 14(1): 81-4.
        [PMID: 18034823]

[16]   Yoo MC, Cho YJ, Kim KI, Ramteke A, Chun YS. The outcome of cementless total hip arthroplasty in
        haemophilic hip arthropathy. Haemophilia 2009; 15(3): 766-73.
        [http://dx.doi.org/10.1111/j.1365-2516.2009.01986.x] [PMID: 19444974]

[17]   Sikkema T, Boerboom AL, Meijer K. A comparison between the complications and long-term
        outcome of hip and knee replacement therapy in patients with and without haemophilia; a controlled
        retrospective cohort study. Haemophilia 2011; 17(2): 300-3.
        [http://dx.doi.org/10.1111/j.1365-2516.2010.02408.x] [PMID: 21070490]

[18]   Wang K, Street A, Dowrick A, Liew S. Clinical outcomes and patient satisfaction following total joint
        replacement in haemophilia23-year experience in knees, hips and elbows. Haemophilia 2012; 18(1):
        86-93.
        [http://dx.doi.org/10.1111/j.1365-2516.2011.02579.x] [PMID: 21649799]

[19] Lee SH, Rhyu KH, Cho YJ, Yoo MC, Chun YS. Cementless total hip arthroplasty for haemophilic arthropathy: follow-up result of more than 10 years. Haemophilia 2015; 21(1): e54-8.
[http://dx.doi.org/10.1111/hae.12544] [PMID: 25296853]

[20] DeLee JG, Charnley J. Radiological demarcation of cemented sockets in total hip replacement. Clin Orthop Relat Res 1976; (121): 20-32.
[PMID: 991504]

[21] Gruen TA, McNeice GM, Amstutz HC. Modes of failure of cemented stem-type femoral components: a radiographic analysis of loosening. Clin Orthop Relat Res 1979; (141): 17-27.
[PMID: 477100]

[22] Brooker AF, Bowerman JW, Robinson RA, Riley LH Jr. Ectopic ossification following total hip replacement. Incidence and a method of classification. J Bone Joint Surg Am 1973; 55(8): 1629-32.
[http://dx.doi.org/10.2106/00004623-197355080-00006] [PMID: 4217797]

[23] Hilliard P, Funk S, Zourikian N, *et al.* Hemophilia joint health score reliability study. Haemophilia 2006; 12(5): 518-25.
[http://dx.doi.org/10.1111/j.1365-2516.2006.01312.x] [PMID: 16919083]

CHAPTER 13

The Management of Foot and Ankle Arthropathy

E. Carlos Rodriguez-Merchan[*]

Department of Orthopedic Surgery, La Paz University Hospital, Madrid, Spain

Abstract: The primary prophylaxis is the best way to protect haemophilic patients from synovitis and arthropathy in foot and ankle. By the replacement of the deficient factor, haemophiliacs requiring orthopedic surgery of the foot and ankle may successfully and safely undergo such type of surgery. Radiosynovectomy is a very effective procedure able to induce the decrease of frequency and intensity of bleedings related to synovitis. On average, the number of haemarthroses may diminishes up to 65%. If three consecutive radiosynovectomy procedures, repeated at six-month intervals, fail to lessen the synovitis, arthroscopy should be performed. In such cases, large osteophytes may develop on the anterior aspect of distal, causing severe pain and impingement. Open or arthroscopic osteophyte removal (queilectomy) should be considered. Achilles tendon lengthening in cases of fixed equinus deformity represents another common procedure in haemophilic subjects. In the case of advanced haemophilic arthropathy of the ankle, the first option is the arthroscopic debridement. In severe cases three further options are available: ankle distraction by means of external fixation (arthrodiastasis), ankle fusion (tibiotalar and/or subtalar), and total ankle replacement.

Keywords: Ankle fusion, Arthropathy, Arthroscopic synovectomy, Conservative treatment, Chemical synovectomy, Foot and ankle, Haemophilia, Rehabilitation, Radiosynovectomy, Removal of osteophytes, Surgical treatment, Total ankle replacement.

INTRODUCTION

In haemophilic patients, the foot (mainly the subtalar joint) and the ankle (tibiotalar joint) are prone to bleedings starting from the age of 2 years, resulting in foot and ankle haemophilic arthropathy [1](Figs. **1** and **2**).

Several deformities affect the tibiotalar and subtalar joints: fixed plantar flexion, related to alteration of the anterior region of the ankle; varus hindfoot, due to a malalignment of the subtalar joint; and ankle valgus rotation, caused by an

---

[*] **Corresponding author E. Carlos Rodriguez-Merchan:** Department of Orthopedic Surgery, La Paz University Hospital, Madrid, Spain; Tel: +32-2 893 24 70; E-mail: ecrmerchan@gmx.es

Christian Carulli (Ed.)

overgrowth of the distal tibial epyphisis during adolescence or progressive arthropathy during maturity [1 - 4]. These conditions may start after a single or recurrent hemarthroses, and are often extremely painful: adequate treatments may induce a full correction of the affected joint. The result of this progression is an antalgic position in equinus or plantar flexion, that eventually becomes fixed.

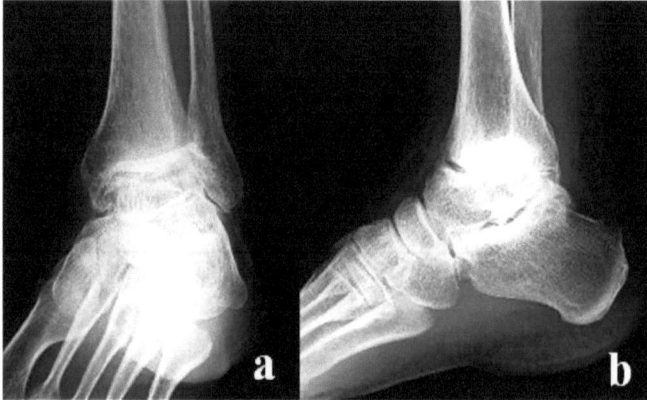

Fig. (1). Radiographs of a haemophilic patient showing severe arthropathy (narrowing of the joint space) of the tibiotalar and subtalar joints: (a) anteroposterior view, (b) lateral view.

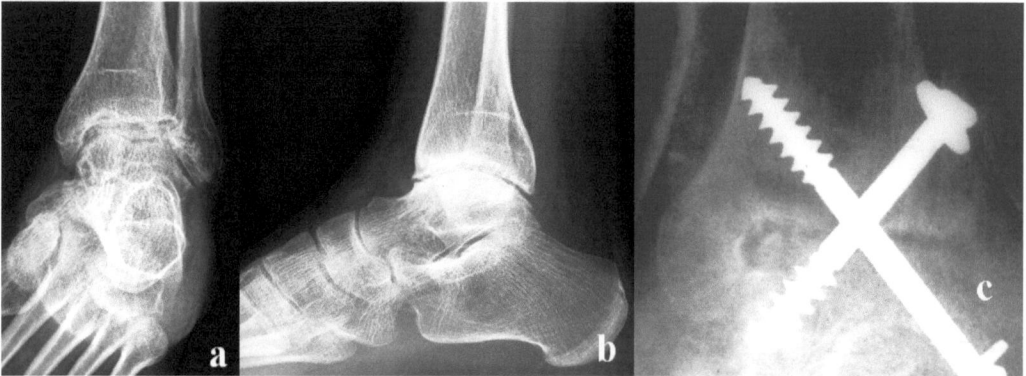

Fig. (2). Radiographs of a haemophilic patient showing severe arthropathy (narrowing of the joint space) of the tibiotalar joint. A tibiotalar fusion by means of two crossed screws was performed due to intense ankle pain: (a) anteroposterior and (b) lateral preoperative radiograph, (c) anteroposterior postoperative view.

Tibiotalar joint is often the first target joint in Haemophilia, with onset of joint bleedings as children start to stand and walk. Advanced ankle arthropathy is common in patients affected by severe Haemophilia since the early adulthood [4 - 8]. Abutting anterior exostoses on the distal tibia and talus usually develop and are associated with equinus deformity [7]. Growth asymmetry can result in a lateral tilt of the distal tibia and valgus malalignment. Patients complaining mild to moderate pain are successfully treated by ankle orthoses (e.g., stirrup air splint). Symptomatic and incapacitated patients, on the other hand, may require further procedures as arthroscopic debridement, arthrodesis, or total ankle replacement (TAR) [1, 5, 9].

In this chapter, the most important therapeutic approaches for the management of haemophilic arthropathy of foot and ankle are reviewed.

CONSERVATIVE TREATMENTS

Conservative treatments are represented by: radiosynovectomy (RS), chemical synovectomy, and rehabilitation (physiotherapy, splints, braces, wedge insoles). Such options should always be attempted prior to surgery [1 - 6, 10 - 17].

Radiosynovectomy

RS associated to primary prophylaxis can help to halt haemophilic synovitis. RS is a relatively simple, virtually painless and inexpensive treatment in case of chronic haemophilic synovitis, even in patients with inhibitors. RS finds its rationale in the necrotic effect on synovial tissue induced by intraarticular injections of a radioactive agent (usually Rhenium-186) (Fig. **3**). Radioactive substances have been for many years used for the treatment of chronic synovitis.

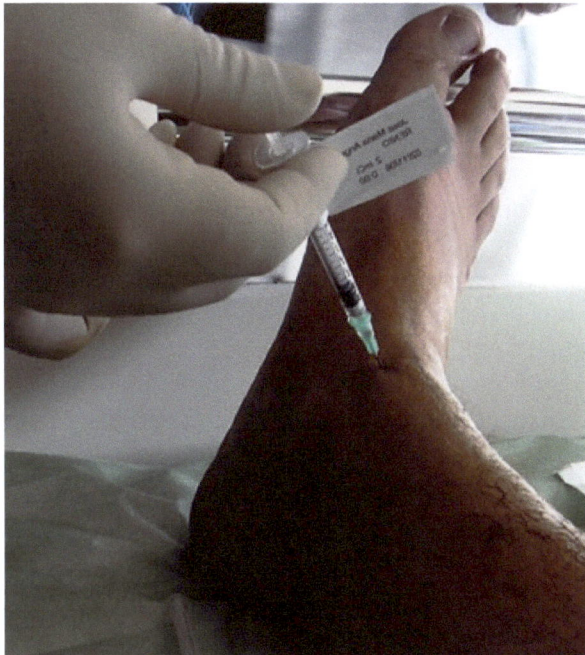

Fig. (3). Clinical view of a radiosynovectomy in a patient with Haemophilia.

The indication for an RS is chronic haemophilic synovitis associated with recurrent hemarthroses, unresponsive to the haematological treatment. Specifically it represents the first efficient procedure to be considered for the ankle, and it can be performed in the outpatient office [13 - 15]. RS may be surely considered an effective, safe, minimally invasive, easy-to-perform, and well tolerated procedure for the treatment of chronic synovitis: it may decrease the number of bleedings up to 65%.

Chemical Synovectomy

Radossi *et al* [16] published their series of 28 haemophilic patients treated by intraarticular injections of rifampicine. Their mean age was 34 years and five patients had inhibitors to factor VIII (three high responders and two low responders). Rifampicine (250 mg) was diluted in 10mL of saline solution and 1-5mL was then injected into the joint once a week for 5 weeks. The follow-up ranged from 6 to 24 months. Thirty-five joints were treated by a total of 169 injections. Twenty-four procedures were considered effective in 19 patients according to the evaluation scales, while six were associated to fair or poor results. In four joints the results were good, while in the two remaining joints the results were poor.

There are two main limitations for the use of rifampicine in the treatment of synovectomy: the procedure is painful, and it should be repeated weekly for many weeks to be effective.

Rehabilitation

The importance of preoperative and postoperative rehabilitation of the ankle in Haemophilia must be emphasized. Children have to utilize the available resources and seek an early consultation with their rehabilitation physician. Several rehabilitative techniques and application have been shown to accelerate recovery, reduce pain, and prevent contractures. Moreover, rehabilitation is important in the functional recovery of the ankle in patients following surgical procedures, and in such cases the specialist should work closely with the orthopedic surgeon [17].

SURGICAL TREATMENT

The most common surgical approaches performed in the ankle are the following: queilectomy, Achilles tendon lengthening, arthroscopic synovectomy, arthroscopic debridement, ankle distraction (arthrodiastasis), tibiotalar and/or subtalar arthrodesis, and TAR [1 - 7, 10 - 13, 18 - 24].

As mentioned before, when RS fails to control synovitis, an arthroscopic synovectomy should be indicated [13 - 15]. Another common procedure to correct a fixed equinus deformity is Achilles tendon lengthening (Fig. **4**) [7].

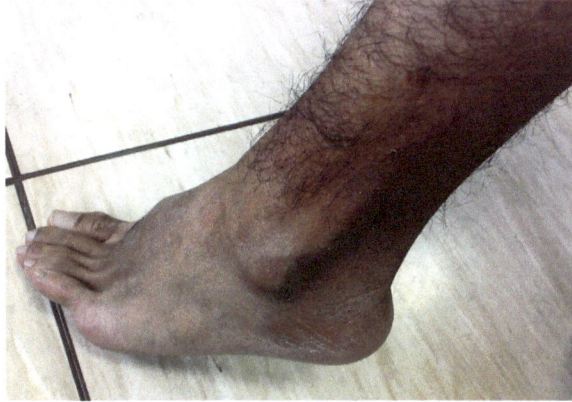

Fig. (4). Clinical view of the foot and ankle of a haemophilic patient showing a severe equinus deformity.

Often a large osteophyte develops on the anterior aspect of the distal tibia causing severe pain and impingement. The surgical removal of the osteophyte by open or arthroscopic queilectomy may be indicated (Fig. **5**). In cases of a significant malalignment in the ankle, a supramalleolar valgus or varus osteotomy may be performed [1, 4].

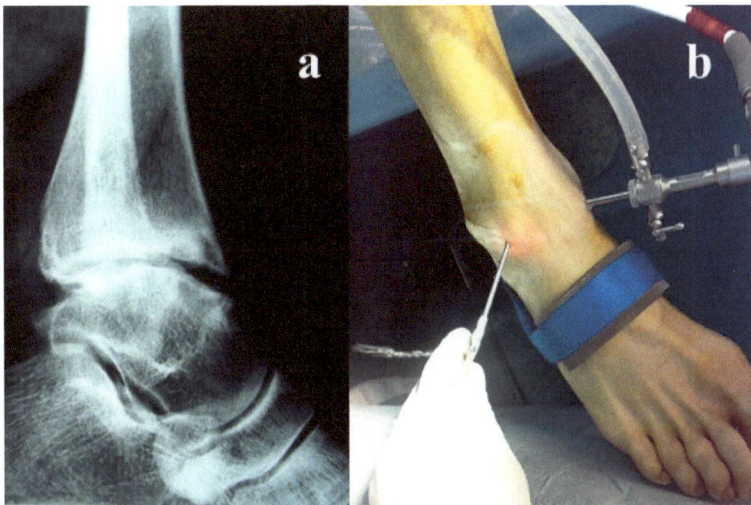

Fig. (5). Haemophilic patient with anterior ankle pain due to a large anterior osteophyte that was arthroscopically removed: (a) lateral preoperative radiograph, (b) intraoperative view of the arthroscopic removal of the osteophyte.

In advanced haemophilic arthropathy, several approaches may be considered: ankle distraction (by means of an external fixator), tibiotalar and/or subtalar arthrodesis Fig. (**6**), or TAR [9, 18, 21 - 24]. The main indications for these are represented by: intractable pain not reduced by alternative treatments, and severe deformity. Ankle arthrodesis has been associated with better long-term results with respect to TAR, that is rarely performed nowadays in haemophilic patients [18, 21, 24].

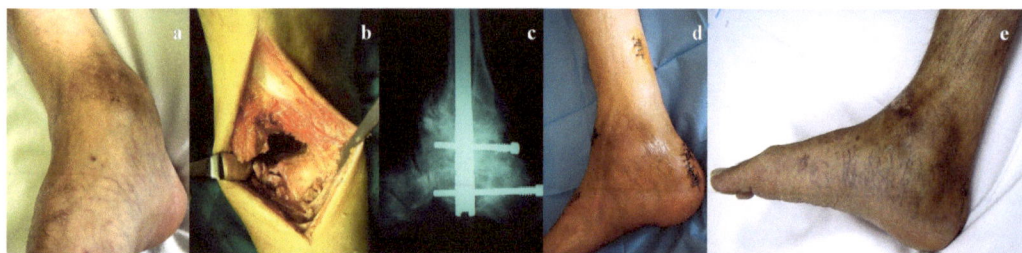

Fig. (6). The ankle of the haemophilic patient of Fig. (**1**) was treated by fusion of the tibiotalar and subtalar joints by means of a retrograde locked intramedullary nail: (a) clinical preoperative view of the ankle; (b) intraoperative view of the ankle fusion; (c) lateral radiograph showing the nail; (d) clinical view just before the removal of surgical staples; (e) clinical view 6 months later after achieving a satisfactory fusion of both joints.

Van Meegeren *et al* reported their experience on three haemophilic patients affected by ankle arthropathy and treated by joint distraction using an Ilizarov external fixator [25]. All patients were very satisfied with the clinical outcomes obtained by this procedure. They reported dramatic improvements for their self-perceived functional ability and autonomy, pain relief, and participation in social life activities. Furthermore, a partial joint mobility was preserved. They concluded that joint distraction may be considered a promising treatment for selected cases of ankle arthropathy related to Haemophilia.

Gamble *et al* [11] reported 10 tibiotalar fusions in eight patients using several techniques. Eight ankles attained fusion and two had painless non-union. Thirty-four tibiotalar fusions were performed at the authors´ center, with one painless non-union. No patients in either series developed infection or had recurrent haemarthrosis at 1- to 18-year follow-up.

Tsailas and Wiedel evaluated the results of internal fixation in haemophilic arthropathy of the ankle and subtalar joint from 1983 to 2006 [9]. Twenty fusions were performed in 13 patients showing advanced arthropathy: in 11 cases an ankle fusion was made; in one case isolated subtalar fusion was performed, while the remainders were combined fusions. Three of the latter underwent a staged subtalar fusion after the index operation. The mean age at the time of the first surgery was 38.7 years, and the mean follow-up was 9.4 years. In most cases, the fusion was achieved by two crossing screws. For the subtalar joint, either staples and screws were used, occasionally extended to the calcaneus. Arthrodesis of the ankle was successful in all but one subject: this patient underwent to a revision obtaining the fusion. There was also one case of painless non-union of the subtalar joint, not scheduled for revision. No recurrent bleeding and no cases of deep infection were recorded. The authors concluded that arthrodesis with cross screw fixation was an effective method for the fusion of the ankle and subtalar joints in patients with Haemophilia.

Mann *et al* described an original technique consisting in the combination of a medial approach to the ankle, medial malleolar osteotomy, bone grafting, and compression with staples [12]. All patients obtained an excellent pain relief and improved function and showed a bony union in the 100% of cases. All functional scores showed a significant improvement after ankle fusion and such technique was considered efficient and reproducible in this population.

Bai *et al* [22] reported the results of a series of ten patients undergoing an arthroscopically assisted ankle arthrodesis for the treatment of end-stage haemophilic arthropathy. The fusion rate was 100% and the average time to fusion was 10.5 weeks. A single case of a superficial wound infection occurred but good to excellent outcomes in 8 subjects (80%) and 2 (20%) fair results were reported. All patients were satisfied.

Tsukamoto *et al* [23] performed three arthroscopic ankle arthrodeses in two patients. The follow-up period ranged from 2 year and 4 months to 6 years and one month. Radiologic union was obtained in all cases, and recurrent joint bleedings stopped or were significantly reduced.

Asencio *et al* [24] reported their series of 21 patients (32 ankles) with haemophilic arthropathy undergoing TAR associated in some cases to additional surgical procedures. The mean follow-up was 4.4 years. The American Orthopaedic Foot and Ankle Society (AOFAS) ankle–hindfoot scale was used to evaluate pain, function, mobility, and alignment. The overall AOFAS score improved from 40.2 before surgery to 85.3 after surgery. The functional score increased from 23.6 to 35.9, and the dorsiflexion from 0.38 to 10.38. At the radiologic study, both tibial and talar components were stable and correctly placed in all ankles, as the alignment was satisfactory. Two patients later underwent to ankle arthrodesis.

The current literature is not definitive concerning the controversy on ankle arthrodesis or TAR in non-haemophilic patients [25]. Regarding Haemophilia, the uncertainty is even greater, as there is very little available literature. Based on all of these data, and on my 40 years of experience treating people with Haemophilia, my advice is to exhaust all types of non-surgical treatment. When surgical treatment is considered absolutely necessary, my recommendation is to preserve as much as possible the joint at all costs by an arthroscopic debridement or an arthrodiastasis with an external fixator, according to each surgeon's preferences. If these techniques fail in Haemophilia, when in doubt on whether to perform fusion or TAR, I would always opt for arthrodesis, as the current results for TAR quite frankly have much room for improvements. It is likely that in the mid-long term, new TAR designs will allow further advancements. On the other hand, it is really hard in Haemophilia to obtain definitive conclusions according to so limited study populations.

Whilst TAR can be a very effective procedure in patients with disabling ankle arthropathy, long-term outcomes may be poor and associated with a high failure rate at approximately 5 years [26]. TAR is of course a major problem in patients with Haemophilia and unlike the knee and the hip, where joint replacement is extremely successful with proven long-term outcomes, the ankle remains a yet unsolved problem.

CONCLUDING REMARKS

Prophylactic replacement therapy and rehabilitation are of paramount importance in order to lessen the development of foot and ankle synovitis and arthropathy. The haematological treatment could avoid the development of haemophilic arthropathy if the concentration of the deficient factor is prevented from falling below 1% with respect to normal values. An early treatment is crucial because the immature skeleton is very sensitive to the complications of Haemophilia as severe structural deficiencies may quickly develop. When synovitis develops in the ankle, radiosynovectomy should be performed before approaching an arthroscopic synovectomy. RS can be repeated up to three times with 6-month intervals. In case of failure or poor outcomes after RS, an arthroscopic synovectomy should be indicated. Only in late stages of tibiotalar and/or subtalar haemophilic arthropathy and severe and incapacitating pain, joint fusions should be carried out. Arthroscopic debridement and arthrodiastasis by means of an external fixator are attractive options to the more commonly used arthrodesis or total ankle arthroplasty.

CONFLICT OF INTEREST

The authors confirm that they have no conflict of interest to declare for this publication.

ACKNOWLEDGEMENTS

Declared none.

REFERENCES

[1] Rodriguez-Merchan EC. Orthopaedic problems about the ankle in hemophilia. J Foot Ankle Surg 2012; 51(6): 772-6.
[http://dx.doi.org/10.1053/j.jfas.2012.06.005] [PMID: 22785085]

[2] Chang TJ, Mohamed S, Hambleton J. Hemophilic arthropathy: considerations in management. J Am Podiatr Med Assoc 2001; 91(8): 406-14.
[http://dx.doi.org/10.7547/87507315-91-8-406] [PMID: 11574642]

[3] Luck JV, Lin JC, Kasper CK, Logan LJ. Orthopaedic management of hemophilic arthropathy. In: Chapman MV, Ed. Chapman's Orthopaedic Surgery. 3rd ed. Philadelphia, PA: Lippincott Williams & Wilkins 2001; pp. 3595-616.

[4] Rodriguez-Merchan EC. The haemophilic ankle. Haemophilia 2006; 12(4): 337-44.
[http://dx.doi.org/10.1111/j.1365-2516.2006.01285.x] [PMID: 16834732]

[5] Rodriguez-Merchan EC. Ankle surgery in haemophilia with special emphasis on arthroscopic debridement. Haemophilia 2008; 14(5): 913-9.
[http://dx.doi.org/10.1111/j.1365-2516.2008.01820.x] [PMID: 18637842]

[6] Pasta G, Forsyth A, Merchan CR, *et al.* Orthopaedic management of haemophilia arthropathy of the ankle. Haemophilia 2008; 14 (Suppl. 3): 170-6.
[http://dx.doi.org/10.1111/j.1365-2516.2008.01720.x] [PMID: 18510538]

[7] Wallny T, Brackmann H, Kraft C, Nicolay C, Pennekamp P. Achilles tendon lengthening for ankle equinus deformity in hemophiliacs: 23 patients followed for 124 years. Acta Orthop 2006; 77(1): 164-8.
[http://dx.doi.org/10.1080/17453670610045867] [PMID: 16534718]

[8] Löfqvist T, Petersson C, Nilsson IM. Radioactive synoviorthesis in patients with hemophilia with factor inhibitor. Clin Orthop Relat Res 1997; (343): 37-41.
[PMID: 9345203]

[9] Tsailas PG, Wiedel JD. Arthrodesis of the ankle and subtalar joints in patients with haemophilic arthropathy. Haemophilia 2010; 16(5): 822-31.
[http://dx.doi.org/10.1111/j.1365-2516.2010.02248.x] [PMID: 20398073]

[10] Panotopoulos J, Hanslik-Schnabel B, Wanivenhaus A, Trieb K. Outcome of surgical concepts in haemophilic arthropathy of the hindfoot. Haemophilia 2005; 11(5): 468-71.
[http://dx.doi.org/10.1111/j.1365-2516.2005.01133.x] [PMID: 16128890]

[11] Gamble JG, Bellah J, Rinsky LA, Glader B. Arthropathy of the ankle in hemophilia. J Bone Joint Surg Am 1991; 73(7): 1008-15.
[http://dx.doi.org/10.2106/00004623-199173070-00007] [PMID: 1908466]

[12] Mann HA, Biring GS, Choudhury MZ, Lee CA, Goddard NJ. Ankle arthropathy in the haemophilic patient: a description of a novel ankle arthrodesis technique. Haemophilia 2009; 15(2): 458-63.
[http://dx.doi.org/10.1111/j.1365-2516.2008.01651.x] [PMID: 19187197]

[13] Rodriguez-Merchan EC, De la Corte-Rodriguez H, Jimenez-Yuste V. Radiosynovectomy in haemophilia: long-term results of 500 procedures performed in a 38-year period. Thromb Res 2014; 134(5): 985-90.
[http://dx.doi.org/10.1016/j.thromres.2014.08.023] [PMID: 25240555]

[14] De la Corte-Rodriguez H, Rodriguez-Merchan EC, Jimenez-Yuste V. Radiosynovectomy in hemophilia: quantification of its effectiveness through the assessment of 10 articular parameters. J Thromb Haemost 2011; 9(5): 928-35.
[http://dx.doi.org/10.1111/j.1538-7836.2011.04246.x] [PMID: 21352468]

[15]   de la Corte-Rodriguez H, Rodriguez-Merchan EC, Jimenez-Yuste V. What patient, joint and isotope characteristics influence the response to radiosynovectomy in patients with haemophilia? Haemophilia 2011; 17(5): e990-8.
[PMID: 21535325]

[16]   Radossi P, Baggio R, Petris U, *et al.* Intra-articular rifamycin in haemophilic arthropathy. Haemophilia 2003; 9(1): 60-3.
[http://dx.doi.org/10.1046/j.1365-2516.2003.00703.x] [PMID: 12558780]

[17]   De la Corte-Rodriguez H, Rodriguez-Merchan EC. The role of physical medicine and rehabilitation in haemophiliac patients. Blood Coagul Fibrinolysis 2013; 24(1): 1-9.
[http://dx.doi.org/10.1097/MBC.0b013e32835a72f3] [PMID: 23103725]

[18]   van der Heide HJ, Nováková I, de Waal Malefijt MC. The feasibility of total ankle prosthesis for severe arthropathy in haemophilia and prothrombin deficiency. Haemophilia 2006; 12(6): 679-82.
[http://dx.doi.org/10.1111/j.1365-2516.2006.01350.x] [PMID: 17083522]

[19]   Greene WB. Synovectomy of the ankle for hemophilic arthropathy. J Bone Joint Surg Am 1994; 76(6): 812-9.
[http://dx.doi.org/10.2106/00004623-199406000-00004] [PMID: 8200887]

[20]   Dunn AL, Busch MT, Wyly JB, Sullivan KM, Abshire TC. Arthroscopic synovectomy for hemophilic joint disease in a pediatric population. J Pediatr Orthop 2004; 24(4): 414-26.
[http://dx.doi.org/10.1097/01241398-200407000-00013] [PMID: 15205625]

[21]   Barg A, Elsner A, Hefti D, Hintermann B. Haemophilic arthropathy of the ankle treated by total ankle replacement: a case series. Haemophilia 2010; 16(4): 647-55.
[PMID: 20331757]

[22]   Bai Z, Zhang E, He Y, Yan X, Sun H, Zhang M. Arthroscopic ankle arthrodesis in hemophilic arthropathy. Foot Ankle Int 2013; 34(8): 1147-51.
[http://dx.doi.org/10.1177/1071100713481775] [PMID: 23478887]

[23]   Tsukamoto S, Tanaka Y, Matsuda T, *et al.* Arthroscopic ankle arthrodesis for hemophilic arthropathy: two cases report. Foot 2011; 21(2): 103-5.
[http://dx.doi.org/10.1016/j.foot.2011.01.001] [PMID: 21295463]

[24]   Asencio JG, Leonardi C, Biron-Andreani C, Schved JF. Short-term and mid-term outcome of total ankle replacement in haemophilic patients. Foot Ankle Surg 2014; 20(4): 285-92.
[http://dx.doi.org/10.1016/j.fas.2014.08.004] [PMID: 25457668]

[25]   Van Meegeren ME, Van Veghel K, De Kleijn P, *et al.* Joint distraction results in clinical and structural improvement of haemophilic ankle arthropathy: a series of three cases. Haemophilia 2012; 18(5): 810-7.
[http://dx.doi.org/10.1111/j.1365-2516.2012.02805.x] [PMID: 22530605]

[26]   Rodriguez-Merchan EC. End-stage haemophilic arthropathy of the ankle: ankle fusion or total ankle replacement. Haemophilia 2014; 20(1): e106-7.
[http://dx.doi.org/10.1111/hae.12323] [PMID: 24354482]

CHAPTER 14

Elbow Arthroplasty

Massimo Ceruso[1,*], **Marco Biondi**[2], **Prospero Bigazzi**[1] and **Sandra Pfanner**[1]

[1] *Hand Surgery and Reconstructive Microsurgery Unit, AOU-Careggi, Florence, Italy*

[2] *Orthopaedic Clinic, University of Florence, Florence, Italy*

Abstract: The elbow is the second most commonly affected joint in haemophilic patients. As for other target joints, the strategy of treatment starts from a medical management, and in case of failure, more specific approaches have to be chosen. Radioactive or chemical synovectomy represent valid options but may not be adequate in moderate arthropathies. In such cases, surgical procedures as arthroscopic or open synovectomy are useful. Advanced haemophilic arthropathy of the elbow may be severely disabling, particularly for younger patients. In these conditions, a total elbow replacement may be a good option. Thanks to modern implant designs and materials, this procedure has shown excellent clinical outcomes and an acceptable survival rate. Nevertheless, it remains a complex surgery and considering the postoperative restrictions and risks, it requires a careful selection of patients.

Keywords: Elbow arthritis, Elbow arthroplasty, Haemophilia, Haemophilic elbow, Stiff elbow, Total elbow replacement.

INTRODUCTION

The elbow is the second most commonly affected joint in haemophilic patients and the most frequent target joint in the upper extremity [1]. Its involvement can be particularly disabling due to its physiological role in positioning the hand in space. In contrast to knees and ankles, however there are limited informations regarding the arthropathy of the elbow in Haemophilia. Longitudinal studies suggest that the arthropathy of elbows may induce severe functional impairments in children since 5 years of age [2]. There is a strong debate on the frequency of the involvement of dominant or non-dominant elbow, even if about half of the patients have a bilateral disease [1, 3 - 5]. The pathophysiology of haemophilic arthropathy starts with recurrent intraarticular bleedings [4], but little is known about the length of the process, frequency, and number of haemarthroses needed to induce the joint compromission [6]. The elbow is exposed to haemathrosis

---

* **Corresponding author Massimo Ceruso:** Hand Surgery and Reconstructive Microsurgery Unit, AOU Careggi, Florence, Italy; Tel: +393356142332; E-mail: cerusom@tin.it

Christian Carulli (Ed.)

firstly due to its anatomical characteristics: it is a diarthrodial hinged joint, as the knee and ankle, with a large amount of synovial tissue, main target of the blood [3, 7, 8]. A concomitant involvement of a joint in the lower legs makes elbow arthropathy more prone to develop disability and symptoms: the use of crutches shifts the elbow from a non-bearing to a bearing one.

CLINICAL SETTINGS AND INDICATIONS

In the acute setting of a haemarthrosis, the joint is swollen, painful, and warm, with limited range of motion (ROM) and strength. The first approach is typically the factor replacement, crucial to induce a partial to full remission. Ice, rest, and pain control are useful to let the elbow returning to a normal condition in days or weeks [9].

Subacute phases of arthropathy are characterized by a persistent joint swelling with decreased motion due to proliferative synovitis. Synovial hyperplasia results in recurrent bleedings. The reduction of such condition is thus the key to prevent recurrence of intraarticular haemorrhages, and the consequent worsening of chondral damage

In chronic stages, haemophilic arthropathy shows osteoarticular changes, cartilage loss, and juxta-articular cysts: ligamentous and capsular fibrosis also develop [10] (Fig. **1**).

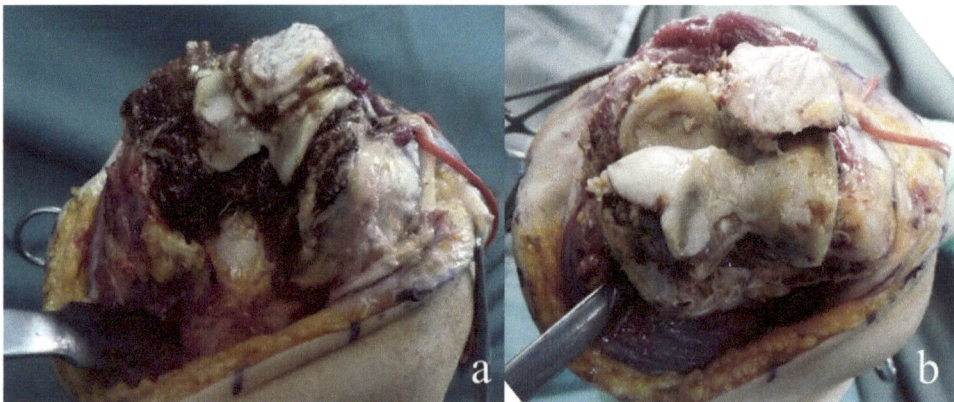

Fig. (1). Intraoperative aspect of the right elbow of a 30-years old haemophilic patient. Synovial proliferation (a) and cartilage erosions (b).

The physical examination of the haemophilic elbow may lead to suspect the presence of synovitis, while deformity and malalignment are evident. Palpation maneuvers help to assess effusion and tenderness. Active and passive ROM is measured and recorded taking care to detect whether limitations are due to a soft tissue interposition or bony impingement. Typically, the first motion to decrease is pronation and supination due to a radio-capitellum involvement, although an extension gap shows a significant reduction related to flexion contractures [11, 12].

Neurologic and vascular examination should be carefully carried out. Peripheral nerve entrapments are relatively frequent in patients with Haemophilia with rates ranging from 4% to 19% [13, 14]. These conditions are generally caused by an extrinsic compression due to intramuscular, intraneural, or intraarticular haemorrhages or pseudotumor.

From a radiological point of view, joint changes in the elbow vary from 25% to 87% [3, 15]. Findings include enlargement of the epiphysis, osteoporosis, and subchondral irregularities. Radial head enlargement or splaying is commonly observed [16] (Fig. **2**).

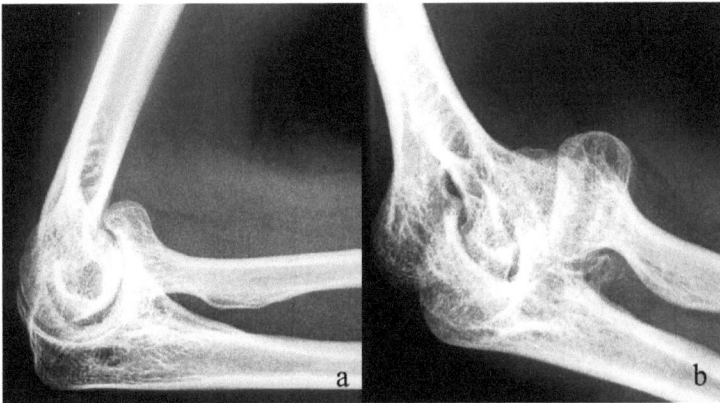

Fig. (2). Radiological signs of haemophilic arthropathy of the elbow: radial head splaying, narrowing of the joint space, articular erosions with chondral irregularity, and subchondral cysts (a). Oblique radial head view showing the predominant involvement of radial side (b).

Obliteration of the capitello-condylar groove, widening of the olecranon fossa, narrowing of the joint, and erosions with cysts are other common radiological signs. Joint deformity, major erosions, and bone fusion develop as advanced findings.

A radiologic study should be obtained, providing AP, lateral, and 45° oblique views MRI is useful to detect early joint changes and synovitis, although it is not routinely necessary. CT scans are helpful for the assessment of bony hypertrophic changes and for the surgical planning (see chapter 6).

SURGICAL OPTIONS

Approaching a haemophilic patient, it is important to consider the number and frequency of bleedings, as well as the pattern and response to factor replacement therapy. Patients with chronic synovitis associated with recurrent haemarthroses (symptomatic or not) may be successfully managed by a surgical synovectomy Fig. (**3**) or chemical/radioactive synoviorthesis (see chapter 8).

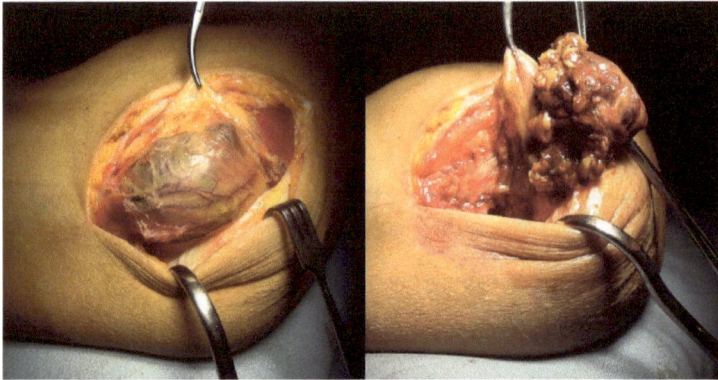

Fig. (3). Open synovectomy of the elbow in a 32-years old haemophilic patient. Intraoperative classical findings are synovial hypertrophy with hemosiderin deposits and articular erosions.

ROM commonly improves after a surgical approach, whereas it rarely does after a synoviorthesis [9, 17]. Both arthroscopic and open synovectomy seem to be successful in limiting bleeding episodes, improving pain and motion [9, 18, 19]. However, the progression of joint erosions does not seem to be halted by synovectomy alone [10, 18]. Recent series reported that open or arthroscopic debridement associated with radial head resection have a beneficial effect on ROM, especially for pronation and supination [20] (Fig. **4**).

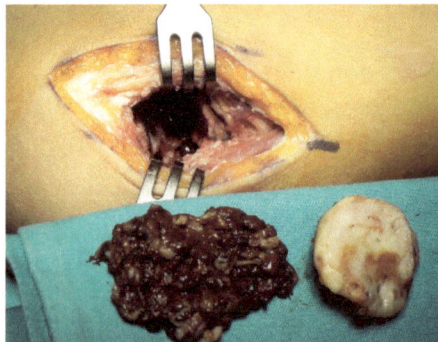

Fig. (4). Open synovectomy of the elbow in a 32-years old haemophilic patient. Intraoperative classical findings are the synovial hypertrophy with haemosiderin deposits and articular erosions.

Such limitation in fact causes a considerable impairment in the daily life activities such as eating and personal hygiene.

On the other hand, in case of advanced, severe arthropathy with fixed ROM involving also flexion and extension, a joint arthroplasty should be considered (Fig. **5**).

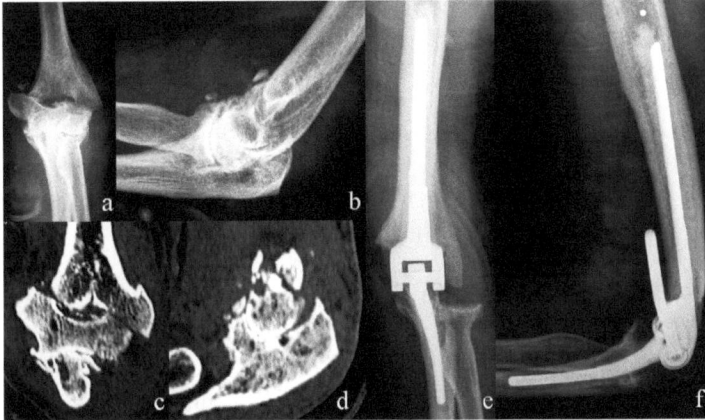

Fig. (5). AP and lateral radiographs of a left elbow showing a supracondylar fracture in advanced haemophilic joint deformity (a,b). TC scan images (c,d). Due to the concomitant severe arthropathy any fixation was excluded. AP and lateral radiographs after a total elbow arthroplasty (e,f).

Little data on the outcome after total elbow arthroplasty (TEA) in Haemophilia are available: most of them are small retrospective series [21 - 32].

Luck and Kasper [28] reviewed their 20-year results of surgical management of severely affected haemophiliacs, reporting only two patients treated by a primary TEA. One was early removed for an early infection, the second showed good outcomes at long term.

Beeton *et al* [27] in their review on the outcome of all joint arthroplasty procedures in haemophiliacs mentioned only two case reports related to an elbow prosthesis.

Kasten and Skinner [29] described only one case of Haemophilia in their large series of TEAs. This was complicated by an aseptic loosening of both components needing a revision surgery.

Chapman-Sheath *et al* [22] reported seven TEAs in 5 patients affected by severe Haemophilia A, with a minimum follow-up of 25 months. Four elbows were managed by the use of unconstrained implants. Three other cases were treated by semiconstrained implants. Complications included one ulnar nerve paralysis, one axillary vein thrombosis, and one late septic loosening (treated by revision with a semiconstrained implant). All patients demonstrated excellent results in terms of pain relief and functional improvement.

Kamineni *et al* [21] described 5 patients undergoing TEA with a mean follow-up of 5.8 years. Three complications were recorded: one case of uncontrollable haemorrhage, one case of deep infection, and one case of persistent pain.

Vochteloo *et al* [31] recently reported a series of 8 TEAs in 5 haemophilic patients. All elbows showed significant functional improvements associated with acceptable survival rates. Revision surgery was performed in 3 elbows: one for a deep infection after a posttraumatic bleeding (44 months after the index operation); one for aseptic loosening of the ulnar component 10 years after TEA; finally, one for an aseptic loosening after 9 years.

Previous series reported high complications rates associated [28]: however, in these experiences, first generation of rigid hinged implants were used, classically more prone to early loosening rates [29]. Recent data suggest good outcomes for TEA in the haemophilic population [30 - 32], although such type of surgery in these patients is at higher risk of complications due to the severe anatomical changes, poor bone quality, and infective comorbidities. Kimineni and colleagues [21] also highlighted several difficulties associated with the intraoperative course in these patients. In one patient, the humeral and ulnar canals were sclerotic and obliterated, and placement of reamers and components required the use of high-speed drills for canal preparation. A second patient had a very small canal requiring additional care for the positioning of the implant.

Infections have been reported as more frequent compared to the general population. Whether these infections are related to HIV infection or self-injection therapy with clotting factor is still a matter of debate [33, 34]. However, antiretroviral therapy has improved the life expectancy of HIV-positive patients.

CHOICE OF IMPLANT AND SURGICAL TECHNIQUE

TEA is a technically demanding procedure in all patients, but generally more complex in haemophilic subjects. Moreover, patients' compliance to post-operative indications and activity restrictions is mandatory. For these reasons only selected and highly collaborative patients should be scheduled for such type of surgery. In addition, complications following TEA can be particularly disabling and revision surgery can be extremely challenging [35, 36]. The most common complications are aseptic loosening, infection, bushing wear, and neurologic lesions [37]. Other complications are implant failure, triceps insufficiency, and surgical wound problems. A clear knowledge of the local anatomy and kinematics, combined to a proper surgical technique help surgeons to reduce these inconveniences.

The choice of the proper implant is crucial. Since the first generation TEA was introduced by Dee in 1972 [38], different designs have been later released. These can be divided into two major groups: linked or unlinked prostheses.

In linked implants, humeral and ulnar components are physically connected. At the beginning this connection was a constrained design with no joint laxity, and leading to early mechanical failures due to an inappropriate mechanical stress transmission through the cement-bone implant interface. The second generation of linked implants was characterized by semiconstrained designs with a sloppy hinge allowing some degree of varus-valgus and prono-supination motions between the components. This allowed a transfer of forces from the implant to the adjacent soft tissues, mimicking the natural relationship of a native elbow, and lowering the rates of failure. The laxity of the hinge is able to reduce the incidence of aseptic loosening, even if its inherent stability is independent from the surrounding capsular and ligamentous structures. For these reasons, a semi-constrained implant can be the proper solution in cases of severe bone and soft tissues alterations, as in Haemophilia Fig. (**6**).

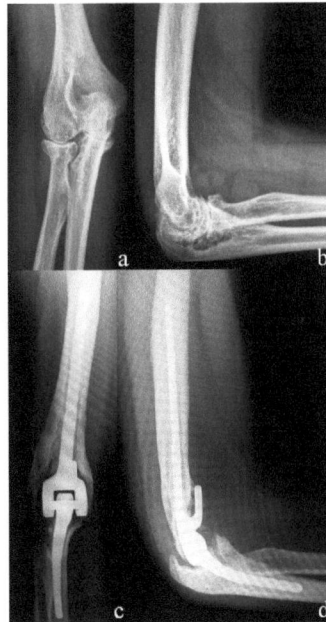

Fig. (6). A right elbow in a 30-years old patient. He complained severe pain, bleedings, and disability in daily life activities. Preoperative radiographs show signs of haemophilic arthropathy: radial head splaying, narrowing of the joint space, articular erosions with chondral irregularity, and subchondral cysts (a,b). X-rays at 4 years after TEA (c,d).

In unlinked implants, humeral and ulnar components are not mechanically linked. The stability of the implant relies on the matching shapes of the bearing surfaces, with the contribute of an adequate bone stock, and soft tissue support. It is less indicated when the elbow anatomy is grossly altered, such as in rheumatoid and haemophilic arthritis.

A proper surgical approach is also important in order to obtain a good exposure not affecting an early postoperative rehabilitation [39]. A posterior approach with a skin incision just medial or lateral to the olecranon is helpful to avoid wound complications (Fig. **7**).

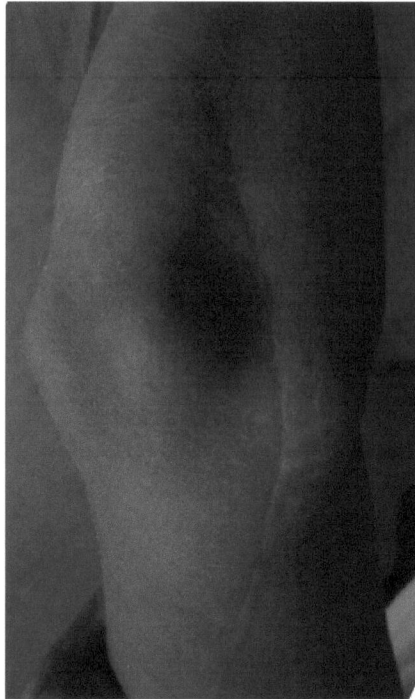

Fig. (7). Skin incision should be performed lateral or medial to the olecranon to avoid excessive wound stress and consequent dehiscence.

Several surgical posterior approaches have been proposed: the common goal is to achieve a wide exposure with preservation of the triceps, avoiding olecranon osteotomy, and respecting the skin coverage [40]. Recent elbow implants allow a triceps-on approach, which offers several advantages: the extensor mechanism is protected, no postoperative ROM restriction is prescribed, and early functional motion is easier to be performed. Disadvantages of such approach are related to the higher complexity compared to other techniques, and a limited exposure of the joint (Fig. **8**).

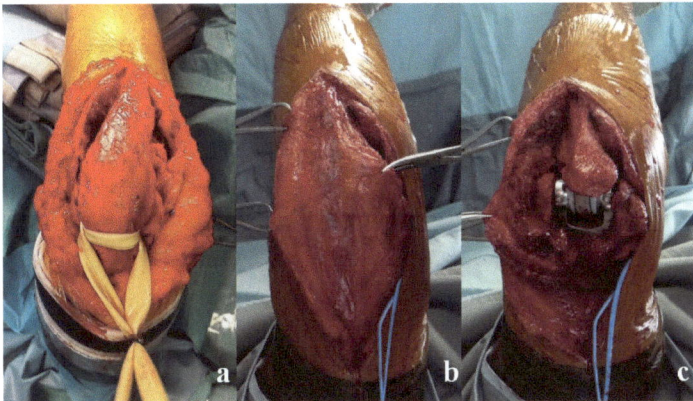

Fig. (8). Surgical approaches for TEA. Triceps-on access (a): the extensor mechanism is left attached to the olecranon, resulting in a more limited exposure but a faster postoperative recovery. Classical posterior Bryan-Morey approach (b,c): reflection of the triceps from medial to lateral, beginning at the medial intermuscular septum and in continuity with the fascia of the forearm and the periosteum. A wide exposure is ensured maintaining the muscle continuity of the extensor mechanism with the forearm fascio-ulnar- periosteal complex.

Olecranon osteotomy, which is a standard procedure in the treatment of articular elbow fractures, should be avoided for the risk of non union, malunion, and residual pain.

The ulnar nerve must be isolated and carefully protected at the beginning of the surgical procedure (Fig. **9**).

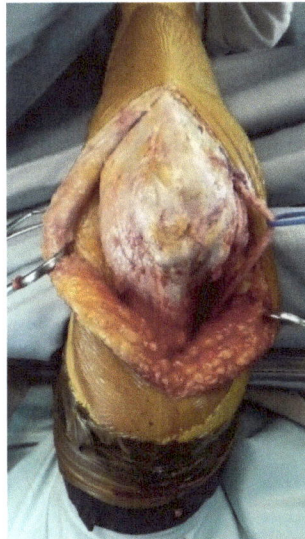

Fig. (9). Ulnar nerve isolation and protection at the beginning of the surgical procedure, and anteriorly transposition at the end of TEA.

Marshall Brooks *et al* [32] reported the ulnar neuropathy as the most common complication after TEA in Haemophilia. In our opinion, anterior subcutaneous ulnar nerve transposition should be performed to avoid complications. A submuscular transposition of the ulnar nerve is not indicated in haemophiliacs considering the high risk of postoperative bleeding in such subjects.

A soft tissues release, including synovectomy, capsulectomy, and removal of heterotopic ossifications and osteophytes, are all required to achieve a full ROM. In the presence of prono-supination deficit due to radial head deformity or proximal radio-ulnar joint impingement, radial head excision should also be performed.

Regarding the humeral osteotomy, resection of condyles does not appear to adversely affect the joint function. Furthermore, if the humeral shortening is less than 2 cm, triceps function will not be compromised [41]. In case of gross deformities, a wide shortening of the humerus is required, and a long-flanged implant with a longer humeral stem is indicated.

Particular care should be taken with the trial implant to detect the "pistoning" of components [42], as the evaluation of articular or heterotopic ossifications impingement during flexion and extension motion should be observed [43]. These findings could predict any future implant failure.

In order to minimize the stress shielding at the bone-implant interface, it is crucial to restore the normal kinematics by a correct alignment of components, replicating the physiological axis of rotation. Malalignment of the humeral component is a prognostic factor for bushing wear. An internal rotation of the humeral component >10° and tight extensors lead to excessive valgus forces. An external rotation >10° and tight flexors contribute to a varus deformity [44]. Figgie *et al* [45] described the proper alignment of the ulnar and humeral implant stem as "implant-medullary canal parallelism".

Preparation of the ulnar shaft is one of the most challenging procedures and should be carefully undertaken. Haemophilic patients often have obliterated canals and thin bone cortices, making unintentional cortical bone penetration more likely to happen.

The final step is the implant cementation. A correct cementing technique requires irrigation of the medullary canal after proper reaming, placement of an intramedullary plug, and use of a cement gun [46]. Irrigation removes all bone debris; intramedullary plug allows pressurization, and prevents any excessive length escaping of the cement; and the use of a cement gun facilitates the uniform filling of the canal.

Regarding the postoperative complications, the failure rate for deep infection of TEA is reported from 3% to 8% [47, 48]. In haemophilic patients, this risk appears to be associated with comorbidities such as HIV and HCV infections. To reduce such risks, the use of an antibiotic-impregnated cement is reasonable [49, 50]. Also, the meticulous management of soft tissues is of paramount importance. A careful haemostasis reduces the risk of postoperative haemorrhages and haematomas, at further high risk of infection and skin necrosis. Superficial and deep drains must be routinely used, as intraoperative and immediate postoperative x-rays performed to assess any malalignment. The postoperative rehabilitation of TEA is early suggested but should not be aggressive. It often requires dedicated and experienced physiotherapists, a precise patients' education, in order to safely perform progressive strengthening and stretching exercises, and upper arm mobilizations. A cast for few days, followed by a removable plaster splint for the first month may be applied.

CONCLUDING REMARKS

Major surgery has become possible in haemophilic patients by the improvements made in the factor replacement therapy. Experiences in elbow arthroplasty have grown in recent decades, and the development of modern implants has expanded its indications. To date, total elbow arthroplasty is a valuable option in the treatment of a severe elbow haemophilic arthropathy of the elbow. It allows an improvement in elbow function and pain relief, with a survival rate comparable to other conditions, such as rheumatoid arthritis. Nevertheless, it is a challenging procedure with postoperative restrictions and risks, thus requiring a careful selection of patients.

CONFLICT OF INTEREST

The authors confirm that they have no conflict of interest to declare for this publication.

ACKNOWLEDGEMENTS

Declared none.

REFERENCES

[1]   Högh J, Ludlam CA, Macnicol MF. Hemophilic arthropathy of the upper limb. Clin Orthop Relat Res 1987; (218): 225-31.
        [PMID: 3568484]

[2]   Adams JE, Reding MT. Hemophilic arthropathy of the elbow. Hand Clin 2011; 27(2): 151-163, v.
        [http://dx.doi.org/10.1016/j.hcl.2011.01.007] [PMID: 21501786]

[3]   Malhotra R, Gulati MS, Bhan S. Elbow arthropathy in hemophilia. Arch Orthop Trauma Surg 2001; 121(3): 152-7.
[http://dx.doi.org/10.1007/s004020000201] [PMID: 11262781]

[4]   Rodríguez-Merchán EC. Effects of hemophilia on articulations of children and adults. Clin Orthop Relat Res 1996; (328): 7-13.
[http://dx.doi.org/10.1097/00003086-199607000-00003] [PMID: 8653981]

[5]   Heim M, Horoszowski H, Martinowitz U, Seligsohn U, Engel J. Haemophiliac hands a three year follow-up study. Hand 1982; 14(3): 333-6.
[http://dx.doi.org/10.1016/S0072-968X(82)80071-5] [PMID: 7152386]

[6]   Fischer K, van der Bom JG, Mauser-Bunschoten EP, *et al.* The effects of postponing prophylactic treatment on long-term outcome in patients with severe hemophilia. Blood 2002; 99(7): 2337-41.
[http://dx.doi.org/10.1182/blood.V99.7.2337] [PMID: 11895765]

[7]   Rodriguez NI, Hoots WK. Advances in hemophilia: experimental aspects and therapy. Pediatr Clin North Am 2008; 55(2): 357-376, viii.
[http://dx.doi.org/10.1016/j.pcl.2008.01.010] [PMID: 18381091]

[8]   Utukuri MM, Goddard NJ. Haemophilic arthropathy of the elbow. Haemophilia 2005; 11(6): 565-70.
[http://dx.doi.org/10.1111/j.1365-2516.2005.01146.x] [PMID: 16236105]

[9]   Verma N, Valentino LA, Chawla A. Arthroscopic synovectomy in haemophilia: indications, technique and results. Haemophilia 2007; 13 (Suppl. 3): 38-44.
[http://dx.doi.org/10.1111/j.1365-2516.2007.01539.x] [PMID: 17822520]

[10]   Post M, Watts G, Telfer M. Synovectomy in hemophilic arthropathy. A retrospective review of 17 cases. Clin Orthop Relat Res 1986; (202): 139-46.
[PMID: 3955942]

[11]   Gamble JG, Vallier H, Rossi M, Glader B. Loss of elbow and wrist motion in hemophilia. Clin Orthop Relat Res 1996; (328): 94-101.
[http://dx.doi.org/10.1097/00003086-199607000-00017] [PMID: 8653985]

[12]   Johnson RP, Babbitt DP. Five stages of joint disintegration compared with range of motion in hemophilia. Clin Orthop Relat Res 1985; (201): 36-42.
[PMID: 4064418]

[13]   Dumontier C, Sautet A, Man M, Bennani M, Apoil A. Entrapment and compartment syndromes of the upper limb in haemophilia. J Hand Surg [Br] 1994; 19(4): 427-9.
[http://dx.doi.org/10.1016/0266-7681(94)90204-6] [PMID: 7964091]

[14]   Katz SG, Nelson IW, Atkins RM, Duthie RB. Peripheral nerve lesions in hemophilia. J Bone Joint Surg Am 1991; 73(7): 1016-9.
[http://dx.doi.org/10.2106/00004623-199173070-00008] [PMID: 1651940]

[15]   MacDonald PB, Locht RC, Lindsay D, Levi C. Haemophilic arthropathy of the shoulder. J Bone Joint Surg Br 1990; 72(3): 470-1.
[PMID: 2341451]

[16]   Wood K, Omer A, Shaw MT. Haemophilic arthropathy. A combined radiological and clinical study. Br J Radiol 1969; 42(499): 498-505.
[http://dx.doi.org/10.1259/0007-1285-42-499-498] [PMID: 5788058]

[17]   Rodriguez-Merchan EC, Goddard NJ. The technique of synoviorthesis. Haemophilia 2001; 7 (Suppl. 2): 11-5.
[http://dx.doi.org/10.1046/j.1365-2516.2001.00103.x] [PMID: 11564138]

[18]   Dunn AL, Busch MT, Wyly JB, Sullivan KM, Abshire TC. Arthroscopic synovectomy for hemophilic joint disease in a pediatric population. J Pediatr Orthop 2004; 24(4): 414-26.
[http://dx.doi.org/10.1097/01241398-200407000-00013] [PMID: 15205625]

[19]   Le Balch T, Ebelin M, Laurian Y, Lambert T, Verroust F, Larrieu MJ. Synovectomy of the elbow in young hemophilic patients. J Bone Joint Surg Am 1987; 69(2): 264-9.
[http://dx.doi.org/10.2106/00004623-198769020-00015] [PMID: 3805089]

[20]   Silva M, Luck JV Jr. Radial head excision and synovectomy in patients with hemophilia. Surgical technique. J Bone Joint Surg Am 2008; 90 (Suppl. 2 Pt 2): 254-61.
[http://dx.doi.org/10.2106/JBJS.H.00577] [PMID: 18829938]

[21]   Kamineni S, Adams RA, ODriscoll SW, Morrey BF. Hemophilic arthropathy of the elbow treated by total elbow replacement. A case series. J Bone Joint Surg Am 2004; 86-A(3): 584-9.
[http://dx.doi.org/10.2106/00004623-200403000-00019] [PMID: 14996887]

[22]   Chapman-Sheath PJ, Giangrande P, Carr AJ. Arthroplasty of the elbow in haemophilia. J Bone Joint Surg Br 2003; 85(8): 1138-40.
[http://dx.doi.org/10.1302/0301-620X.85B8.13986] [PMID: 14653595]

[23]   Chantelot C, Feugas C, Ala Eddine T, Migaud H, Gueguen G, Fontaine C. [Kudo non-constrained elbow prosthesis for inflammatory and hemophilic joint disease: analysis in 30 cases]. Rev Chir Orthop Repar Appar Mot 2002; 88(4): 398-405.
[PMID: 12124540]

[24]   Martinson A. Elbow arthroplasty in haemophilic arthritis. Thromb Haemost 1977; 38: 357.

[25]   Phillips AM, Ribbans WJ, Goddard NJ. Ipsilateral total shoulder and elbow prosthetic replacement in a patient with severe haemophilia B. Haemophilia 1995; 1(4): 270-3.
[http://dx.doi.org/10.1111/j.1365-2516.1995.tb00088.x] [PMID: 27214636]

[26]   Surace A, Pietrogrande V. Total replacement of knee and elbow in hemophilia: three cases. Int Surg 1983; 68(1): 85-8.
[PMID: 6853091]

[27]   Beeton K, Rodriguez-Merchan EC, Alltree J. Total joint arthroplasty in haemophilia. Haemophilia 2000; 6(5): 474-81.
[http://dx.doi.org/10.1046/j.1365-2516.2000.00443.x] [PMID: 11012688]

[28]   Luck JV Jr, Kasper CK. Surgical management of advanced hemophilic arthropathy. An overview of 20 years experience. Clin Orthop Relat Res 1989; (242): 60-82.
[PMID: 2650951]

[29]   Kasten MD, Skinner HB. Total elbow arthroplasty. An 18-year experience. Clin Orthop Relat Res 1993; (290): 177-88.
[PMID: 8472447]

[30]   Wang K, Street A, Dowrick A, Liew S. Clinical outcomes and patient satisfaction following total joint replacement in haemophilia23-year experience in knees, hips and elbows. Haemophilia 2012; 18(1): 86-93.
[http://dx.doi.org/10.1111/j.1365-2516.2011.02579.x] [PMID: 21649799]

[31]   Vochteloo AJ, Roche SJ, Dachs RP, Vrettos BC. Total elbow arthroplasty in bleeding disorders: an additional series of 8 cases. J Shoulder Elbow Surg 2015; 24(5): 773-8.
[http://dx.doi.org/10.1016/j.jse.2015.01.004] [PMID: 25745827]

[32]   Marshall Brooks M, Tobase P, Karp S, Francis D, Fogarty PF. Outcomes in total elbow arthroplasty in patients with haemophilia at the University of California, San Francisco: a retrospective review. Haemophilia 2011; 17(1): 118-23.
[http://dx.doi.org/10.1111/j.1365-2516.2010.02373.x] [PMID: 20738412]

[33]   Powell DL, Whitener CJ, Dye CE, Ballard JO, Shaffer ML, Eyster ME. Knee and hip arthroplasty infection rates in persons with haemophilia: a 27 year single center experience during the HIV epidemic. Haemophilia 2005; 11(3): 233-9.
[http://dx.doi.org/10.1111/j.1365-2516.2005.01081.x] [PMID: 15876268]

[34]   Ragni MV, Crossett LS, Herndon JH. Postoperative infection following orthopaedic surgery in human immunodeficiency virus-infected hemophiliacs with CD4 counts < or = 200/mm3. J Arthroplasty 1995; 10(6): 716-21.
[http://dx.doi.org/10.1016/S0883-5403(05)80065-8] [PMID: 8749751]

[35]   Toulemonde J, Ancelin D, Azoulay V, Bonnevialle N, Rongieres M, Mansat P. Complications and revisions after semi-constrained total elbow arthroplasty: a mono-analysis of one hundred cases. Int Orthop 2015; 97(10): 1377-84.
[PMID: 26435264]

[36]   Kim JM, Mudgal CS, Konopka JF, Jupiter JB. Complications of total elbow arthroplasty. J Am Acad Orthop Surg 2011; 19(6): 328-39.
[http://dx.doi.org/10.5435/00124635-201106000-00003] [PMID: 21628644]

[37]   Little CP, Graham AJ, Carr AJ. Total elbow arthroplasty: a systematic review of the literature in the English language until the end of 2003. J Bone Joint Surg Br 2005; 87(4): 437-44.
[http://dx.doi.org/10.1302/0301-620X.87B4.15692] [PMID: 15795188]

[38]   Dee R. Total replacement arthroplasty of the elbow for rheumatoid arthritis. J Bone Joint Surg Br 1972; 54(1): 88-95.
[PMID: 5011749]

[39]   Wilkinson JM, Stanley D. Posterior surgical approaches to the elbow: a comparative anatomic study. J Shoulder Elbow Surg 2001; 10(4): 380-2.
[http://dx.doi.org/10.1067/mse.2001.116517] [PMID: 11517370]

[40]   McKee M. Posterior surgical approaches to the elbow: a comparative anatomic study. J Shoulder Elbow Surg 2003; 12(2): 204.
[http://dx.doi.org/10.1067/mse.2002.126213] [PMID: 12728930]

[41]   McKee MD, Pugh DM, Richards RR, Pedersen E, Jones C, Schemitsch EH. Effect of humeral condylar resection on strength and functional outcome after semiconstrained total elbow arthroplasty. J Bone Joint Surg Am 2003; 85-A(5): 802-7.
[http://dx.doi.org/10.2106/00004623-200305000-00005] [PMID: 12728028]

[42]   Cheung EV, ODriscoll SW. Total elbow prosthesis loosening caused by ulnar component pistoning. J Bone Joint Surg Am 2007; 89(6): 1269-74.
[http://dx.doi.org/10.2106/00004623-200706000-00015] [PMID: 17545430]

[43]   Ramsey ML, Adams RA, Morrey BF. Instability of the elbow treated with semiconstrained total elbow arthroplasty. J Bone Joint Surg Am 1999; 81(1): 38-47.
[http://dx.doi.org/10.2106/00004623-199901000-00006] [PMID: 9973052]

[44]   Schuind F, ODriscoll S, Korinek S, An KN, Morrey BF. Loose-hinge total elbow arthroplasty. An experimental study of the effects of implant alignment on three-dimensional elbow kinematics. J Arthroplasty 1995; 10(5): 670-8.
[http://dx.doi.org/10.1016/S0883-5403(05)80214-1] [PMID: 9273381]

[45]   Figgie HE III, Inglis AE, Mow C. A critical analysis of alignment factors affecting functional outcome in total elbow arthroplasty. J Arthroplasty 1986; 1(3): 169-73.
[http://dx.doi.org/10.1016/S0883-5403(86)80027-4] [PMID: 3559591]

[46]   Faber KJ, Cordy ME, Milne AD, Chess DG, King GJ, Johnson JA. Advanced cement technique improves fixation in elbow arthroplasty. Clin Orthop Relat Res 1997; (334): 150-6.
[PMID: 9005908]

[47]   Wolfe SW, Figgie MP, Inglis AE, Bohn WW, Ranawat CS. Management of infection about total elbow prostheses. J Bone Joint Surg Am 1990; 72(2): 198-212.
[http://dx.doi.org/10.2106/00004623-199072020-00007] [PMID: 2303506]

[48]　Yamaguchi K, Adams RA, Morrey BF. Infection after total elbow arthroplasty. J Bone Joint Surg Am 1998; 80(4): 481-91.
[http://dx.doi.org/10.2106/00004623-199804000-00004] [PMID: 9563377]

[49]　Aldridge JM III, Lightdale NR, Mallon WJ, Coonrad RW. Total elbow arthroplasty with the Coonrad/Coonrad-Morrey prosthesis. A 10- to 31-year survival analysis. J Bone Joint Surg Br 2006; 88(4): 509-14.
[http://dx.doi.org/10.1302/0301-620X.88B4.17095] [PMID: 16567787]

[50]　Morrey BF, Adams RA. Semiconstrained arthroplasty for the treatment of rheumatoid arthritis of the elbow. J Bone Joint Surg Am 1992; 74(4): 479-90.
[http://dx.doi.org/10.2106/00004623-199274040-00003] [PMID: 1583042]

CHAPTER 15

Revision Surgery in the Lower Limb of Haemophilic Patients

Massimo Innocenti, Christian Carulli* and Roberto Civinini

Orthopaedic Clinic, University of Florence, Florence, Italy

Abstract: The management of a failed orthopaedic implant is potentially complex in haemophilic patients. Several critical aspects have to be considered ranging from a tailored haematological care and rehabilitative period to high technically demanding surgical procedures and type of implants needed for the management of the compromised joint. Hip and knee are the most involved joints needing a substitution after a prosthetic failure. All these interventions are delicate and expensive, particularly when the failure is not a simple aseptic loosening but it is represented by an infection or a case with severe bone defects, pseudotumours, and soft tissue mortification. Only specific facilities and specialized teams may be able to manage such these conditions in a safe manner.

Keywords: Ankle arthroplasty, Aseptic loosening, Haemophilia, Hip arthroplasty, Infection, Knee arthroplasty, Revision, Salvage surgery.

INTRODUCTION

A *revision* is defined as the substitution of one or more components of a failed orthopaedic implant. Several mechanisms may induce a failure of a prosthesis, and then needing a revision. The most frequent causes of failure are: aseptic loosening and wear, infection, and instability. Lower more than upper limbs are affected by these clinical issues [1 - 5]. During last decades, given the increasing mean age of the population and the consequent more active general way of life, we are assisting to a worsening of chronic diseases. This is particularly true for degenerative articular pathologies as Osteoarthritis, specifically in hips and knees. The result is that a larger number of surgical procedures (primary total hip and knee arthroplasties) have been recently performed worldwide with respect to the past [1, 4 - 6]. The more the number of procedures, the more the rate of complications: an increasing number of failures are consequently expected [6, 7].

---

* **Corresponding author Christian Carulli:** Orthopaedic Clinic, University of Florence, Florence, Italy; Tel: 0039 055 794 8200; Email: christian.carulli@unifi.it

In the haemophilic population, a joint replacement is generally performed in very young patients, often less than 40 years old. In this setting and differently from adult-elderly subjects affected by Osteoarthritis, the main mechanism of failure of an orthopaedic implant has been considered the septic loosening [8 - 13] (Fig. **1**).

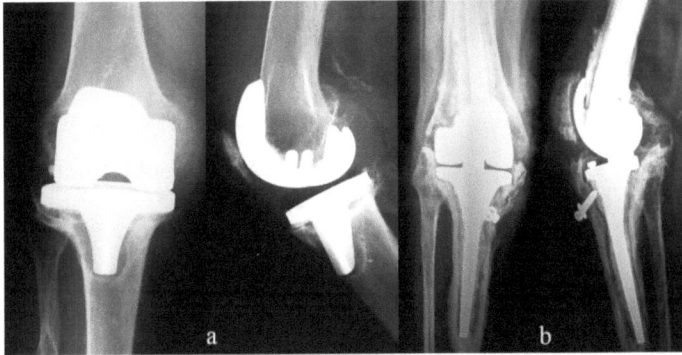

Fig. (1). Comparison between the classic radiologic aspect of a failure of primary cemented knee implants in patients affected by Osteoarthritis (a: aseptic loosening in a 74 years-old female) and Haemophilic arthropathy (b: septic loosening in a 53-years old male).

Several generations of haemophiliacs suffered for infections after orthopaedic procedures with dramatic rates of incidence reported in different series [8, 9, 11, 12]. The second common cause of failures is represented by the aseptic loosening related to bleedings after surgery [8, 9, 11, 12, 14 - 17](Fig. **2**).

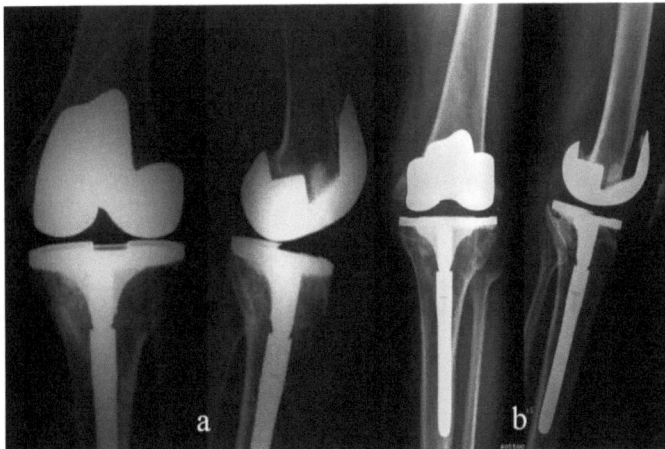

Fig. (2). Typical radiologic aspect of a TKA in a 42 years-old haemophilic patient **(a)** failed after recurrent bleedings 4 years after the index operation **(b)** . Of noting, the cemented femoral component and tibial baseplate, and the cementless tibial keel and stem. This is the modern ideal fixation of components in young haemophilic patients.

No clear data are reported regarding wear and pure mechanical failures. Differently from the past, the modern evaluation of clinical results is based not only on relief from symptoms and restoration of functional ability but also on the longest survivorship of the implants. Thus, it would be necessary to consider also the survival rates of orthopaedic implants in very young patients [18].

RISK FACTORS & CLINICAL SETTINGS

As mentioned, most failures in Haemophilia are related to infections more than aseptic loosening or instability. Several factors are likely involved: a higher prevalence of pre-existing joint damage due to recurrent haemarthrosis before surgery; the consistent risk of subclinical haemarthroses in subjects after a joint replacement; and the growing number of joint replacements performed in this population in the last decades. Historically, co-infections in haemophilic patients have been addressed as important risk factors [19 - 27]. Most failures have been related to co-infections in patients treated by clotting factor products before 1990. The main co-infections have been represented by hepatitis B and C, and HIV.

Hepatitis B and C seem nowadays not to be significant as potential infectious risks, despite the prevalence of hepatitis C has been reported as 80–100% in the haemophilic population and in about 80% of these subjects a chronic hepatitis developed [20 - 23]. HIV infection is considered a strong risk factor for septic sequelae in Haemophilia. Ragni *et al.* reported a survey on the US haemophilia centers to determine the incidence of postoperative infections in HIV-positive haemophiliacs with CD4 counts of ≤ 200 mm³ undergoing orthopaedic surgery. Among 115 centers a postoperative infection occurred in 10 (15.1%) of 66 patients undergoing 74 orthopaedic procedures within 6 months following surgery [24]. Joint arthroplasty has shown a 10 times higher risk of postoperative infection with respect to other forms of surgery (arthroscopy, osteotomy, joint fusion) with a percentage of 26.5% *vs.* 2.5%. Phillips *et al.* similarly reported a higher risk of postoperative bacterial and opportunistic infections in HIV-positive haemophilic patients undergoing orthopaedic surgery: however no significant difference between the number of CD4 lymphocyte in HIV-positive patients undergoing surgery was found when compared to HIV-positive subjects not undergoing surgery [25]. Moreover, the overall rate of prosthetic joint infection after arthroplasty in haemophiliacs especially if HIV-positive has been reported as higher than the non-haemophilic population [23, 26 - 29]. Thomason *et al.* published a series of 15 HIV-positive haemophiliacs undergoing 23 TKAs with 4 infective failures (2 early, 2 late) at a mean follow-up of 7.5 years [26]. Rodriguez-Merchan and Wiedel reported their series of 26 HIV-positive patients (37 TKAs) with at least 200mm³ CD4 count at a mean follow-up of 9.6 years. They recorded a total of 28 complications, with 5 failures related to infections (one case of a superficial infection managed by irrigation, antibiotics, and debridement; three deep infections treated by major surgery) and 2 two aseptic loosening [27]. Ashrani *et al.* reported an overall incidence rate of joint infections of 83/100.000 cases per year in a 7-years period, ranging from 26 to 129 cases per 100,000 person-years annually. The incidence of septic arthritis in haemophilic patients was 15–40 times higher than the reported incidence in the general population, 3–4 times higher than Rheumatoid Arthritis, and similar to that reported in patients with prosthetic joints [28]. Unger *et al.* reported about their series of 15 patients (26 TKAs) affected by HIV that at a mean follow-up of 6.4 years presented a high rate of complications (haemarthrosis, stiffness, varus or valgus deformity, inhibitors development) but no septic loosening [29]. It is nowadays accepted that a very symptomatic and altered joint arthropathy in HIV-positive patients with a CD4 count of $\geq 200mm^3$ and a not conclamate AIDS should be the minimum criteria to plan a major orthopaedic procedure [23, 30]: respecting these indications, a clinical success is expected without an increased risk for complications similar to haemophiliacs without co-infections [15].

Haemophilia type-A is more severe than type-B in terms of bleeding rate, development of inhibitors, progression of the arthropathy, and severity of symptoms [31 - 34]. Similarly, subjects affected by Haemophilia A seems to be prone to develop more severe arthropathies and a higher number of postoperative complications after orthopaedic surgery with respect to Haemophilia B [7, 11, 12, 32]. Moreover, patients with Haemophilia A showed a lesser survivorship due to a higher rate of complications compared to Haemophilia B subjects [32].

Haemophilic patients with inhibitors are mostly prone to develop complications (haemarthrosis, aseptic and septic loosening) after an arthroplasty compared to haemophiliacs without inhibitors since a higher tendency to undergo bleedings [7, 31, 35, 36]. Recurrent postoperative bleedings and permanence of free blood in an operated joint may induce two different mechanisms of failure. Blood and its components may activate an acute inflammation with involvement of cells and cytokines acting as trigger for bone resorption at the bone-component counterface. This may lead to osteolysis and early loosening of the implant [11, 12, 31]. This condition usually realizes with a typical interval of months, characterized by persisting and increasing pain, functional limitation, perceived instability, and necessity of devices as crutches or canes. In haemophilic subjects, a specific pattern of aseptic failure of an implant is the formation of *pseudotumours*, masses characterized by areas of destructured bone and fibrous tissue in bone segments (femur, tibia) close to the prosthetic components. This is the result of recurrent bleedings or persistency of blood in zones of osteolysis in which inflammation does not resume. In such these cases, components loosening realizes and periprosthetic bone becomes weak not able to support the weightbearing. Patients complain pain and progressive functional impairment, needing support by devices as canes or crutches earlier than a simple loosening (Fig. **3**).

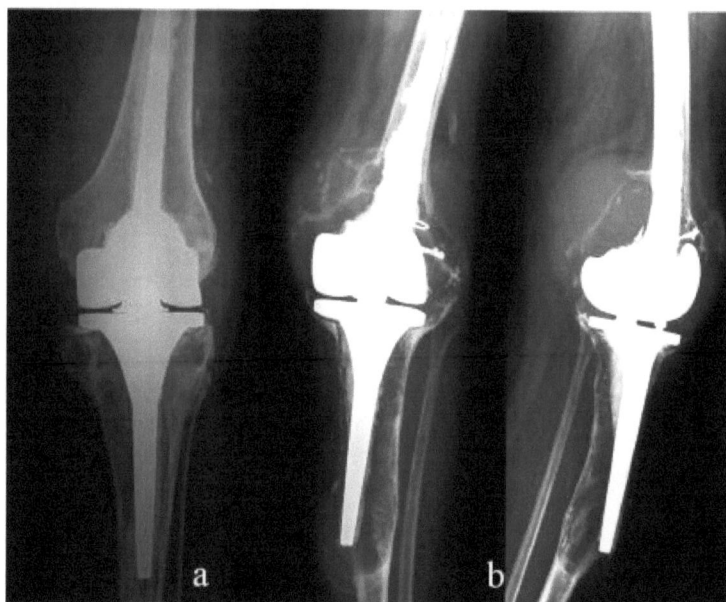

Fig. (3). Primary TKA in a 37 years-old haemophiliac with all cemented components **(a)** . Nine years after surgery, severe aseptic failure with gross instability and formation of pseudotumours on the distal femur and the metadiaphyseal portion of tibia.

On the other side, blood in a joint is an ideal pabulum for bacterial contamination, thus an infection may develop inducing a septic failure. Generally, a TKA or THA infection in haemophilic patients does not differ from non-haemophilic patients. However, if it occurs in HIV co-infected haemophiliacs, serious life-threatening conditions characterized by a septic status may realize [29]. The time interval of such this complication is variable from days to months, depending on the acute, subacute, or chronic onset of the joint infection [29, 36]. Moreover, in a small percentage of haemophilic patients it is not uncommon that a knee or hip deep infection may quickly evolve in a severe compromission of soft tissues, with a large swelling, a sinus tract, and even skin necrosis. An infected pseudotumour may add a further complication in an already severe clinical setting (Fig. **4**).

Recent studies have found that blacks, hispanics and age >30 years were associated with increased risk for septic arthritis among patients with Haemophilia. The reasons for these differences are not to date entirely clear, but it is possible that minorities have decreased access to health care compared with whites and may also undergo to a delay in seeking medical attention for either haemarthrosis or localized or systemic infection. Moreover, Hispanics and blacks generally have a worse functional status than Caucasians across all ages regardless of inhibitor status [37 - 39]. These may represent a further risk factor for complications after a joint replacement, and has to be kept in mind by the Haemophilia teams.

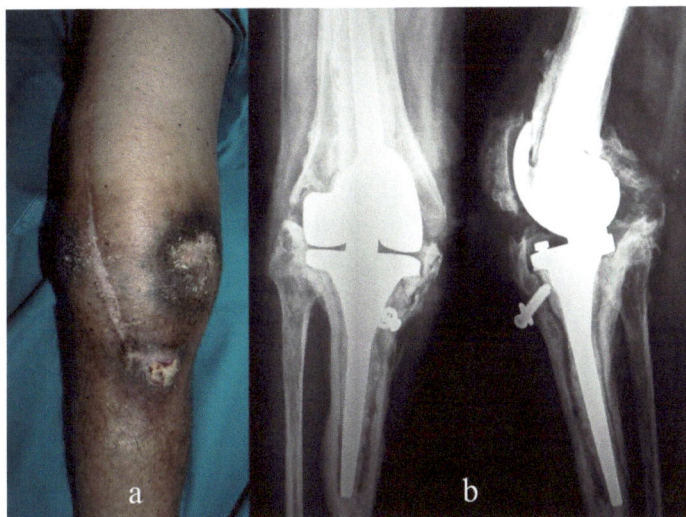

Fig. (4). Clinical **(a)** and radiographic **(b)** aspects of an infected cemented primary TKA with long stems and high constraint in a 53-years old male affected by severe Haemophilia A with high-titre inhibitors. To note the severe soft tissue mortification and the active sinus tract.

Finally, immune modulated and biologic therapies have been recently introduced to control HIV or to induce a negativization of hepatitis C [40]. In case of a joint replacement, subjects should be consider the risk of infections facing these treatments. A multidisciplinary evaluation, a clear and specific informed consent, and a strict control by the orthopaedic surgeon, haematologist, and infectious disease specialist should be strongly considered to prevent or to detect early complications.

DIAGNOSTIC ASPECTS

Diagnosis of a THA or TKA failure in haemophiliacs is performed as for other orthopaedic patients. Clinical signs, blood examinations, synovial fluid analysis, imaging, and exclusion of other causes are generally sufficient to confirm the suspect and to plan a revision. Radiolucent lines and areas of osteolysis should be evaluated and detected by a standard radiographic follow-up (usually 1-3-6-12 months after surgery; then yearly evaluation). The presence of not or slowly progressive radiolucency zones have been reported in several series around acetabular cups, femoral stems, or femoral and tibial components [7, 11, 41, 42] at a mean follow-up of less than 10 years. Mostly of these reported radiographic alterations were asymptomatic and few cases effectively needed a revision.

In case of pseudotumours, a MRI with contrast or a bone scan by marked leucocytes is suggested to exclude any actual tumoral condition, given the particular cancer-like aspect of most masses around hips and knees. A further biopsy in specific cases may be indicated as an exclusion criteria.

TREATMENT OPTIONS

As mentioned, despite the presence of radiolucent lines and osteolysis in several series after a THA or TKA at the mid- to long-follow-up, mostly of the haemophilic patients do not complain symptoms or actually need any revision of their implants. In such cases, it is reasonable a more strict radiographic and orthopaedic evaluation to detect any further worsening. Some cases may benefit of the brand new strategies that are arising in the last years and associated with encouraging results despite there is still lack of full evidence. Examples of these treatments are pharmacological substances acting as promoter of bone metabolism [43] and the physical therapy improving the local bone metabolism in the sense of ingrowth more than resorption [44].

In case of significant progressive radiolucencies or severe osteolysis associated with symptoms, revision surgery is mandatory, particularly in younger subjects. In most cases, by a close cooperation between haematologists and orthopaedics, and a tailored haematological treatment, it is possible to perform a revision similarly to a standard revision. Furthermore, general perioperative risks are fewer given the young mean age of the subjects candidate to this procedure.

Three are the most common settings of failures of an implant of the lower limb in haemophilic patients: the aseptic loosening related to recurrent bleedings; the septic loosening; and the severe failure with soft tissue mortifications associated or not with pseudotumours. The following is a brief overview of these specific cases.

In case of an aseptic failure, revision of one or more component is required. The use of modular knee and hip systems have recently simplified this condition. However, old generation implants as used during the '80s and '90s do not usually allow a simple preoperative or intraoperative setting. Often a full revision is needed. Nowadays, we consider mandatory the use of a modern modular knee or hip systems, in order to facilitate a future revision in case of failure: this is dramatic important particularly for younger patients. Nonetheless, in cases of severe joint destruction, there is a remarkable necessity to adapt the implant to the altered anatomy of a joint with a failed prosthesis. The availability of wedges, stems, cones, offsets in the knee, or wedges, insert, necks, and heads in the hip represents an useful tool to face any bone defects or potential instability during surgery (Fig. **5**).

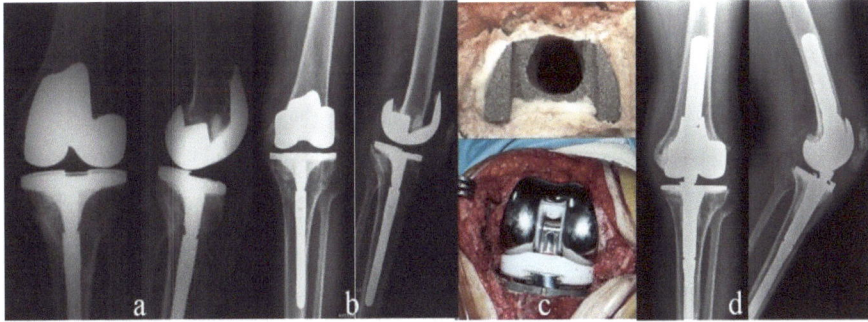

Fig. (5). Radiologic history of the case presented in Fig. (**2**). Primary TKA in a 42 years-old haemophilic patient with high-titre inhibitors (**a**) . Four years after TKA, aseptic loosening with mechanical failure of the femoral component and in the posterior aspect of the tibial baseplate induced by recurrent bleedings (**b**) . The availability of a modern modular knee system allowed the revision with the use of a "cone" in the femoral side to fulfil the severe bone loss, and a high constraint ensured a stability of the implant (**c**) . Radiographic aspect 4 years after revision (**d**) .

Often in revision THA and rarely in revision TKA bone loss management has to be planned. As for others type of patients, bone loss may easily be filled by bone grafts (autologous, homologous, synthetic) and various techniques (impaction grafting, engineered bone grafts by stem cells or Platelet Rich Plasma-PRP, bulky grafts) or in combination with modular parts of the implant (wedges, cones, inserts) [45 - 47] (Fig. **6**). However, very few reports in literature deal with these kind of approaches in Haemophilia.

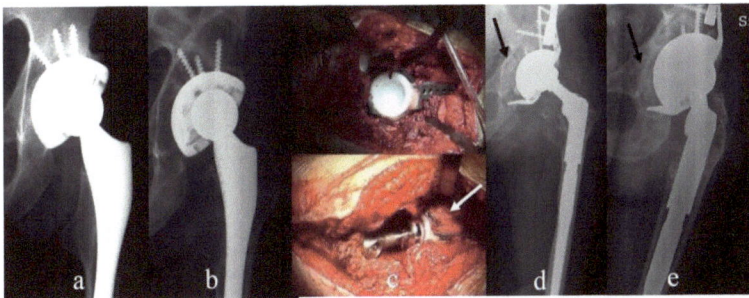

Fig. (6). Ceramic-on-PolyEthylene primary THA in a 41-years old subject affected by Haemophilia A with inhibitors (**a**) . Five years later, aseptic loosening with gross osteolysis in the acetabular and femoral components (**b**) . Revision with a trabecular metal cage, heterologous bone grafts enriched by autologous stem cells concentrate (white arrow), and a Metal-on-PolyEthylene coupling (**c**) . Postoperative x-rays at 6 months (**d**) and two years after surgery (**e**) with evidence of progressive osseointegration of bone grafts.

In case of a septic failure, the setting may be more complex, in particular in patients with sinus tract, dehiscence, or skin alterations. The two-stage revision is to date considered the gold standard for the management of a failed infected implant. However, in case of large sinus tract or skin defect, a staged or simultaneous surgical step with skin coverage by a local or free flap may be necessary (Fig. 7).

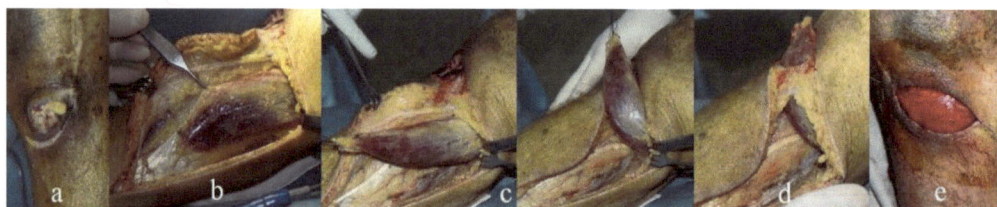

Fig. (7). Sinus tract in an infected knee implant of a haemophilic patient with inhibitors (a) . The first surgical step were the soft tissue debridement and dissection of the ipsilateral gemellus medialis (b) . Then the flap was isolated and rotated (c) and passed by a subcutaneous tunnel until reaching the loss of substance (d) . The final aspect of the flap after the positioning (e) .

Timing for the first of two stages and for the second stage is generally equivalent to non-haemophilic patients. The use of modern generation modular knee or hip systems is clearly convenient. Specifically, it is not uncommon the use of a *"megaprosthesis"*, that consists in an implant indicated to substitute a large segment of a bone, in its epiphysis, metaphysis, and even its diaphysis (Fig. **8**) [48, 49]: its use is common in oncologic surgery, after large bone resections. Of noting, that this choice is technically demanding, needs a longer surgical timing, a larger dissection and tissues exposition, and finally it is correlated to mechanical complications more than standard primary and revision implants. Instability is more frequent for this kind of prostheses, particularly for hips, where an abduction bracing is mandatory after surgery for several weeks. The use of megaprosthesis in knee surgery is generally easier than in the hip, but often correlated to limited range of motion of the joint and prolonged rehabilitation protocols.

Finally, cases of failures and development of pseudotumours or aggressive acute septic failures are settings particularly challenging. In such cases, we should talk about *"salvage surgery"* more than "revision surgery". High rates of complications and expected not brilliant clinical outcomes are very common and patients and their relatives should be clearly informed. In our opinion, this kind of surgery when feasible should be reserved to young subjects as an attempt to avoid the other surgical approaches (joint fusion, amputation). In case of further failure, the option to face a more aggressive and "no-return" surgery is possible. On the other hand, we suggest a joint fusion or an amputation in adult or elderly haemophiliacs affected by this severe failure in order to quickly return to a more functional condition without facing further surgical procedures.

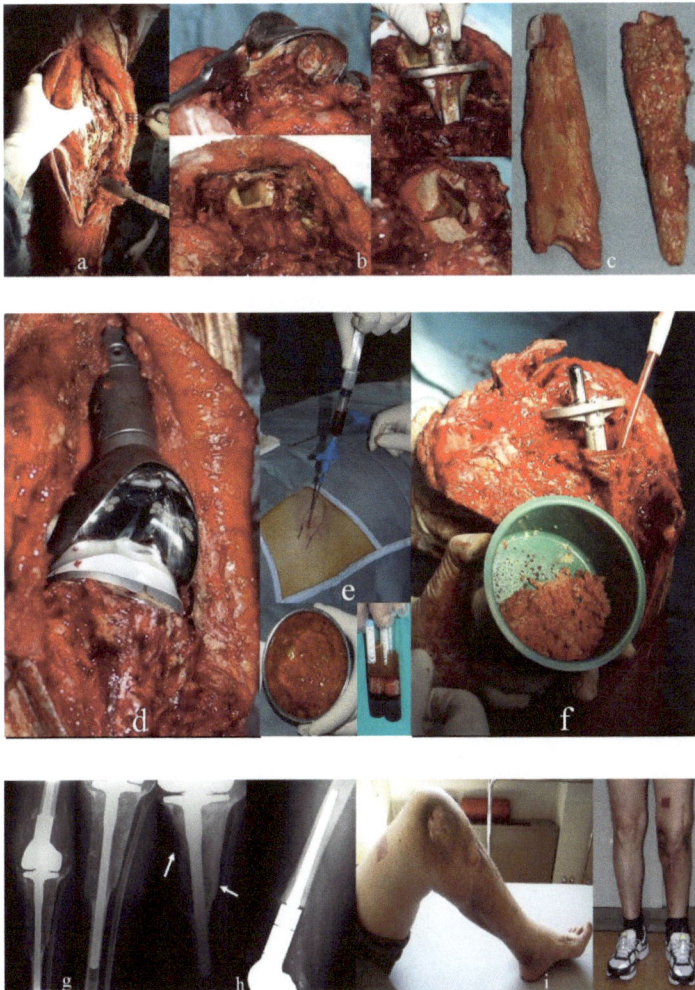

Fig. (8). Revision of a failed primary right TKA in a haemophilic patient with inhibitors **(a)** . Loose components **(b)** and cement removal **(c)** . Implant of a megaprostheses characterized by a cemented stem in the femoral side **(d)** , a cementless tibial component with long porous stem, and heterologous bone grafts enriched by autologous PRP and stem cells concentrate harvested by ipsilateral iliac crest (e and f). Radiologic follow-up at one month (g) and two years **(h)** . Of noting, the progressive enlargement of tibial corticals and resorption of heterologous bone grafts substituted by own bone (white arrows). Clinical aspect of the operated leg after 4 years **(i)** .

As mentioned in chapter 11, many haemophilic patients affected by severe knee arthropathy have been and in some cases still now are treated by primary TKAs with high constraint and cemented long-stemmed implants (Fig. **3a**) [29, 50 - 52].

This solution has been proposed in several cases to ensure a better postoperative stability and to dissipate all forces in the femoral and tibial diaphysis more than on the tibial insert. Typical indications have been represented by: severe tibial or femoral bone loss, excessive valgus or varus deformity, and noteworthy flexion contractures. However, most of these implants showed a very short survivorship with early loosening on the tibial baseplate and femoral component: wide zones of osteolysis and progressive radiolucencies have been reported with failure of the entire implants (Figs. **3b** and **4b**). At the time of revision, cement removal and bone defects represent the most challenging steps, particularly in young subjects (Figs. **8b** and **8c**). The typical setting in such cases is a gross bone loss and asymmetric flexion and extension gaps to be filled with modern modular revision implants and bone substitutes (Figs. **8e** and **8f**). Offsets for stems are crucial in order to restore an adequate balance between flexion and extension gaps, and to allow a recovery of the joint line close to the physiological (Fig. **9**) [53].

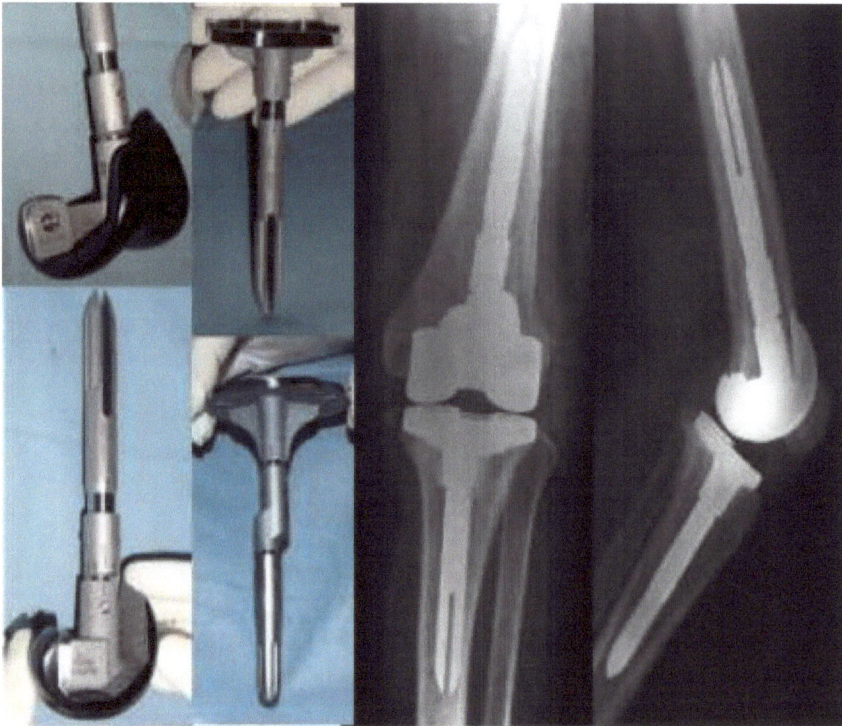

Fig. (9). Example of a modern revision knee implant. Oxidized zirconium femoral component is indicated in young subjects to ensure the lowest wear and the longest survivorship of the implant. Porous fluted stems are useful to allow a biological bone ingrowth. Finally, offsets are mandatory to adapt the implant to the peculiar anatomy of such these patients.

Tissue engineering techniques have recently gained interest in the field of reconstructive surgery also in Orthopaedics [45]. The management of large bone defects and the need to ensure the better osseointegration of metal components to bone has induced many surgeons to adopt autologous stem cell concentrations, PRP combined with bone grafts or synthetic bioceramics to enhance the local metabolism of the host bone. The coupling of such these *"biological composites"* with modern high osteoinductive and osteoconductive implant surfaces seems to be very encouraging and efficient in the integration of metal components to the host bone (Figs. **8g** and **8h**) [46].

Rehabilitation after a revision surgery has to follow the basic principles of the management of a joint after multiple surgery but with the close collaboration between with dedicated figures as physical therapists, physiotherapists, orthopaedic surgeons, haematologists, and nurses. No protocols but tailored approaches have to be considered for each patients, as tailored is the haematological prophylaxis during rehabilitative pathways.

Joint fusion and amputation, once strongly considered as surgical options in severe cases, have nowadays lesser indications than before [50, 54]. However they still are indicated as the last attempt to save the limb after the failure of other surgical approaches (Fig. **10**). Joint fusion remains a discussed choice in the late stages of ankle arthropathy, being indicated mostly for adult or elderly subjects as an alternative for an ankle replacement when approaching an arthropathy [55]. It is mandatory after a failure of a previous ankle replacement given the good clinical outcomes even if resulting in a fixed joint [54]. Amputation followed by the wearing of an artificial prosthesis is today the indication for failures of any kind of medical and surgical procedures in patients with severe involvement of soft and hard tissues or in cases of failing multiple surgeries.

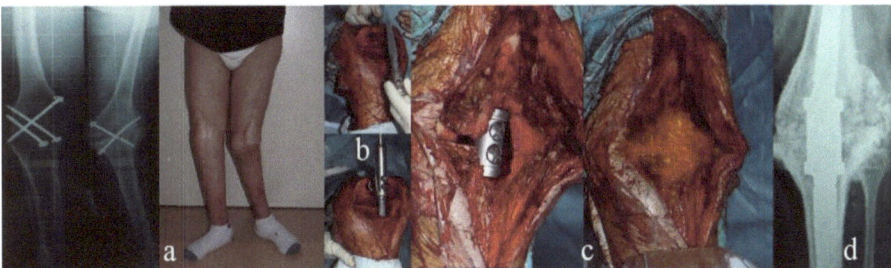

Fig. (10). Forty-eight years old haemophilic patient with an atraumatic mechanical failure of the fusion on his left knee performed 6 years before **(a)** . Intraoperative pictures showing the preparation for a new joint fusion by an cementless intramedullary nail and a biological composite (b and c). Radiologic follow-up at two years **(d)** .

The management of a failed THA or TKA implant in haemophilic subjects is clearly high demanding. The complexity lies not only in the preoperative multidisciplinary evaluation of a patient complaining a failed implant, but also in the medical expenses due to the haematological prophylaxis, the orthopaedic implant, and the costs for the hospital stay, usually prolonged with respect to standard revision settings. The prolonged hospitalization is in our opinion mandatory for a double purpose: it ensures the monitoring of critical patients, at risk for postoperative bleedings and infections; for the necessity of a long and often slow/soft rehabilitation, balancing a progressive functional recovery without exposing to further haemarthrosis a frail joint.

This requires the identification of specific facilities in which a multidisciplinary expertise may take care of this kind of patients and in which the opportunity to face such these costs is acceptable in an efficient manner and without uneconomical wastes.

CONCLUDING REMARKS

The management of a failed hip or knee implant is potentially complex in haemophilic patients. Several aspects have to be considered: the delicate haematological care and the related very high costs; the necessity of a modern modular implant, in order to adapt the prostheses to the patients and not vice versa; the several local settings of the patients that may be affect by an aseptic loosening, by a deep infection, and in some cases by a severe bone and soft tissue mortification; the need of a closed multidisciplinary monitoring and of a surveillance over the usually long rehabilitative care; and the consequent prolonged hospitalization.

Only specific facilities and specialized teams may be able to manage such these conditions.

CONFLICT OF INTEREST

The authors confirm that they have no conflict of interest to declare for this publication.

ACKNOWLEDGEMENTS

Declared none.

REFERENCES

[1]   Sharkey PF, Hozack WJ, Rothman RH, Shastri S, Jacoby SM. Insall Award paper. Why are total knee arthroplasties failing today? Clin Orthop Relat Res 2002; (404): 7-13.
[http://dx.doi.org/10.1097/00003086-200211000-00003] [PMID: 12439231]

[2]	Fitzgerald SJ1, Trousdale RT. Why knees fail in 2011: patient, surgeon, or device? Orthopedics 2011; 9(34(9)): e513-5.

[3]	Lombardi AV Jr, Berend KR, Adams JB. Why knee replacements fail in 2013: patient, surgeon, or implant? Bone Joint J 2014; 96-B(11) (Suppl. A): 101-4.
	[http://dx.doi.org/10.1302/0301-620X.96B11.34350] [PMID: 25381419]

[4]	Sharkey PF, Lichstein PM, Shen C, Tokarski AT, Parvizi J. Why are total knee arthroplasties failing today--has anything changed after 10 years? J Arthroplasty 2014; 29(9): 1774-8.
	[http://dx.doi.org/10.1016/j.arth.2013.07.024] [PMID: 25007726]

[5]	Biemond JE, Venkatesan S, van Hellemondt GG. Survivorship of the cementless Spotorno femoral component in patients under 50 years of age at a mean follow-up of 18.4 years. Bone Joint J 2015; 97-B(2): 160-3.
	[http://dx.doi.org/10.1302/0301-620X.97B2.34926] [PMID: 25628276]

[6]	Carulli C, Villano M, Bucciarelli G, Martini C, Innocenti M. Painful knee arthroplasty: definition and overview. Clin Cases Miner Bone Metab 2011; 8(2): 23-5.
	[PMID: 22461811]

[7]	Solimeno LP, Perfetto OS, Pasta G, Santagostino E. Total joint replacement in patients with inhibitors. Haemophilia 2006; 12 (Suppl. 3): 113-6.
	[http://dx.doi.org/10.1111/j.1365-2516.2006.01267.x] [PMID: 16684005]

[8]	Sikkema T, Boerboom AL, Meijer K. A comparison between the complications and long-term outcome of hip and knee replacement therapy in patients with and without haemophilia; a controlled retrospective cohort study. Haemophilia 2011; 17(2): 300-3.
	[http://dx.doi.org/10.1111/j.1365-2516.2010.02408.x] [PMID: 21070490]

[9]	Rodriguez-Merchan EC. Total knee replacement in haemophilic arthropathy. J Bone Joint Surg Br 2007; 89(2): 186-8.
	[http://dx.doi.org/10.1302/0301-620X.89B2.18682] [PMID: 17322432]

[10]	Magone JB, Dennis DA, Weis LD. Total knee arthroplasty in chronic hemophilic arthropathy. Orthopedics 1986; 9(5): 653-7. [Short term].
	[PMID: 3714579]

[11]	Kelley SS, Lachiewicz PF, Gilbert MS, Bolander ME, Jankiewicz JJ. Hip arthroplasty in hemophilic arthropathy. J Bone Joint Surg Am 1995; 77(6): 828-34. [A>b].
	[PMID: 7782355]

[12]	Heeg M, Meyer K, Smid WM, Van Horn JR, Van der Meer J. Total knee and hip arthroplasty in haemophilic patients. Haemophilia 1998; 4(5): 747-51. [A>B].
	[http://dx.doi.org/10.1046/j.1365-2516.1998.00183.x] [PMID: 9873881]

[13]	Hicks JL, Ribbans WJ, Buzzard B, *et al.* Infected joint replacements in HIV-positive patients with haemophilia. J Bone Joint Surg Br 2001; 83(7): 1050-4.
	[http://dx.doi.org/10.1302/0301-620X.83B7.11242] [PMID: 11603522]

[14]	Park JJ, Slover JD, Stuchin SA. Recurrent hemarthrosis in a hemophilic patient after revision total knee arthroplasty. Orthopedics 2010; 11(33(10)): 771.

[15]	Solimeno LP, Mancuso ME, Pasta G, Santagostino E, Perfetto S, Mannucci PM. Factors influencing the long-term outcome of primary total knee replacement in haemophiliacs: a review of 116 procedures at a single institution. Br J Haematol 2009; 145(2): 227-34.
	[http://dx.doi.org/10.1111/j.1365-2141.2009.07613.x] [PMID: 19236610]

[16]	Zingg PO, Fucentese SF, Lutz W, Brand B, Mamisch N, Koch PP. Haemophilic knee arthropathy: long-term outcome after total knee replacement. Knee Surg Sports Traumatol Arthrosc 2012; 20(12): 2465-70. [ahead of print].
	[http://dx.doi.org/10.1007/s00167-012-1896-7] [PMID: 22293897]

[17]   Duffy GP, Trousdale RT, Stuart MJ. Total knee arthroplasty in patients 55 years old or younger. 10- to 17-year results. Clin Orthop Relat Res 1998; (356): 22-7.
[http://dx.doi.org/10.1097/00003086-199811000-00005] [PMID: 9917663]

[18]   Carulli C, Martini C, Matassi F. Primary Total Knee Arthroplasty in Haemophilia: a long-term experience with modern implants. Podium presentation at the 14th International Musculoskeletal Congress of Haemophilia. Belfast (UK). 2015.

[19]   Wilde JT. HIV and HCV coinfection in haemophilia. Haemophilia 2004; 10(1): 1-8.
[http://dx.doi.org/10.1046/j.1351-8216.2003.00828.x] [PMID: 14962214]

[20]   Mauser-Bunschoten EP, Bresters D, van Drimmelen AA, *et al.* Hepatitis C infection and viremia in Dutch hemophilia patients. J Med Virol 1995; 45(3): 241-6.
[http://dx.doi.org/10.1002/jmv.1890450302] [PMID: 7539831]

[21]   Posthouwer D, Mauser-Bunschoten EP, Fischer K, Makris M. Treatment of chronic hepatitis C in patients with haemophilia: a review of the literature. Haemophilia 2006; 12(5): 473-8.
[http://dx.doi.org/10.1111/j.1365-2516.2006.01317.x] [PMID: 16919076]

[22]   Brettler DB, Alter HJ, Dienstag JL, Forsberg AD, Levine PH. Prevalence of hepatitis C virus antibody in a cohort of hemophilia patients. Blood 1990; 76(1): 254-6.
[PMID: 2114186]

[23]   Rodriguez-Merchan EC. HIV and HCV coinfected haemophilia patients: what are the best options of orthopaedic treatment? Haemophilia 2006; 12 (Suppl. 3): 90-101.
[http://dx.doi.org/10.1111/j.1365-2516.2006.01264.x] [PMID: 16684002]

[24]   Ragni MV, Crossett LS, Herndon JH. Postoperative infection following orthopaedic surgery in human immunodeficiency virus-infected hemophiliacs with CD4 counts < or = 200/mm3. J Arthroplasty 1995; 10(6): 716-21.
[http://dx.doi.org/10.1016/S0883-5403(05)80065-8] [PMID: 8749751]

[25]   Phillips AM, Sabin CA, Ribbans WJ, Lee CA. Orthopaedic surgery in hemophilic patients with human immunodeficiency virus. Clin Orthop Relat Res 1997; (343): 81-7.
[PMID: 9345211]

[26]   Thomason HC III, Wilson FC, Lachiewicz PF, Kelley SS. Knee arthroplasty in hemophilic arthropathy. Clin Orthop Relat Res 1999; (360): 169-73.
[http://dx.doi.org/10.1097/00003086-199903000-00020] [PMID: 10101322]

[27]   Rodriguez-Merchan EC, Wiedel JD. Total knee arthroplasty in HIV-positive haemophilic patients. Haemophilia 2002; 8(3): 387-92.
[http://dx.doi.org/10.1046/j.1365-2516.2002.00610.x] [PMID: 12010439]

[28]   Ashrani AA, Key NS, Soucie JM, Duffy N, Forsyth A, Geraghty S. Septic arthritis in males with haemophilia. Haemophilia 2008; 14(3): 494-503.
[http://dx.doi.org/10.1111/j.1365-2516.2008.01662.x] [PMID: 18298584]

[29]   Unger AS, Kessler CM, Lewis RJ. Total knee arthroplasty in human immunodeficiency virus-infected hemophiliacs. J Arthroplasty 1995; 10(4): 448-52.
[http://dx.doi.org/10.1016/S0883-5403(05)80144-5] [PMID: 8523002]

[30]   Colvin R. Hemophilia and HIV standard of care. Common Factor 1997; 11(11): 10-1.
[PMID: 11364844]

[31]   Rodriguez-Merchan EC, De La Corte H. Orthopaedic surgery in haemophilic patients with inhibitors: a review of the literature In: Rodriguez-Merchan EC, Goddard NJ, Lee CA, Eds. Musculoskeletal aspect of Haemophilia. Blackwell Science Ltd 2000.

[32]   Tagariello G, Iorio A, Santagostino E, *et al.* Italian Association Hemophilia Centre (AICE). Comparison of the rates of joint arthroplasty in patients with severe factor VIII and IX deficiency: an index of different clinical severity of the 2 coagulation disorders. Blood 2009; 23(114): 779-84. [http://dx.doi.org/10.1182/blood-2009-01-195313]

[33]   Nagel K, Walker I, Decker K, Chan AK, Pai MK. Comparing bleed frequency and factor concentrate use between haemophilia A and B patients. Haemophilia 2011; 17(6): 872-4. [http://dx.doi.org/10.1111/j.1365-2516.2011.02506.x] [PMID: 21342368]

[34]   Mannucci PM, Franchini M. Is haemophilia B less severe than haemophilia A? Haemophilia 2013; 1(19): 499-502.

[35]   Ludlam C. Identifying and managing inhibitor patients requiring orthopaedic surgery - the multidisciplinary team approach. Haemophilia 2005; 11 (Suppl. 1): 7-10. [http://dx.doi.org/10.1111/j.1365-2516.2005.01152.x] [PMID: 16219043]

[36]   Carcao M, Lambert T. Prophylaxis in haemophilia with inhibitors: update from international experience. Haemophilia 2010; 16 (Suppl. 2): 16-23. [http://dx.doi.org/10.1111/j.1365-2516.2009.02198.x] [PMID: 20132334]

[37]   Aledort LM, Dimichele DM. Inhibitors occur more frequently in African-American and Latino haemophiliacs. Haemophilia 1998; 4(1): 68. [http://dx.doi.org/10.1046/j.1365-2516.1998.0146c.x] [PMID: 9873872]

[38]   Leissinger C, Cooper DL, Solem CT. HTRS Investigators. Assessing the impact of age, race, ethnicity and inhibitor status on functional limitations of patients with severe and moderately severe haemophilia A. Haemophilia 2011; 17(6): 884-9. [http://dx.doi.org/10.1111/j.1365-2516.2011.02509.x] [PMID: 21447095]

[39]   Carpenter SL, Michael Soucie J, Sterner S, Presley R. Hemophilia Treatment Center Network (HTCN) Investigators. Increased prevalence of inhibitors in Hispanic patients with severe haemophilia A enrolled in the Universal Data Collection database. Haemophilia 2012; 18(3): e260-5. [http://dx.doi.org/10.1111/j.1365-2516.2011.02739.x] [PMID: 22250850]

[40]   Mancuso ME, Rumi MG, Aghemo A, *et al.* Hepatitis C virus/human immunodeficiency virus coinfection in hemophiliacs: high rates of sustained virologic response to pegylated interferon and ribavirin therapy. J Thromb Haemost 2009; 7(12): 1997-2005. [http://dx.doi.org/10.1111/j.1538-7836.2009.03624.x] [PMID: 19799716]

[41]   Miles J, Rodríguez-Merchán EC, Goddard NJ. The impact of haemophilia on the success of total hip arthroplasty. Haemophilia 2008; 14(1): 81-4. [PMID: 18034823]

[42]   Yoo MC, Cho YJ, Kim KI, Ramteke A, Chun YS. The outcome of cementless total hip arthroplasty in haemophilic hip arthropathy. Haemophilia 2009; 15(3): 766-73. [http://dx.doi.org/10.1111/j.1365-2516.2009.01986.x] [PMID: 19444974]

[43]   Carulli C, Civinini R, Matassi F, Villano M, Innocenti M. The use of anti-osteoporosis drugs in total knee arthroplasty. Aging Clin Exp Res 2011; 23(2) (Suppl.): 38-9. [PMID: 21970917]

[44]   Massari L, Caruso G, Sollazzo V, Setti S. Pulsed electromagnetic fields and low intensity pulsed ultrasound in bone tissue. Clin Cases Miner Bone Metab 2009; 6(2): 149-54. [PMID: 22461165]

[45]   Carulli C, Matassi F, Civinini R, Innocenti M. Tissue engineering applications in the management of bone loss. Clin Cases Miner Bone Metab 2013; 10(1): 22-5. [PMID: 23858306]

[46]   Matassi F, Botti A, Sirleo L, Carulli C, Innocenti M. Porous metal for orthopedics implants. Clin Cases Miner Bone Metab 2013; 10(2): 111-5. [PMID: 24133527]

[47]   van Loon CJ, Wijers MM, de Waal Malefijt MC, Buma P, Veth RP. Femoral bone grafting in primary and revision total knee arthroplasty. Acta Orthop Belg 1999; 65(3): 357-63.
[PMID: 10546358]

[48]   Stumpf UC, Eberhardt C, Kurth AA. Orthopaedic limb salvage with a mega prosthesis in a patient with haemophilia A and inhibitors - a case report. Haemophilia 2007; 13(4): 435-9.
[http://dx.doi.org/10.1111/j.1365-2516.2007.01476.x] [PMID: 17610563]

[49]   Sunnassee Y, Wan R, Shen Y, Xu J, Southern EP, Zhang W. Preliminary results for the use of knee mega-endoprosthesis in the treatment of musculoskeletal complications of haemophilia. Haemophilia 2015; 21(2): 258-65.
[http://dx.doi.org/10.1111/hae.12541] [PMID: 25377302]

[50]   Rana NA, Shapiro GR, Green D. Long-term follow-up of prosthetic joint replacement in hemophilia. Am J Hematol 1986; 23(4): 329-37.
[http://dx.doi.org/10.1002/ajh.2830230405] [PMID: 3788961]

[51]   Kjaersgaard-Andersen P, Christiansen SE, Ingerslev J, Sneppen O. Total knee arthroplasty in classic hemophilia. Clin Orthop Relat Res 1990; (256): 137-46.
[PMID: 2114246]

[52]   Legroux-Gérot I, Strouk G, Parquet A, Goodemand J, Gougeon F, Duquesnoy B. Total knee arthroplasty in hemophilic arthropathy. Joint Bone Spine 2003; 70(1): 22-32.
[http://dx.doi.org/10.1016/S1297-319X(02)00008-8] [PMID: 12639614]

[53]   Innocenti M, Matassi F, Carulli C, Soderi S, Villano M, Civinini R. Joint line position in revision total knee arthroplasty: the role of posterior femoral off-set stems. Knee 2013; 20(6): 447-50.
[http://dx.doi.org/10.1016/j.knee.2013.05.012] [PMID: 23790671]

[54]   Rodriguez-merchan EC, Goddard NJ. Chapter 10: Joint debridement, alignment osteotomy and arthrodesis. In: Rodriguez-Merchan EC, Goddard NJ, Lee CA, Eds. Musculoskeletal aspect of Haemophilia. Blackwell Science 2000.

[55]   Daniels TR, Younger AS, Penner M, *et al.* Intermediate-term results of total ankle replacement and ankle arthrodesis: a COFAS multicenter study. J Bone Joint Surg Am 2014; 96(2): 135-42.
[http://dx.doi.org/10.2106/JBJS.L.01597] [PMID: 24430413]

CHAPTER 16

Postoperative Rehabilitation

Pietro Pasquetti, Lorenzo Apicella*, Elisa Pratelli and Giuseppe Mangone

Rehabilitation Unit, Azienda Ospedaliero-Universitaria Careggi, Florence, Italy

Abstract: The proposal of a comprehensive rehabilitation program after major orthopaedic surgery, specifically Total Hip Arthroplasty (THA) and Total Knee arthroplasty (TKA), is a key event in the management of patients affected by haemophilia arthropathy. Rehabilitative protocols should be carried out by a multidisciplinary team. This is a modern approach consists of three main stages: preoperative evaluation and education, in-hospital rehabilitation, and out-patient rehabilitation. The primary purposes are the control of pain, the recovery and maintenance of range of movement, and the muscle strengthening. In-hospital rehabilitation usually starts the day after surgery, using specific protocols in order to gradually counteract joint stiffness and pain. After the discharge haemophilic patients should improve their training with task-oriented exercises. An adequate and individually-tailored rehabilitation program could optimize the result of major orthopaedic surgery, improving the functional ability of haemophiliacs, and resulting in a better quality of life.

Keywords: Continuous passive motion, Haemophilia, Proprioception, Rehabilitation, Total knee arthroplasty, Total hip arthroplasty.

INTRODUCTION

Orthopaedic surgery in haemophilic patients (HP) showed significant advancements after the introduction of factor concentrates [1]. Another key event in the management of such patients was the improvement of a comprehensive rehabilitation program after major orthopaedic surgery, particularly Total Hip Arthroplasty (THA) and Total Knee arthroplasty (TKA) [2]. Some considerations in the postoperative management of HP are mandatory:

- Generally, HP are young and affected by more severe joint alterations than non haemophiliacs [3]. Similarly, in the postoperative setting, HP have more functional requests with respect to the general population undergoing major orthopaedic surgery;

---

* **Corresponding author Lorenzo Apicella:** Rehabilitation Unit, Azienda Ospedaliero-Universitaria Careggi, Florence, Italy; Tel: +39 055 7948382; Email: lorenzo.apicella@gmail.com

Christian Carulli (Ed.)

- Postoperative physiotherapy has several purposes: early recovery of range of motion (ROM), muscle strength, and proprioception [4];
- Reconditioning of motor patterns has to be as much as possible complete in order to improve the functional ability minimizing the risk of future bleeding episodes;
- Postoperative recovery of HP is often limited due to the involvement of several other target joints, particularly in the lower limb [5];
- The best result is achieved by close communication and cooperation between physiatrists, physical therapists, and surgeons, coupled with the generally high motivations of patients The concept of the multidisciplinary team (MT) is crucial [6];
- Also a preoperative relationship between MT and the patient may improve the feeling and influence the outcomes. By this knowledge, the MT has the opportunity to evaluate the functional status, bleeding pattern, and the muscles conditions of the patient [7];
- Treatment goals, timelines, and all aspects of rehabilitation should be discussed before surgery [8].

Postoperative rehabilitative protocols after major orthopaedic procedures in HP have been rarely investigated, due to the fact that Haemophilia is a rare disease, and few centres usually deal with such conditions. The few reported protocols vary from one centre to another [9, 10]. Moreover, rehabilitative protocols have to be specific and tailored for each HP.

The following is the overview of the rehabilitative aspects related to Total Knee Arthroplasty (TKA) and Total Hip Arthroplasty (THA).

TOTAL KNEE ARTHROPLASTY

The knee is the most involved target joint and TKA is a valid treatment for severe, end-stage cases of arthropathy [11, 12]. The medical community agrees on the brilliant outcomes of TKA in terms of pain relief, functional recovery, deformity correction, and patient's quality of life (QoL) [13 - 15].

The ideal indications for TKA in a patient affected by Haemophilia are persistent pain and impaired function as a result of extensive erosion of the joint surfaces, and a severely restricted range of motion [16](See Chapter 11). Functional impairment, often subjectively referred as 'joint stiffness', is objectively measured by the loss of ROM. Stiffness is defined as an inadequate ROM that results in functional limitations in activities of daily life [17, 18]. Despite all the advancements in surgical techniques, implant design, haematological care, and postoperative management, stiffness continues to be a relatively common complication for haemophilic patients after TKA.

Preoperative ROM is the most important variable influencing the postoperative ROM. Thus, the presence of a significant flexion contracture and/or poor passive flexion is highly correlated with a poor postoperative ROM. Also a preoperative physical and muscular conditioning may improve the functional recovery or, if not performed, predict some limits in the postoperative rehabilitation. As well, an early knee mobilization after TKA is as soon as possible encouraged both in flexion and in extension [19].

It is possible to underline different stages in rehabilitation after TKA in HP: preoperative evaluation and education; in-hospital rehabilitation; out-patient rehabilitation.

Preoperative Evaluation and Education

During the preoperative assessment, the MT should perform a complete evaluation of all target joints (ROM, muscular strength, local conditions, evaluation scales), discussing the patient's expectations after surgery [2, 20]. In some reviews [21 - 23] several authors concluded that preoperative physiotherapy may not be effective for the outcomes. In other studies, however, individually tailored, multidisciplinary preoperative rehabilitation was suggested to reduce the hospital stay in selected patients with comorbidities or limited social supports [21].

In-Hospital Rehabilitation

After surgery, the first stage of rehabilitation is started directly in the orthopedic ward (Table **1**). The primary objectives are: control of pain, recovery of ROM, and muscle strengthening [19]. In selected cases and depending on the pain, the day of surgery patient could immediately turn on his side and move actively the knee. The patient should also start with ankle flexion/extension exercises. In order to guarantee a correct postural alignment, the horizontal decubitus in the bed is alternated with the semi-sitting position, tilting the head of the bed up to 45°. Pain could be controlled by the use of cryotherapy or painkillers. To prevent bleeding complications, each session of physiotherapy should be preceded by an infusion of the deficient clotting factor.

On the first day after surgery, passive flexion and extension exercises can be performed by the physiotherapist; autonomous active and continuous passive mobilization (CPM) exercises may be realized manually or by dedicated devices. Knee mobilization should start from a limited ROM (10°- 40°) and gradually increased to 0°- 90° in the first week [24]. After TKA, the flexion improves quickly and reaches a plateau within a few months, while the extension requires more time to be achieved [25]. It is crucial that patients understand the importance of continuing exercises also after hospital discharge. Knees with haemophilic arthropathy are characterized by the presence of arthrofibrosis that limits ROM by forming bands of scar tissue between the quadriceps mechanism and the distal femur. The patellofemoral mobility decreases, and the medial and lateral gutters often scar down. When the knee flexes, these bands of scar tissue prevent the excursion of the quadriceps mechanism finally limiting the motion [26]. Therefore, patellofemoral mobilization must be initiated as soon as possible.

Table 1. In-hospital rehabilitation protocol after Total Knee Arthroplasty.

1ˢᵗ day after surgery	- Patient could immediately turn on his side and move actively the knee depending on the pain - Local cryotherapy for 15-20 minutes, 3\4 times a day - Painkiller under medical prescription **Exercises:** - Ankle flexion/extension, calf pump (active exercises), with or without elastic band, slow movements; maintain positions for 5–10 s - Knee flexion/extension: passive exercise, or continue passive motion (CPM). *If performed, CPM should be started from 10°-40°; gradually increased to 0°-90° in the first week* - Active knee flexion/extension with ROM 0°-40° - Isometric contractions of quadriceps, gluteus and adductors muscles position maintenance for 5–10 s, with gradual increase - Straight leg elevation with extended knee under physiotherapist control
2ⁿᵈ day after surgery	- Local cryotherapy for 15-20 minutes, 3\4 times a day - Painkiller under medical prescription **Exercises:** - Same as above - Slowly increase of CPM and active flexion exercises - Isometric contractions of abductor and adductor muscles - Recovery of seat position **In seat position:** - Knee flexion and extension exercises, with the help of the physiotherapist - Auto-assisted exercises **Gait:** - Training with aids (crutches) with gradual progression of weightbearing
3ʳᵈ day after surgery	- Local cryotherapy for 15-20 minutes, 3\4 times a day - Painkiller under medical prescription **Exercises:** - Same as above - Slowly increase of CPM and active flexion exercises - Gait exercises with crutches with partial weightbearing Exercises in prone position: - Passive knee extension - Knee flexion, gradual motion increase with the help of the physiotherapist depending on pain - If tolerated quadriceps electrostimulation

(Table 1) contd.....

4th day after surgery	- Local cryotherapy for 15-20 minutes, 3\4 times a day - Painkiller under medical prescription **Exercises:** - Same as above - Slowly increase CPM degrees and active flexion degrees - Gait with crutches with partial weightbearing
Other steps	- From 9th day stairs training with aids - From 3rd week close kinetic chain exercises - From 3rd week use of stationary bike - From 3rd week proprioceptive exercises - Hydrotherapy at scar healing

CPM is a postoperative method aimed to aid a functional recovery after orthopaedic surgery. CPM is made by a device used to gently flex and extend the knee joint passively without the need of any voluntary muscle contraction. The use of CPM is actually controversial [27 - 29]; however it appears to be strongly helpful in the first stages of the rehabilitation, mainly in presence of postoperative pain [29]. A Cochrane review concluded that CPM combined with physical therapy may shorten the hospital stay, decrease the number of postoperative manipulations, and reduce the use of analgesics [30]. In the first few days following surgery, CPM is also useful to minimize the haemarthrosis and the periarticular oedema. If CPM is used through a greater ROM where tissues tension is greater, the pumping effect in the periarticular tissues is predicted to have a greater impact on soft tissue [29].

Starting from the first day after surgery isometric contractions of quadriceps, gluteus, and adductors muscles should be performed. Several studies [31] revealed that quadriceps strength was the physical parameter most significantly reduced following TKA, and never regained when compared to the contralateral limb. Furthermore, quadriceps strength was the most highly correlated parameter associated with the functional performance. Additionally, some authors [32] documented that the isometric strength of leg extensors was weaker in a group of HP by 32–38% compared to a healthy control group. A balanced strength training program therefore appears to be important for HP after TKA.

On the second day after surgery, HP can assume the seated position and, in absence of complications, start a partial weightbearing with aids and in a carefully manner under physiotherapist surveillance. Because of the quadriceps inhibition, the use of a walker or crutches is necessary. A training with aids should be performed with a gradual progression of weightbearing: frame from the first week after surgery, 50% weightbearing with two crutches from the 7th to the 20th days, and 70% weightbearing with one crutch from the 20th day. Full weightbearing is usually allowed from the 25th to the 30th day. Crutches may be dropped after 45 days: the decision of discharging the patient involves all components of MT.

In several cases it is possible to associate a physical therapy. "Low Level Laser therapy" could be used to achieve a faster recovery from oedema and soft tissues haematoma. Electrical stimulation of quadriceps muscle is a complementary tool for the muscle strengthening in association to active exercises [33].

Out-Patient Rehabilitation

At home HP needs a rigorous rehabilitation program. To prevent bleeding complications, each session of physiotherapy should be preceded by an infusion of clotting factor according to the schedule released from the haematologist.

Sessions will be focused on the continuity of ROM exercises for flexion and extension, proprioceptive exercises, and alternating specific muscle strengthening in "open kinetic chain" (OKC) and in "closed kinetic chain" (CKC)(Table **2**). Kinetic chain terminology has been introduced to describe the strengthening exercises for lower limbs. During CKC exercises, the foot is fixed and motion at the knee is accompanied by the motion at the hip and ankle joints in a predictable manner [34]. There are a variety of progressive CKC exercises focused on cardiopulmonary rehabilitation, such as stationary bicycling and stepper device, as well as on strength recovery (lateral set-ups, stair climbing, leg press and mini-squats). CKC exercises result in increased joint compressive forces, increased joint congruency and stability, decreased shear forces, stimulation of proprioceptors, and enhanced dynamic stability [35, 36].

Table 2. Examples of exercises suggested to patients after TKA in their daily home-rehabilitation program (*partially adapted from: Kathy Mulder. Exercises for people with Haemophilia, published by the World Federation of Hemophilia, 2006*).

Start: Sit with legs out straight (or lie on back). *Exercise:* Bend hip and knee, and slide heels towards body. Then straighten knees by sliding heels away from body. Repeat several times. *Goal:* Try to get the back of the knee as close to the surface as possible. Also try to bend the knee as much as the other knee can bend.	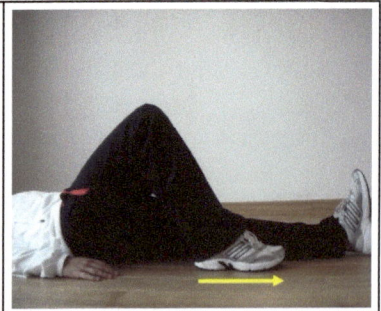

(Table 2) contd.....

Start: Sit on chair. Support the weight of the affected leg with the other leg if necessary. ***Exercise:*** Allow the knee to bend as much as is comfortable, then straighten the leg as far as possible. ***Goal:*** Try to bend a bit more each time.	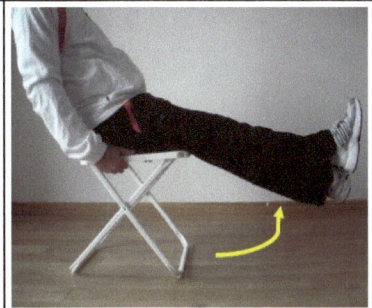
Note: If the person has difficulty lying on his stomach, it may be necessary to place a pillow under the waist so that the hip is more comfortable, or a pad under the thigh to take pressure off the knee cap. ***Start:*** Lie on stomach. ***Exercise:*** Bend knee and try to touch heel to buttocks. Assist with the other leg if necessary. Then straighten the leg as far as possible. ***Goal:*** Bend the knee as much as knee could bend before bleedings.	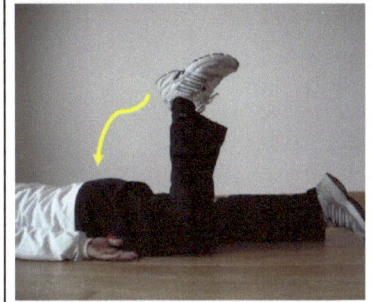
Start: Lie in a comfortable position. ***Exercise:*** Move foot up and down, in and out. Practice drawing shapes or letters of the alphabet with the foot, keeping the rest of the leg still. ***Goal:*** Full ankle motion equal to the opposite ankle or baseline.	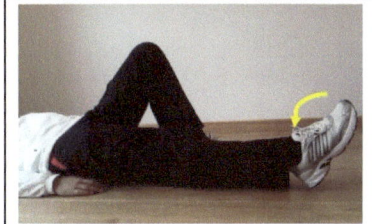
Strength:	
Start: Lie on back with a roll under the knee. ***Exercise:*** Tighten the muscle at front of the thigh, extend the knee and lift the heel. Hold for several seconds, then relax. Repeat until the muscle feels tired. ***Goal:*** Straighten the knee completely or as straight as the knee could go before the most recent bleeding. Compare to the other knee or the baseline assessment.	
Start: Sit on a chair with the knee bent. ***Exercise:*** Extend the knee, lifting the foot off the floor as far as possible. Hold for several seconds, then slowly return foot to floor. Repeat until the muscle feels tired. ***Goal:*** As above, straighten the knee completely or as straight as it could go before the most recent bleeding. Increase repetitions. Compare contralateral or the baseline assessment.	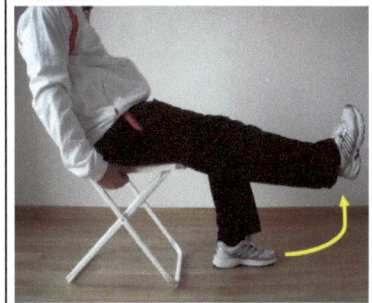

(Table 2) contd.....

Start: Sit on chair. Cross the ankle of the uninjured leg over the ankle of the affected leg. ***Exercise:*** Press ankles together as hard as possible. Hold for several seconds, then relax. Repeat with the knee bent at different angles. Repeat until the muscle feels tired. ***Goal:*** As above, straighten the knee completely or as straight as it could go. Continue until the affected leg can exert a strong pressure, equal to the unaffected leg.	
Proprioception:	
Start: Stand on the affected leg. ***Exercise:*** Maintain balance. ***Goal:*** Practice until balance can be maintained for 30 seconds.	
Start: Stand on the affected leg with eyes closed. ***Exercise***: Maintain balance with eyes closed as long as possible. ***Goal:*** Practice until balance can be maintained with eyes closed for 30 seconds.	
Start: Stand on the affected leg on an unstable surface (*e.g.*, pillow, block of foam). ***Exercise:*** Maintain balance. ***Goal:*** Practice until balance can be maintained for 30 seconds.	
Start: Stand on the affected leg on an unstable surface and close eyes. ***Exercise:*** Maintain balance with eyes closed as long as possible. ***Goal:*** Practice until balance can be maintained with eyes closed for 30 seconds.	

In contrast, in OKC exercises the foot is mobile and motion at the knee occurs independently from the motion at the hip and ankle joints [34]. OKC exercises lead to increased distraction and rotational forces, activation of muscular mechanoreceptors, and greater concentric acceleration and eccentric deceleration forces. These are characteristics typical of 'non-weightbearing' activities [35]. OKC activities for the knee may include exercises to improve strength or ROM. Resisted OKC exercises may be applied manually to the knee, as in proprioceptive neuromuscular facilitation, or through an external resistance using a leg-extension device. OKC exercises should be performed later respect to CKC activities in the rehabilitation program.

Proprioception is defined as the unconscious perception of movement and spatial orientation arising from stimuli within the body itself. Maintenance of postural balance includes a complex sensorial process involving articular mechanoreceptors, the vestibular and the visual systems. Sensorial and motor informations are then processed in the central nervous system. Finally, there is a motor response involving various muscle groups, including those around ankles, thighs, trunk, and neck [34]. A subject undergoing TKA may experience an impaired balance both in the sensory and motor level. The position of the center of gravity relative to the base of support may not be accurately sensed because of the destruction of knee mechanoreceptors following surgery. The automatic movements required to bring the center of gravity to a balanced position may be compromised as a result of quadriceps inhibition.

In the haemophilic population, preexisting proprioceptive deficits may also be present [37]. A specialized training for the proprioception performance may therefore be helpful to compensate any coordination deficits [32].

Hydrotherapy could be useful and can be started as soon as the surgical scar heals. The buoyancy of the water allows assisted, active, and resisted exercises while providing a sense of security [38]. Using buoyant principles, the aquatic environment can provide a gradual transition from no to full weightbearing exercises. Additionally, the tactile stimulation from the turbulence generated during movements provides a feedback that aids the proprioception [38]. Also, the warmth of the water aids in relaxing muscles and reducing pain. Psychologically, hydrotherapy may also increase the confidence as the patient experiences an increased walking ability, stretching or strengthening activities in the water [19].

TOTAL HIP ARTHROPLASTY

Hip arthropathy is less common in comparison with knee, elbow and ankle arthropathy in haemophilic patients [39]. One possible reason is that haemarthroses occurs less frequently in the hip given its relative poor amount of synovial tissue with respect to other target joints. If arthropathy is severe, a THA may be required. Research on outcomes of THA is fewer than TKA and limited to smaller case series [40, 41] (see Chapter 12). THA in patients with Haemophilia, as for other hip diseases, may offer a significant pain relief and improved function, even if there is a higher rate of complications that lead to revisions in 20–57% of patients [42]. It is possible to underline different stages in rehabilitation after TKA in hip: preoperative setting, in-hospital rehabilitation, and out-patient rehabilitation.

Preoperative Setting

During the preoperative assessment, the MT should perform a complete evaluation of all joints (ROM, strength, local conditions, evaluation scales). This preoperative evaluation also provides the opportunity for the patient and MT to discuss about postoperative expectations [20]. A specific objective of THA is the education about restricted movements of hip immediately after surgery (in particular to avoid hip adduction and external rotation, flexion >90°), and a training on the use of crutches [43].

In–Hospital Rehabilitation

After surgery the first stage of rehabilitation could be started directly in the orthopedic ward (Table **3**). To prevent bleeding complications, each session of physiotherapy should be preceded by infusion of clotting factor. Primary objectives are the reduction of pain, recovery of a minimal ROM, and an initial muscle strengthening. The day of surgery pain could be alleviated by the use of cryotherapy or painkillers. In-bed, in order to guarantee a correct postural alignment, the horizontal decubitus may be alternated with the semi-sitting position by tilting the head of the bed up to 45°. Lower limbs are spread apart by the use of an abductor pillow and the foot of the operated limb maintained oriented toward the ceiling. Internal rotation of the leg and intersection of lower limbs is prohibited. The patient could also start with ankles flexion/extension exercises [3].

Table 3. In-hospital rehabilitation protocol after Total Hip Arthroplasty.

1st day after surgery	- The patient could immediately turn on his side and move actively the hip, as tolerated - Local cryotherapy for 15-20 minutes, 3\4 times a day - Painkiller under medical prescription **Exercises:** - Ankle flexion/extension, calf pump (active exercises), with or without elastic band, slow movements; maintain positions for 5–10 s - Hip mobilizations in flexion-extension, passive manual techniques undertaken by the physiotherapist. Hip flexion should gradually start from a limited ROM of 10°-45° - Hip mobilization in abduction by passive manual techniques at a maximum of 30° - Isometric contractions of quadriceps, gluteus and adductors muscles for 5–10 s, with gradual increase - Straight leg elevation with extended knee by physiotherapist's assistance

(Table 3) contd.....

2nd day after surgery	- Local cryotherapy for 15-20 minutes, 3\4 times a day - Painkiller under medical prescription **Exercises:** - Same as above - Slowly increase of active flexion and abduction exercises - Isometric contractions of abductor and adductor muscles - Recovery of the seat position In seat position: - Knee flexion and extension exercises with the physiotherapist - Auto-assisted exercises
3rd day after surgery	- Local cryotherapy for 15-20 minutes, 3\4 times a day - Painkiller under medical prescription - Orthostatic readaptation by exercises of load transfer in lateral and anteroposterior **Exercises:** - Same as above - Slowly increase of active flexion and abduction exercises - Isometric exercises against resistance of the therapist for the abductors and adductors
4th day after surgery	- Local cryotherapy for 15-20 minutes, 3\4 times a day - Painkillers under medical prescription ***Gait:*** - Training with aids (two crutches) with gradual progression of weightbearing **Exercises:** - Same as above - Slowly increase of CPM and active flexion exercises - Gait with crutches with partial weightbearing
Other steps	- From 9th day stairs training with aids - From 3rd week close kinetic chain exercises - From 3rd week use of cyclette - From 3rd week proprioceptive exercises - Hydrotherapy as soon as the scar healing allows

On the first day after surgery, patients should start isometric contractions of the gluteus: series of 3-5 sessions to be repeated 3 to 5 times a day. Patients should carry on isometric contractions of the quadriceps muscle, slowly contracting the anterior thigh muscles, pushing the knee against the bed and pulling on the toe. Such contractions should be maintained for at least 10 seconds then released for at least 15 seconds: 3 to 5 series of exercises to be repeated 3-5 times a day. Hip mobilizations in flexion and extension can be performed by passive manual techniques undertaken by the physiotherapist. Hip flexion should gradually start from a limited ROM of 10°- 45° by sliding the heel on the sheet, and keeping the knee facing the ceiling. Hip abduction can be performed by passive manual techniques undertaken by the physiotherapist: on the first day it should reach at a maximum ROM of 30° [43].

On the second day after surgery, the same program should be proposed, followed by sitting in position in the bed for 1 hour at least three times a day, if tolerated. The sitting position should be on the side corresponding to the operated limb taking the operated limb out of bed with the help of the physiotherapist, followed by the healthy limb. Hip flexion may thus reach a ROM of 80°-90°, as the knee could reach a 90° flexion and the trunk erected by a support of a chair or pillows. It is important not to exceed 90° of hip flexion. In such position, the patient is encouraged to perform some exercises as active flexion and extension of the knee, alternating the contraction of one gluteus to the other [43].

On the third day after surgery, exercises should be repeated with a gradual increasing of ROM for flexion and extension. Patient should start isometric exercises against resistance of the therapist for the abductor and adductor muscles. These exercises should be performed only in the presence of the operator. Patients should carry on an orthostatic re-adaptation with partial weightbearing by means of exercises of load transfer in lateral and anteroposterior: this would progressively improve the self-conscience of the weight to be transferred on the operated limb. Then the recovery of the orthostatic position by the use of two crutches and assistance of the operator should be yielded. In standing position, the patient should perform some simple exercises, such as hip and knee flexion, and hip abduction [24].

From the 4th to the 10thday after surgery, the patient should improve his gait ability, using closed shoes and over a nonslip surface. Initially the therapist should teach how to walk by two crutches with a "three times" scheme: crutches-operated limb/healthy limb (put forward the crutches, carry on the operated limb at the level of crutches, and then the healthy limb beyond the crutches).

In order to learn the sitting position, the patient should use a chair with armrests for the support during the transition from sitting to standing position, always keeping his feet parallel during the movement: it has to be avoided an excessive forward flexion of the trunk and a hip flexion >90°. Training with aids should be performed with gradual progression of weightbearing: a frame might be used from the first postoperative week, with 50% of weightbearing with two crutches from the day 7 to 20, and 70% of weightbearing with 1 crutch from the 20th day. Full weightbearing is generally allowed from the 30th day. A physical therapy with laser therapy (Low Level Laser) may be used to treat oedema or soft tissues haematoma. Electrical stimulation of quadriceps muscle is a complementary tool for the muscle strengthening when added to active exercises [33].

Out-Patient Rehabilitation

As after TKA, HP after THA should follow a tailored and progressively intense rehabilitation program. To prevent bleedings, each session should be preceded by an infusion of clotting factor. Sessions should be focused on ROM exercises for flexion and extension, proprioceptive exercises, and alternating specific muscle strengthening in CKC and OKC.

For the first three months, patients should be discouraged to cross their legs and assume a squatting position on heels. It could be useful for one to two months to use a pillow on the chair during the night, and to use chairs with high armrests. Patients should use suitable hikes for toilet and bidet for the first two months. A lateral decubitus on the operated side during night is allowed once achieved the complete healing of the surgical wound. Specialized training for the proprioception performance may therefore be helpful to compensate any deficit [32].

Hydrotherapy could be also useful and started after healing of the scar. As mentioned before after TKA, water exercises offer a safe rehabilitation and sense of security [38].

CONCLUDING REMARKS

A comprehensive rehabilitative program proposed by a multidisciplinary team is the key to optimize the results of major orthopaedic surgery in patients affected by Haemophilia. Rehabilitation should be based on shared protocols, and at the same time specific and individualized for each patient, in order to improve the functional ability, finally ensuring a better quality of life.

CONFLICT OF INTEREST

The authors confirm that they have no conflict of interest to declare for this publication.

ACKNOWLEDGEMENTS

Declared none.

REFERENCES

[1]   de Kleijn P, Sluiter D, Vogely HCh, Lindeman E, Fischer K. Long-term outcome of multiple joint procedures in haemophilia. Haemophilia 2014; 20(2): 276-81.
        [http://dx.doi.org/10.1111/hae.12285] [PMID: 24533953]

[2]   Lobet S, Pendeville E, Dalzell R, *et al.* The role of physiotherapy after total knee arthroplasty in patients with haemophilia. Haemophilia 2008; 14(5): 989-98.
        [http://dx.doi.org/10.1111/j.1365-2516.2008.01748.x] [PMID: 18582230]

[3]   De Kleijn P, Blamey G, Zourikian N, Dalzell R, Lobet S. Physiotherapy following elective orthopaedic procedures. Haemophilia 2006; 12 (Suppl. 3): 108-12.
        [http://dx.doi.org/10.1111/j.1365-2516.2006.01266.x] [PMID: 16684004]

[4]   Forsyth A, Zourikian N. How we treat: Considerations for physiotherapy in the patient with haemophilia and inhibitors undergoing elective orthopaedic surgery. Haemophilia 2012; 18(4): 550-3.
[http://dx.doi.org/10.1111/j.1365-2516.2012.02755.x] [PMID: 22934294]

[5]   Teitel JM, Carcao M, Lillicrap D, *et al.* Orthopaedic surgery in haemophilia patients with inhibitors: a practical guide to haemostatic, surgical and rehabilitative care. Haemophilia 2009; 15(1): 227-39.
[http://dx.doi.org/10.1111/j.1365-2516.2008.01840.x] [PMID: 18752535]

[6]   Heijnen L, Dirat G, Chen L, *et al.* The role of the physiatrist in the haemophilia comprehensive care team in different parts of the world. Haemophilia 2008; 14 (Suppl. 3): 153-61.
[http://dx.doi.org/10.1111/j.1365-2516.2008.01743.x] [PMID: 18510536]

[7]   Stephensen D. Rehabilitation of patients with haemophilia after orthopaedic surgery: a case study. Haemophilia 2005; 11 (Suppl. 1): 26-9.
[http://dx.doi.org/10.1111/j.1365-2516.2005.01151.x] [PMID: 16219047]

[8]   Mancuso CA, Sculco TP, Wickiewicz TL, *et al.* Patients expectations of knee surgery. J Bone Joint Surg Am 2001; 83-A(7): 1005-12.
[http://dx.doi.org/10.2106/00004623-200107000-00005] [PMID: 11451969]

[9]   Canadian Hemophilia Society. Standards of Physiotherapy Care and Assessment 2009.

[10]   Blamey G, Forsyth A, Zourikian N, *et al.* Comprehensive elements of a physiotherapy exercise programme in haemophiliaa global perspective. Haemophilia 2010; 16 (Suppl. 5): 136-45.
[http://dx.doi.org/10.1111/j.1365-2516.2010.02312.x] [PMID: 20590873]

[11]   Mulder K, Llinás A. The target joint. Haemophilia 2004; 10 (Suppl. 4): 152-6.
[http://dx.doi.org/10.1111/j.1365-2516.2004.00976.x] [PMID: 15479389]

[12]   Rodriguez-Merchan EC. Total joint arthroplasty: the final solution for knee and hip when synovitis could not be controlled. Haemophilia 2007; 13 (Suppl. 3): 49-58.
[http://dx.doi.org/10.1111/j.1365-2516.2007.01553.x] [PMID: 17822522]

[13]   NIH Consensus Development Conference on Total Knee Arthroplasty. National Institutes of Health Consensus Development Conference Statement 2003.

[14]   Scalone L, Mantovani LG, Mannucci PM, Gringeri A. Quality of life is associated to the orthopaedic status in haemophilic patients with inhibitors. Haemophilia 2006; 12(2): 154-62.
[http://dx.doi.org/10.1111/j.1365-2516.2006.01204.x] [PMID: 16476090]

[15]   Solovieva S. Clinical severity of disease, functional disability and health-related quality of life. Three-year follow-up study of 150 Finnish patients with coagulation disorders. Haemophilia 2001; 7(1): 53-63.
[http://dx.doi.org/10.1046/j.1365-2516.2001.00476.x] [PMID: 11136382]

[16]   Silva M, Luck JV Jr. Long-term results of primary total knee replacement in patients with hemophilia. J Bone Joint Surg Am 2005; 87(1): 85-91.
[PMID: 15634817]

[17]   Bong MR, Di Cesare PE. Stiffness after total knee arthroplasty. J Am Acad Orthop Surg 2004; 12(3): 164-71.
[http://dx.doi.org/10.5435/00124635-200405000-00004] [PMID: 15161169]

[18]   Strauss AC, Goldmann G, Schmolders J, *et al.* Impact of Preoperative Knee Stiffness on the Postoperative Outcome after Total Knee Arthroplasty in Patients with Haemophilia. Z Orthop Unfall 2015; 153(5): 526-32.

[19]   Viliani T, Zambelan G, Pandolfi C, *et al.* In-patient rehabilitation in haemophilic subjects with total knee arthroplasty. Haemophilia 2011; 17(5): e999-e1004.
[PMID: 21535326]

[20]   McDonald S, Hetrick S, Green S. Pre-operative education for hip or knee replacement. Cochrane Database Syst Rev 2004; 1(1): CD003526.
[PMID: 14974019]

[21]   Beaupre LA, Lier D, Davies DM, Johnston DB. The effect of a preoperative exercise and education program on functional recovery, health related quality of life, and health service utilization following primary total knee arthroplasty. J Rheumatol 2004; 31(6): 1166-73.
[PMID: 15170931]

[22]   Ackerman IN, Bennell KL. Does pre-operative physiotherapy improve outcomes from lower limb joint replacement surgery? A systematic review. Aust J Physiother 2004; 50(1): 25-30.
[http://dx.doi.org/10.1016/S0004-9514(14)60245-2] [PMID: 14987189]

[23]   Mitchell C, Walker J, Walters S, Morgan AB, Binns T, Mathers N. Costs and effectiveness of pre- and post-operative home physiotherapy for total knee replacement: randomized controlled trial. J Eval Clin Pract 2005; 11(3): 283-92.
[http://dx.doi.org/10.1111/j.1365-2753.2005.00535.x] [PMID: 15869558]

[24]   De Kleijn P, Fischer K, Vogely HCh, Hendriks C, Lindeman E. In-hospital rehabilitation after multiple joint procedures of the lower extremities in haemophilia patients: clinical guidelines for physical therapists. Haemophilia 2011; 17(6): 971-8.
[http://dx.doi.org/10.1111/j.1365-2516.2011.02527.x] [PMID: 21457409]

[25]   Atilla B, Caglar O, Pekmezci M, Buyukasik Y, Tokgozoglu AM, Alpaslan M. Pre-operative flexion contracture determines the functional outcome of haemophilic arthropathy treated with total knee arthroplasty. Haemophilia 2012; 18(3): 358-63.
[http://dx.doi.org/10.1111/j.1365-2516.2011.02695.x] [PMID: 22103453]

[26]   Maloney WJ. The stiff total knee arthroplasty: evaluation and management. J Arthroplasty 2002; 17(4) (Suppl. 1): 71-3.
[http://dx.doi.org/10.1054/arth.2002.32450] [PMID: 12068410]

[27]   McInnes J, Larson MG, Daltroy LH, *et al.* A controlled evaluation of continuous passive motion in patients undergoing total knee arthroplasty. JAMA 1992; 268(11): 1423-8.
[http://dx.doi.org/10.1001/jama.268.11.1423] [PMID: 1512910]

[28]   Crowe J, Henderson J. Pre-arthroplasty rehabilitation is effective in reducing hospital stay. Can J Occup Ther 2003; 70(2): 88-96.
[http://dx.doi.org/10.1177/000841740307000204] [PMID: 12704972]

[29]   De Kleijn P, Blamey G, Zourikian N, Dalzell R, Lobet S. Physiotherapy following elective orthopaedic procedures. Haemophilia 2006; 12 (Suppl. 3): 108-12.
[http://dx.doi.org/10.1111/j.1365-2516.2006.01266.x] [PMID: 16684004]

[30]   Milne S, Brosseau L, Robinson V, *et al.* Continuous passive motion following total knee arthroplasty. Cochrane Database Syst Rev 2003; 2(2): CD004260.
[PMID: 12804511]

[31]   Mizner RL, Petterson SC, Snyder-Mackler L. Quadriceps strength and the time course of functional recovery after total knee arthroplasty. J Orthop Sports Phys Ther 2005; 35(7): 424-36.
[http://dx.doi.org/10.2519/jospt.2005.35.7.424] [PMID: 16108583]

[32]   Hilberg T, Herbsleb M, Puta C, Gabriel HH, Schramm W. Physical training increases isometric muscular strength and proprioceptive performance in haemophilic subjects. Haemophilia 2003; 9(1): 86-93.

[33]   Stevens JE, Mizner RL, Snyder-Mackler L. Neuromuscular electrical stimulation for quadriceps muscle strengthening after bilateral total knee arthroplasty: a case series. J Orthop Sports Phys Ther 2004; 34(1): 21-9.
[http://dx.doi.org/10.2519/jospt.2004.34.1.21] [PMID: 14964588]

[34] Lutz GE, Palmitier RA, An KN, Chao EY. Comparison of tibiofemoral joint forces during open-kinetic-chain and closed-kinetic-chain exercises. J Bone Joint Surg Am 1993; 75(5): 732-9.
[http://dx.doi.org/10.2106/00004623-199305000-00014] [PMID: 8501090]

[35] Prentice WE. Open-*versus* closed-kinetic chain exercises in rehabilitation In: Prentice WE, Voight MI, Eds. Techniques in Musculoskeletal Rehabilitation. USA: McGraw-Hill 2001.

[36] Palmitier RA, An KN, Scott SG, Chao EY. Kinetic chain exercise in knee rehabilitation. Sports Med 1991; 11(6): 402-13.
[http://dx.doi.org/10.2165/00007256-199111060-00005] [PMID: 1925185]

[37] Buzzard BM. Proprioceptive training in haemophilia. Haemophilia 1998; 4(4): 528-31.
[http://dx.doi.org/10.1046/j.1365-2516.1998.440528.x] [PMID: 9873788]

[38] Erler K, Anders C, Fehlberg G, Neumann U, Brücker L, Scholle HC. [Objective assessment of results of special hydrotherapy in inpatient rehabilitation following knee prosthesis implantation]. Z Orthop Ihre Grenzgeb 2001; 139(4): 352-8.
[http://dx.doi.org/10.1055/s-2001-16923] [PMID: 11558055]

[39] Rodriguez-Merchan EC. Total joint arthroplasty: the final solution for knee and hip when synovitis could not be controlled. Haemophilia 2007; 13 (Suppl. 3): 49-58.
[http://dx.doi.org/10.1111/j.1365-2516.2007.01553.x] [PMID: 17822522]

[40] Wang K, Street A, Dowrick A, Liew S. Clinical outcomes and patient satisfaction following total joint replacement in haemophilia23-year experience in knees, hips and elbows. Haemophilia 2012; 18(1): 86-93.
[http://dx.doi.org/10.1111/j.1365-2516.2011.02579.x] [PMID: 21649799]

[41] Carulli C, Felici I, Martini C, *et al.* Total Hip Arthroplasty in Haemophilic Patients with Modern Cementless Implants. J Arthroplasty 2015; 30(10): 1757-60.
[http://dx.doi.org/10.1016/j.arth.2015.04.035] [PMID: 25998131]

[42] Löfquist T, Sanzén L, Petersson C, Nilsson IM. Total hip replacement in patients with hemophilia. Acta Orthop Scand 1996; 4: 747-51.

[43] Kelley SS, Lachiewicz PF, Gilbert MS, Bolander ME, Jankiewicz JJ. Hip arthroplasty in hemophilic arthropathy. J Bone Joint Surg Am 1995; 77(6): 828-34.
[http://dx.doi.org/10.2106/00004623-199506000-00003] [PMID: 7782355]

Frontiers in Arthritis, 2017, *Vol. 2*, 229-239

CHAPTER 17

Complications of the Orthopaedic Surgery in Haemophilia

Luigi Piero Solimeno[1], **Mattia Alessio Mazzola**[2] and **Gianluigi Pasta**[1,*]

[1] *Fondazione IRCCS Ca' Granda Ospedale Maggiore Policlinico, Milan, Italy*
[2] *Orthopaedic Clinic, University of Genoa, Genoa, Italy*

Abstract: The knowledge regarding the management of complications related to orthopaedic surgery in Haemophilia is still limited due to the lack of published data and several concerns about the possible catastrophic damage to patients. A quote of 12% to 17% of haemophilic patients need a hospital admission to undergo orthopaedic surgery and more than one procedure is often needed for some subjects. Complications in haemophilic patients occur from 2% to 66% and are strictly related to the severity of disease, type of orthopaedic procedure, and patient comorbidities.

Bleeding, haematoma, wound complications, infection, inhibitors development, deep venous thromboembolism, and intraoperative fractures are the most frequently reported complications. The management of complications of the orthopaedic surgery in haemophiliacs is a challenging task, requiring complex treatment performed in a highly specialized centre by a multidisciplinary team.

Keywords: Bleeding, Complications, Fractures Haemophilia, Haematoma, Infection, Inhibitors, Orthopaedic surgery.

INTRODUCTION

In recent decades, the availability of safe and effective clotting factors concentrates had a strong impact on the natural history of Haemophilia, reducing the incidence of arthropathy and allowing surgeons to perform a greater number of orthopaedic procedures. Despite the use of the replacement therapy, surgery in patients with Haemophilia remains challenging. Clinical guidance on treatment during orthopaedic procedures in this population are strongly recommended to prevent or minimize any related complications [1]. Many orthopaedic surgeons still hesitate to perform surgeries for haemophilic arthropathy because of the higher risk of complications. However, orthopaedic surgery should be restricted to

* **Corresponding author Gianluigi Pasta:** Fondazione IRCCS Ca' Granda, Milan, Italy; Tel: 00393332539893; E-mail: gianluigi.pasta@policlinico.mi.it

Christian Carulli (Ed.)

patients with severe joint damage and when conservative treatments have failed [2].

Hepatitis C virus (HCV) and human immunodeficiency virus (HIV), have been mediated by unheated plasma-derived factor concentrates, and discouraged most of the orthopaedic surgeons from performing surgery. Moreover, antiretroviral therapies increased the risk of metabolic syndrome, diabetes, renal insufficiency, and cardiovascular disease exposing patients to additional generic complications [3].

Nevertheless, 12% to 17% of haemophilic patients usually need a hospital admission to perform orthopaedic surgery, and more than one procedure is often requested by several subjects.

Complications in haemophiliacs occur from 2% to 66% and are strictly related to several factors: severity of disease, type of orthopaedic procedure, and patient comorbidities [4, 5].

The management of complications of orthopaedic surgery in Haemophilia is still debated due to the lack of published data and several concerns about the possible catastrophic damages to patients.

The knowledge of preoperative factors affecting the incidence of perioperative complications is crucial to safely perform surgery in such patients.

Surgery must be performed by an experienced surgeon, under a tailored haematological prophylaxis, and in a specialized center, in order to manage the proper daily replacement therapy. This multidisciplinary approach is essential to ensure a surgical success [2].

SPECIFIC COMPLICATIONS OF THE ORTHOPAEDIC SURGERY IN HEMOPHILIA

Bleeding

Bleeding is the most common complication during orthopaedic surgery in haemophilic patients.

A satisfactory control of haemostasis is achieved in most patients but bleeding complications are observed in 3% to 20% of treated patients and it is more frequent in case of major orthopaedic procedures [6 - 8], and in inhibitor than non-inhibitor patients. Published data have demonstrated that a proper replacement therapy can provide an adequate and well-tolerated perioperative and postoperative haemostatic coverage for a variety of major orthopaedic procedures in patients with Haemophilia. Although a surgical haemostasis can be achieved by the use of tourniquet and infusion of factor concentrates at the adequate dose, our recommendation for surgeons is always to have availability of local intraoperative haemostatic agents (*i.e.* fibrin glue, absorbable hemostatic sponge) [9].

Blood Loss

The decline in haemoglobin levels and transfusion requirement tend to be greater in haemophiliacs than in the general population [7].

Blood loss is often associated with total hip and knee replacements. The median blood loss, and postoperative drainage is reported to be respectively 1350 mL and 500 mL in Total Hip Arthroplasty (THA) and 625 mL and 600 mL in Total Knee Arthroplasty (TKA). The median red blood cell transfusion volume in THA is reported to be 5 U (0-14), and 2 U (0-18) in TKA [10].

The success rate for haemostasis response during and after surgery is very high and the reported results are "excellent" or "good" in major and minor surgical procedures [11].

Haematoma

Haematoma related to arthroscopic surgery has been described in two papers and is considered as a rare event. Arthroscopic surgery may be certainly considered as a low risk procedure associated with satisfactory outcomes. The only relative disadvantage is the poor management of postoperative bleedings and the risk of additional haemarthroses [12]. In 1998, Heim reported two expansive haematomas at the arthroscopic portal and in 1992, he described an arterovenous fistula following a knee arthroscopy [13].

In order to avoid these complications, we recommend to highlight all the arterials, venous, and nervous landmarks by a dermographic marker pen before performing the standard arthroscopic portals.

On the other hand, the incidence of postoperative intraarticular haematoma following a joint replacement is higher (up to 7.7%) than in non-haemophilic population. This complication is usually managed by additional doses of coagulative factors replacement, and a delayed beginning of the rehabilitation. A surgical evacuation is rarely necessary and not always recommended. An accurate monitoring of the evolution of haematoma is necessary to early identify local signs of infection.

Wound Complications

Wound complications can be devastating. Patient-specific risk factors are described in the literature (diabetes mellitus, peripheral vascular disease, rheumatoid arthritis, immune-modifying medications, smoking and obesity) [14]. It has also been demonstrated in animal models that bleeding disorders including Haemophilia may affect the wound healing [15]. On one hand proper wound healing requires coagulation with strong thrombin generation resulting in fibrin formation. On the other hand, poor haemostasis, renal or liver disease, and immunodeficiency were reported to be systemic factors that may compromise wound healing in total joint replacement [3].

Wound complications in Haemophilia are described in 3.4-3.8% of total joint replacements occurring from 20 to 30 days after surgery.

Various type of wound complications have been described including superficial and full-thickness soft-tissue necrosis. The management of these complications is demanding and secondary infection and fistula are the most frightening consequences if the treatment is delayed.

Superficial soft-tissue necrosis (<30mm) generally requires wound debridement with or without secondary closure. Larger defects (>30 mm) often are managed by soft tissues coverage with flaps as described by Zhai *et al.* [10]. Vacuum assisted wound closure may also improve blood supply enhancing the wound healing [16].

In case of full-thickness necrosis, prosthetic components can be exposed and prompt irrigation and debridement are strongly recommended. In these cases, a secondary closure is often unsuccessful, and a vascularized tissue transfer seems to be the unique solution [17].

Although no specific preoperative risk factors affecting the incidence of delayed wound healings are described in the literature, a meticulous surgical technique optimizes the wound healing potential.

We strictly recommend to achieve a good haemostasis in haemophilic patients especially with inhibitor, and a stable immunological status of HIV-seropositive patients.

Infection

The infection of a total joint replacement is a fearful complication that generally requires the surgical removal of the infected implant by a one-stage or two-stage exchange procedure associated with prolonged courses of intravenous or oral antimicrobial therapy. This event leads to an increase in both direct and indirect costs, resulting in a 400-600% growth in healthcare outlay.

Septic arthritis causes a great despondency and physical suffering to patients, sometimes involving the irreversible loss of joint function. Specific treatments of prosthetic joint infection in haemophilic patients are explained in detail in chapter 15.

The use of prostheses is associated with an increase in the risk of postoperative infection; arthroplasty appears to have a 10 times greater risk of infection than other procedures [18, 12]. In elective orthopedic surgery, we can expect in patients without comorbidities (such as HIV and/or HCV), an infection rate varying from 0.67% to 12.4%. Revision procedures following aseptic loosening are also increasing, and the infection rate in revision surgery in these cases is even higher (2-20%) [19]. In haemophilic patients the risk of postoperative infection is significantly higher than the non-haemophilic population, ranging from 7% to 26.5% in case of TKA [19, 20].

Inhibitors represent the main risk factor for infection. Several factors may justify the increased infectious risk in inhibitor patients: the prolonged surgical time due to end-stage arthropathies may induce an intraoperative contamination; bleeding or delayed wound healing may predispose to a microbial overgrowth; finally, the use of central venous catheters (often needed for frequent or continuous infusion) represents a specific risk factor for the development of bacteraemia [7] (Fig. **1**).

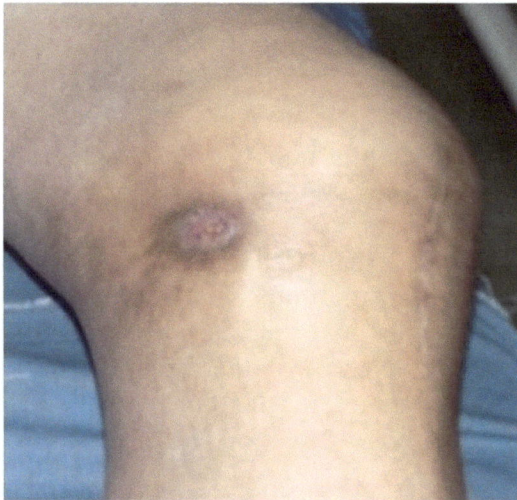

Fig. (1). Cutaneous fistula in a patient with inhibitors and porth-a-cath.

We recommend the inhibitor eradication before orthopaedic elective surgery given that it may result in a 30% lower incidence of infectious complications.

Hence, therapeutic strategies to eradicate or drastically reduce any inhibitor titer (as immune-tolerance induction or immune-absorption) may have a potential role prior to elective TKA in this subgroup of patients [7].

A septic arthritis in haemophilic patients should be considered when an episode of apparent haemarthrosis fails to promptly respond to the treatment by coagulation factor concentrates and joint immobilization. Severe haemarthrosis may cause slight pyrexia but, if the fever exceeds 38°C and is accompanied by rigors, a septic arthritis should be suspected [21].

Most authors agree that in the non-hemophilic population early infections are the most common prosthetic joint infections, but in patients with Haemophilia late infections prevail. The median time is approximately 2 years. Presence of inhibitors, continuous factors infusion, cementless implants, and a surgeon with less than 20 years of experience are associated with an increased risk of infection [7].

The short-term intravenous antibiotic prophylaxis, starting 30-60 min before skin incision, is recommended. A chemoprophylaxis reduces the incidence of postoperative joint infections. First or second generation cephalosporins and/or glycopeptides are the first-line antibiotics. Cefazolin (2 g I.V. 30–60 min prior to surgery followed by 0,5–1 g I.V. every 6–8 hours for 24 hours postoperatively) and/or vancomycin (1g I.V. single dose) should be administered [22]. To our knowledge the choice of Vancomycin in addition to cephalosporins in haemophiliacs is recommended because the higher MRSA infection risk.

Inhibitor Development

Not all patients with Haemophilia undergoing a replacement therapy develop inhibitors: however, a cumulative inhibitor risk increases with age. In severe Haemophilia A, 30-36% of patients develop inhibitors. For Haemophilia B the cumulative risk is lower (8%) than Haemophilia A [23]. Specific genetic risk factors for the development of inhibitors have been identified [24] but older patients with mild Haemophilia are at increased risk for inhibitors development following intensive factor replacement therapies for orthopaedic procedures. Patients should be carefully monitored for the presence of inhibitors related to factor exposure [23].

The main treatment option for eradicating inhibitors is the regular infusion of large doses of FVIII for many months to induce the so called "tolerance". This treatment is time consuming and extremely expensive with a success rate of 60–70% in most series [24].

Desmopressin may be contraindicated in mild Haemophilia with inhibitors due to an increased risk of myocardial infarction following its intravenous infusion [23].

Patients with inhibitors developing perioperative bleeding episodes or undergoing orthopaedic surgery are typically treated by rVIIa or aPCC (see Chapter 19). Risk of thrombotic complications associated with the use of bypassing agents should be considered in the ageing population with Haemophilia [25].

Venous Thromboembolism

The correction of the haemostatic defect in Haemophilia through perioperative use of coagulative factor concentrates theoretically increases the risk of venous thromboembolism (VTE) similarly to the general population [26]. However, the routinary use of pharmacologic VTE prophylaxis in patients with Haemophilia remains controversial and variable.

The concern for bleeding complications in this population has led to a variation of the VTE prophylaxis [27], and the paucity of randomized controlled trials exclude the development of evidence-based guidelines.

The actual incidence of VTE after total joint arthroplasty in patients with Haemophilia is unknown, and no clinical trials comparing the use of pharmacological prophylaxis *versus* placebo are available [26].

Haemophilia centers base their protocols on current state of knowledge and expert opinion. To the best of our knowledge the incidence of symptomatic VTE is very low. The routinary use of mechanical compression associated with the pharmacological VTE prophylaxis considered in selected high-risk patients (fractures, malignancies, other comorbidities) is a reasonable approach [28].

We recommend the use of knee-high compression stockings in every patient, and sequential compression devices and pharmacological prophylaxis only in selected cases.

Intraoperative Fractures

Haemophilic patients are predisposed to fractures during surgery because muscle wasting and osteoporosis affect bones that result more fragile and prone to fracture.

Fractures may realize in long bones but are more frequent at the periarticular zone or in the diaphysis of long bones. The haemophilic bone develops structural changes secondary to subperiosteal or intraosseous bleeding producing cysts or pseudotumours. Lower limb bones, especially the femur, are the common sites of fracture [29].

In case of fracture it is mandatory to maintain the level of the deficient factor to a value of 30–40% in the first 2–3 weeks after surgery.

In order to avoid iatrogenic fractures, the orthopaedic surgeon must pay a meticulous attention in the components' positioning. Surgeons must also remember that haematomas tend to be larger in volume than in non-haemophilic population, and may be the cause of compartment syndromes and neurovascular damages [30]. Moreover, it is very important to have a deep knowledge of the surgical anatomy of the upper and lower extremities to perform an adequate decompression in case of emergency conditions.

Management of intraoperative fractures in haemophilic patients must include the correct choice of stabilization as for periprosthetic fractures during a joint replacement in any kind of patients (Fig. **2**).

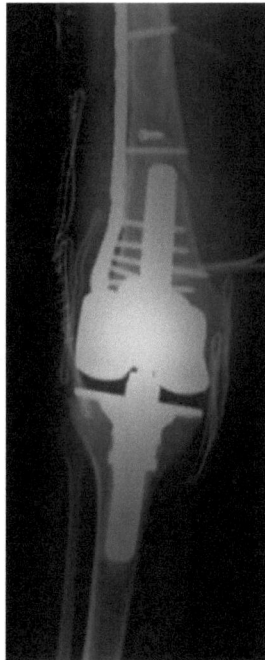

Fig. (2). Intraoperative periprosthetic femoral fracture and its treatment.

Specific steps for haemophiliacs are the prevention of bleeding and an early mobilization of the limb to prevent atrophy, in order to promote a return to the better functional outcome.

Vascular Injuries

One of the most common causes of haemarthrosis following joint replacement surgery or arthroscopic procedure in Haemophilia is the development of a pseudoaneurysm. An unrecognized injury of the periarticular vessels is the cause of this complication. Failed diagnosis and treatment may lead to subsequent recurrent bleedings. Endovascular treatments offer a minimally invasive treatment option in such cases [31].

CONCLUDING REMARKS

The management of complications of the orthopaedic surgery in haemophiliacs is a challenging task, requiring complex treatments performed in highly specialized centers by a multidisciplinary team, trained and experienced in this type of pathology, including an orthopaedic surgeon, anaesthesiologist, and haematologist.

CONFLICT OF INTEREST

The authors confirm that they have no conflict of interest to declare for this publication.

ACKNOWLEDGEMENTS

Declared none.

REFERENCES

[1]   Ingerslev J, Hvid I. Surgery in hemophilia. The general view: patient selection, timing, and preoperative assessment. Semin Hematol 2006; 43(1) (Suppl. 1): S23-6.
[http://dx.doi.org/10.1053/j.seminhematol.2005.11.024] [PMID: 16427380]

[2]   Lobet S, Hermans C, Lambert C. Optimal management of hemophilic arthropathy and hematomas. J Blood Med 2014; 5(5): 207-18.
[http://dx.doi.org/10.2147/JBM.S50644] [PMID: 25378964]

[3]   Hirose J, Takedani H, Koibuchi T. The risk of elective orthopaedic surgery for haemophilia patients: Japanese single-centre experience. Haemophilia 2013; 19(6): 951-5.
[http://dx.doi.org/10.1111/hae.12209] [PMID: 23746133]

[4]   Di Minno MN, Ambrosino P, Franchini M, Coppola A, Di Minno G. Arthropathy in patients with moderate hemophilia a: a systematic review of the literature. Semin Thromb Hemost 2013; 39(7): 723-31.
[http://dx.doi.org/10.1055/s-0033-1354422] [PMID: 24022804]

[5]   Serban M, Poenaru D, Patrascu J, *et al.* Risks and challenges of orthopaedic invasive interventions in haemophilia in a low-resource country. A single-center experience. Hamostaseologie 2014; 34 (Suppl. 1): S30-5.
[http://dx.doi.org/10.5482/HAMO-14-01-0007] [PMID: 25382767]

[6] Shapiro AD, Akins S. Cooper. Long-term outcomes from orthopaedic surgery in haemophilia: are we measuring success and documenting and assessing complications? Haemophilia 2014; 20: e359-75.
[http://dx.doi.org/10.1111/hae.12504] [PMID: 25039933]

[7] Solimeno LP, Mancuso ME, Pasta G, Santagostino E, Perfetto S, Mannucci PM. Factors influencing the long-term outcome of primary total knee replacement in haemophiliacs: a review of 116 procedures at a single institution. Br J Haematol 2009; 145(2): 227-34.
[http://dx.doi.org/10.1111/j.1365-2141.2009.07613.x] [PMID: 19236610]

[8] Siboni SM, Biguzzi E, Pasta G, et al. Management of orthopaedic surgery in rare bleeding disorders. Haemophilia 2014; 20(5): 693-701.
[http://dx.doi.org/10.1111/hae.12387] [PMID: 24612427]

[9] Rodriguez-Merchan EC. Local fibrin glue and chitosan-based dressings in haemophilia surgery. Blood Coagul Fibrinolysis 2012; 23(6): 473-6.
[http://dx.doi.org/10.1097/MBC.0b013e3283555379] [PMID: 22688558]

[10] Zhai JL, Weng XSh, Peng HM, Sun TW, Zhou L. Common complications after arthroplasty in patients with haemophiliaa Chinese experience. Haemophilia 2015; 21(3): e230-2.
[http://dx.doi.org/10.1111/hae.12633] [PMID: 25649826]

[11] Santagostino E, Lentz SR, Misgav M, et al. Safety and efficacy of turoctocog alfa (NovoEight®) during surgery in patients with haemophilia A: results from the multinational guardian™ clinical trials. Haemophilia 2015; 21(1): 34-40.
[http://dx.doi.org/10.1111/hae.12518] [PMID: 25273984]

[12] Poenaru DV, Pătraşcu JM, Andor BC, Popa I. Orthopaedic and surgical features in the management of patients with haemophilia. Eur J Orthop Surg Traumatol 2014; 24(5): 685-92.
[http://dx.doi.org/10.1007/s00590-013-1361-4] [PMID: 24297373]

[13] Heim M. Orthopaedic surgery in hemophilia. the tel Hashomer experience. Haemophilia 1998; 4: 8-10.

[14] Galat DD, McGovern SC, Larson DR, Harrington JR, Hanssen AD, Clarke HD. Surgical treatment of early wound complications following primary total knee arthroplasty. J Bone Joint Surg Am 2009; 91(1): 48-54.
[http://dx.doi.org/10.2106/JBJS.G.01371] [PMID: 19122078]

[15] Hoffman M. Animal models of bleeding and tissue repair. Haemophilia 2008; 14 (Suppl. 3): 62-7.
[http://dx.doi.org/10.1111/j.1365-2516.2008.01729.x] [PMID: 18510524]

[16] Webb LX. New techniques in wound management: vacuum-assisted wound closure. J Am Acad Orthop Surg 2002; 10(5): 303-11.
[http://dx.doi.org/10.5435/00124635-200209000-00002] [PMID: 12374481]

[17] Hallock GG. Salvage of total knee arthroplasty with local fasciocutaneous flaps. J Bone Joint Surg Am 1990; 72(8): 1236-9.
[http://dx.doi.org/10.2106/00004623-199072080-00017] [PMID: 2204633]

[18] Campoccia D, Montanaro L, Arciola CR. The significance of infection related to orthopedic devices and issues of antibiotic resistance. Biomaterials 2006; 27(11): 2331-9.
[http://dx.doi.org/10.1016/j.biomaterials.2005.11.044] [PMID: 16364434]

[19] Sikkema T, Boerboom AL, Meijer K. A comparison between the complications and long-term outcome of hip and knee replacement therapy in patients with and without haemophilia; a controlled retrospective cohort study. Haemophilia 2011; 17(2): 300-3.
[http://dx.doi.org/10.1111/j.1365-2516.2010.02408.x] [PMID: 21070490]

[20] Caviglia HA, Solimeno LP, Eds. Orthopedic Surgery in Patients with Hemophilia. Springer 2008.
[http://dx.doi.org/10.1007/978-88-470-0854-0]

[21]   Rodriguez-Merchan EC. Total knee arthroplasty in patients with haemophilia who are HIV-positive. J Bone Joint Surg Br 2002; 84(2): 170-2.
[http://dx.doi.org/10.1302/0301-620X.84B2.13015] [PMID: 11922355]

[22]   Prokuski L. Prophylactic antibiotics in orthopaedic surgery. J Am Acad Orthop Surg 2008; 16(5): 283-93.
[http://dx.doi.org/10.5435/00124635-200805000-00007] [PMID: 18460689]

[23]   Zawilska K, Podolak-Dawidziak M. Therapeutic problems in elderly patients with hemophilia. Pol Arch Med Wewn 2012; 122: 567-76.

[24]   Tunstall O, Astermark J. Strategies for reducing inhibitor formation in severe haemophilia. Eur J Haematol 2015; 94 (Suppl. 77): 45-50.
[http://dx.doi.org/10.1111/ejh.12501] [PMID: 25560794]

[25]   Darby SC, Keeling DM, Spooner RJ, *et al.* UK Haemophilia Centre Doctors Organization. The incidence of factor VIII and factor IX inhibitors in the hemophilia population of the UK and their effect on subsequent mortality. J Thromb Haemost 2004; 2: 1047-54.
[http://dx.doi.org/10.1046/j.1538-7836.2004.00710.x] [PMID: 15219185]

[26]   Perez Botero J, Spoon DB, Patnaik MS, *et al.* Incidence of symptomatic venous thromboembolism in patients with hemophilia undergoing joint replacement surgery: a retrospective study. Thromb Res 2015; 135(1): 109-13.
[http://dx.doi.org/10.1016/j.thromres.2014.11.010] [PMID: 25434629]

[27]   Pradhan SM, Key NS, Boggio L, Pruthi R. Venous thrombosis prophylaxis in haemophiliacs undergoing major orthopaedic surgery: a survey of haemophilia treatment centres. Haemophilia 2009; 15(6): 1337-8.
[http://dx.doi.org/10.1111/j.1365-2516.2009.02084.x] [PMID: 19702632]

[28]   Pruthi RK, Heit JA, Green MM, *et al.* Venous thromboembolism after hip fracture surgery in a patient with haemophilia B and factor V Arg506Gln (factor V Leiden). Haemophilia 2000; 6(6): 631-4.
[http://dx.doi.org/10.1046/j.1365-2516.2000.00431.x] [PMID: 11122387]

[29]   Rodriguez-Merchan EC. Bone fractures in the haemophilic patient. Haemophilia 2002; 8(2): 104-11.
[http://dx.doi.org/10.1046/j.1365-2516.2002.00628.x] [PMID: 11952845]

[30]   Rodriguez-Merchan EC, Caviglia H, Perez-Bianco R, Beeton KS. Principles of surgery in haemophilic patients: guidelines for developing countries. In: Heijnen L, Ed. Comprehensive Haemophilia Care in Developing Countries Lahore: Ferozsons (Pvt) Ltd. Sohail, MT 2001; pp. 75-85.

[31]   Rodriguez-Merchan EC, Ymenez-Juste V, Gomez-Cardero P, Rodriguez T. Severe postoperative haemarthrosis following a total knee replacement in a hemophiliac patient caused by a pseudoaneurysm: early treatment with arterial embolization. Haemophilia 2014; 20: 86-9.
[http://dx.doi.org/10.1111/hae.12286]

CHAPTER 18

Microsurgery and Plastic Surgery in Haemophilia

Giulio Menichini[1]**, Dario Melita**[1,*]**, Federico Cipriani**[1]**, Antonio Amenta**[2] **and Marco Innocenti**[1]

[1] *Plastic Surgery and Reconstructive Microsurgery Unit, University of Florence, Florence, Italy*

[2] *Plastic Surgery and Reconstructive Microsurgery Unit, University of Messina, Messina, Italy*

Abstract: Microsurgery is increasing popularity among plastic surgeons, creating new alternative solutions for patients that until few years ago only had amputation as final option. Muscles are supplied by several vascular pedicles and the knowledge of their anatomy may allow the use of myocutaneos islands and a rotation on its axis (propeller flap), or a complete detaching from the rest of the body (free flap) and its anastomosis with a recipient vessel to cover soft tissue defects. These procedures are very similar in patients affected by Haemophilia: the only specific issue in such patients is the attention paid to the maintenance of an adequate vascularization that represents the key for the survival of any type of flap.

Keywords: free flaps, Haemophilia, Microsurgery, plastic surgery, propeller flaps.

INTRODUCTION

Patients with haematological disorders usually represent a significant challenge of unappreciated complexity for plastic and reconstructive surgeons. The key for a successful outcome is a close cooperation between plastic surgeon, orthopedic surgeon, haematologist, and infectious disease specialist for a strict follow-up of patients' before and after surgery. This section focuses on the general principles of surgical management of haemophilic patients, pointing out indications, new successful microsurgery techniques, and tip and tricks for such patients. To date, there are no published studies investigating the correct management of haemophilic patients in order to reduce complications and maximize outcomes.

PRINCIPLES IN PLASTIC SURGERY

Regardless of defect's area, size, and shape, the surgeon's task is to choose the correct method for its closure or reconstruction in a single stage. Following the

* **Corresponding author Dario Melita:** Plastic and Reconstructive Microsurgery Unit, University of Florence, Florence, Italy; Tel: 00393336835043; E-mail: melitadario@gmail.com

Christian Carulli (Ed.)

so-called "reconstructive ladder", surgeons have to deserve the best repair technique, starting from the simplest reconstructive method, as skin grafts or local tissue transfer, then progressing to more complex strategies, such as pedicled or free flaps. In particular, free tissue transfers can improve patient's expectancy for a normal daily routine by ensuring a full-thickness cover of damaged tissues by transferring well-vascularized tissues, without loss of function from the donator site. In addition, patients very often show a recovery of daily life activities, such as the gait or legs functional ability in the perioperative period, if compared with delayed or no reconstructions.

HISTORY OF FLAPS IN PLASTIC SURGERY

The history of plastic surgery corresponds to the evolution of flaps. Because of the limited knowledge of specific patterns of reliability of blood supply, historically surgeons started to harvest random flap based on strict length-to-width ratios to avoid necrosis, but limiting dimensions and mobility especially for wound coverage in the lower leg. Firstly described by McGregor and Jackson in 1972 [1], axial pattern flap entails the detriment of a main artery to gain better results [2 - 6]. Muscolocutaneous flaps increased their popularity since first description by Ger in 1966 [7] and Orticochea in 1972 [8] because of their reliability [9]. Fasciocutaneous flaps, because of their lack of extension for distal third of the leg coverage [10 - 13], were suggested in selected cases although Ponten in 1981 proved that by including the deep fascia in a cutaneous flap, they could be raised without respecting the length-to-width ratio, even if anatomical basis were investigated later [14 - 17].

The unreliability of fasciocutaneous flap for wound coverage of the lower third of the leg is reported by Chatre and Quaba, with an elevated incidence of necrosis (about 25% of cases) [13].

New impulse to flap design was given by the discovery of *angiosomes*, defined as a well-defined anatomical territory with a complete vascular network supplied by a main artery and vein, partly linked by anastomosis to the surrounding angiosomes [18 - 20].

Taylor and Pan [21] set the first milestone for the use of perforator flaps in the lower leg by proving that a damage to deep fascia creates a new vascular network in all directions. Later works by Koshima and Soeda [22] and Kroll and Rosenfield [23] set the starting point for perforator flaps-based reconstruction.

To reconstruct lower leg and foot, free perforators flap taken from different anatomical regions (such as anterolateral thigh perforator flap [11, 24, 25], tensor fasciae latae muscle perforator flap [11, 26], inferior epigastric artery perforator flap [27], thoracodorsal artery perforator flap [28 - 30], medial sural artery perforator flap [11, 31]) were considered as first surgical option since reliability and safety of local perforator flaps was proven, as showed in literature.

Perforasomes, firstly identified by Saint-Cyr and his coworkers and later discussed by Geddes *et al.* [32], increased the interest for harvesting new or improving perforator flaps, exploiting their dynamic potential in lower leg [33 - 36]. Due to a strictly connected vessel network [35], the harvest of a single perforator flap stimulates a hyperperfusion, as described by Rubino *et al* [37], allowing larger dimension flaps because of new enrollment of interconnected vessels.

Perforator flaps have many advantages such as: less donor site morbidity, a satisfying blood flow for musculocutaneous flap, restore of the anatomy with like-to-like reconstruction, primary closure (in most of the cases), faster and easier technique compared to free flaps harvest [6, 10, 13, 34, 36, 38 - 41].

Hyakusoku *et al.* [42], in 1991, was the first to develop the concept of propeller flap by using a subcutaneous pedicled flap with a rotation of 90°. Hallock [43], instead, was the first one who defined the term of propeller flap with a perforator flap with a skeletonized pedicle rotated of 180°. Only in 2009, at the First Tokyo Meeting on Perforator and Propeller Flaps [44] was reached the last definition of propeller flap as a perforator flap designed as a skin island with two paddles of various dimensions (equal or different) based on the permitted rotation of the pedicle for at least 90 to 180 degrees. Teo [45] in 2006 meticulously described the proper technique to harvest propeller flaps in lower leg reconstruction.

After first works have been published in literature [11 - 13, 17 - 21, 26, 46 - 50], an increasing number of microsurgeons became interested in pedicled perforator flap, by evaluating perforator arteries, to reconstruct lower leg [6, 10 - 13, 25 - 28, 31, 33 - 37, 39, 41, 44, 45, 51 - 56]. Despite many advantages are present, complication rates of propeller perforator flap and free flaps are similar, mostly due to partial or total necrosis for venous congestion [10, 13, 36, 44, 52, 53, 55]. This problem is partly solved by supercharging the venous network with the suture of a concomitant subcutaneous vein [36, 38, 44, 57].

To improve the chance of an efficient mobility of the flap, Teo suggested to add 1cm to the distance between the distal edge of the defect and the flap [45] and 0,5cm to the width, with the pedicle released from muscular branches for 2cms at least (also around the venae comitantes). To assess the proper vascularization, flap must rest in its original position for fifteen minutes after tourniquet is released.

Since major risks for microsurgical reconstruction is due to vascular complications, mostly because of buckling and rotation of the pedicle, Wong *et al.* [58] suggested to dissect 1mm perforators of at least 3cms. Nowadays, perforasomes concept [35] modified the ideal dimension of a perforator flaps: fifteen years ago to maintain a proper vascularity and reduce the risk of vascular complications, the ideal length of perforator flap was the distance between two perforators [59 - 61], while now, because of hyperperfusion [35], single-perforator flaps are reliable, since higher pressure in larger vessels open new linking vessels [62]. Perforators arteries, despite initial blood flow reduced compared to main arteries, showed an increased perfusion rate once flap is harvested [37, 63].

There is an obvious indirect relationship among the number of perforators and the dimension of the anatomical district vascularized by each perforator [11]. Perforators derived from the posterior tibial artery are fewer but larger compared to perforators derived from peroneal and anterior tibial arteries [20].

It is mandatory to decide the dimension of the flap according to the size of the perforators for a safe dissection of the flap. Panse *et al.* [63] tried to describe the connection between the length of the lower leg and the length of the flap to avoid necrosis founding a necrosis complication rate 6 times higher if the length of the flap is one-third of the length of the limbs.

There are many methods described for preoperative identification of the perforators such as color Doppler, usefull to identify the internal diameter of the perforator, handheld Doppler, used to identify the perforator [62, 64 - 66], Duplex ultrasound, MRI angiography, arteriography and high resolution CT: however, no imaging may deserve informations about the possibility of flap harvesting [41].

The use of fluorescein was popularized as a method to define intraoperatively the safe dimensions of the flap, even if it showed to under predict its viability [41, 67, 68]. Also the use of indocyanine green near-infrared angiography was proposed as a more accurate method [41, 69 - 71].

An alternative method to reduce complications is to use "perforators plus flap" technique [41, 72, 73]. This procedure consists in the design of the flap based on one perforator and to keep its base attached with the donor site, in order to improve vascular supply and venous drainage.

The description and the respect of vascular axis and angiosomes is mandatory to prevent flap necrosis [36].

Proximally to the joints the vascular axis is directed distally from them, so it's important that the long axis of the flap is directed in the same way. Other procedures were proposed as a flap delay, but they are affected by a long lasting treatment before getting acceptable results [36, 41, 44, 61, 72, 74]. In 1983, Asko-Seljavaara [75] was the first one who introduced the concept of *freestyle* perforator flap, based on any major perforator vessel. This new technique could be applied to pedicled perforator flap in order to give more choices of reconstruction [76].

Quaba *et al.* [77] in 1990 in the hand and in 2006 in lower leg, described the concept of "ad hoc" perforator flap that was similar to the freestyle one, but the origin of the source vessel and their anatomical variation were considered irrelevant [10, 77].

Quaba and Quaba [10] customize the flap on a potential donor site close to the defect to be covered by detecting a reliable perforator using a Doppler probe. Later, Mardini *et al.* [78] and Wei and Mardini [79] modified the previous technique to obtain a safer harvest of the flap by incising a single edge of the flap and then dissecting the perforator previously identified by a preoperative Doppler examination.

The same authors described a similar technique to harvest local perforator flaps [80] and various authors described their experience in harvesting freestyle perforators flap in different anatomical districts [81 - 85]. Georgescu *et al.* [38, 84] and Matei *et al.* [85] described the harvest of several perforator flaps in the forearm not using a preoperative identification of the perforator, since many cases showed a wrong identification of the perforator itself by using a handheld Doppler signal, and proved that microsurgical dissection of the vessel with a single incision of the flap is higher reliable. This approach, similar to Asko-Seljavaara's technique for initial identification of source vessels, was sustained by Lee [86] and Matei *et al.* [85] and can be applied for harvesting propeller flaps in the lower leg, where anterior and posterior tibial arteries are superficial.

INDICATIONS IN HAEMOPHILIA

The following are the typical indications for a microsurgical reconstruction in patients affected by Haemophilia and other bleeding disorders:

• Chronic wound dehiscence after haematoma
• Severe damage of soft tissues unresponsive to previous medical and surgical treatments
• Reconstruction after surgical pseudotumor excision
• Reconstruction after tumor excision and wide tissue demolition
• Wound dehiscence following surgeries, *i.e.* orthopedic procedures

Every case needs an individual analysis by a multidisciplinary team, in order to achieve the best reconstructive option.

DISTAL LOWER LEG RECONSTRUCTION BY PROPELLER FLAPS

Reconstruction of distal lower leg and foot defects, with or without exposure of tendons, bones and hardware, with propeller perforator flaps is a new success for microsurgery because of their reliability and safety proved by long-term clinical practice [53, 87].

Anatomical Considerations

Perforators, sufficiently capable to guarantee flap survival, arise from lower leg major vessels (posterior and anterior tibial artery - PTA, ATA, peroneal artery, popliteal artery, and descending genicular artery - DGA). The mean number of perforators, as described by Geddes *et al* [32], is 30±13 with a medium calibre of 0.7±0.2mm, with the skin of leg and knee covering 34% of lower extremity integument. Vascular territories, in number of five, are divided into a series of four longitudinal rows organized inside the intermuscular septa of the lower leg [32, 34].

Saphenous artery, a superficial branch derived from DGA, supplies medial aspect of the knee, the pes anserinus and the gastrocnemius muscle (medial head) and anastomoses with ATA anteriorly, with the sural artery posteriorly and with the PTA inferiorly. Popliteal artery supplies the popliteal area and the posterior region of the distal leg in its superior portion by superficial and deep sural branches. The deep medial and lateral sural arteries supply the gastrocnemius, soleus, and plantaris muscles.

A single musculocutaneous perforator usually origins from the lateral portion of gastrocnemius muscle, while from the inferior and medial aspect of medial head generally 2-3 perforators emerge, but the number may vary depending on the presence of the superficial sural arteries, usually one lateral and one medial. The latter, with a diameter of 1 mm, is the most relevant because escorted with small saphenous vein, sural and medial sural cutaneous nerves. The previously mentioned vessels find anastomoses with PTA inferiorly, DGA medially and ATA and peroneal laterally. A great portion (about 10%) of integument of lower leg, tibia, soleus, FDL and tibialis posterior muscles is supplied by PTA, largest branch derived from popliteal artery. The number of perforators is still debated in literature, with some authors counting from 3 to 5 perforators [40, 50] while Geddes *et al.* [32] described up to 10±4 cutaneous perforators, with a mean diameter of 1mm [32, 40, 50, 88]. In the middle third of the lower leg, between soleus and FDL, perforators diameter is usually larger, between 1 to 5mm [34, 89].

Some authors found that the largest representation of perforators are from 5 to 14 cm above the internal malleolus [10, 40, 50]. Three clusters were discovered by Schaverien and Saint-Cry [34] (4 to 9cm, 13 to 18cm, and 21 to 26cm from the intermalleolar line), everyone with the 23% of the total number of perforators and at least one perforator in each cluster in 80% of cases. Perforators with bigger diameter are in the proximal two-thirds, and sometimes in the peroneal septum [48].

Most of the perforator are septocutaneous [34, 89]: a relatively constant one is found approximately 5cm above the medial malleolus [16]. Muscolocutaneous perforators are well represented through the medial, posterior and lateral aspects.

The descending genicular artery anastomoses with the upper perforators and over the tibial crest with perforators of anterior tibial artery [32]. Distally they give their contribution to the network of the ankle, with branches from the anterior tibial artery and peroneal artery [6]. In the distal part, 1-2 perforators arise from ATA right above extensor retinaculum with two major branches (anteromedial and anterolateral) to supply the anterior area over both malleola [6]. At the ankle level, vessels derived from peroneal artery and PTA are linked [6].

A variable number, usually from 3 to 7, of muscolo- and septocutaneous perforators, located posteriorly to the fibula [52] and with a mean diameter of 0.8 ± 0.2mm [32, 48, 88, 90, 91] arises from peroneal artery and provides, partly with PTA, about 5% of the integument of lower leg (including lateral leg and Achilles tendon skin cover, fibula and peroneal muscles).

Higher concentration of perforators can be found in the middle third of the leg, about from 13 to 18cm proximally to the lateral malleolus [34]. The musculocutaneous perforators can be detected usually in the context of soleus and/or peroneus longus muscle, while septocutaneous perforators are more distally based, in the septum between peroneus brevis and flexor hallucis longus [34]. After its passage anteriorly to the interosseous membrane, about 5cm above the lateral malleolus, a perforator (with constantly large diameter) splits itself into a descendant and an ascendant branch [6, 32]. The latter one get connected with SPA while the descending anastomoses with ATA (anterolateral branches).

SURGICAL TECHNIQUE

A proper coverage for a wound localized on the knee region is challenging for the reconstructive surgeon. Local options are quite limited in terms of size and arc often restricted by their arc of rotation. However, free flaps may increase the length and complexity of surgery. Whenever possible, salvage of the knee is highly advocated, as above-the-knee amputation is associated with a high complication rate and increase in energy expenditure for the patient. It is well established that muscle flaps are best indicated to fill the dead space when present. Moreover, the high vascular volume of these flaps may serve as a carrier for antibiotics locally. Since the anterior surface of the knee requires soft, flexible and thin tissue, fasciocutaneous flaps are the preferred choice because they perfectly match these characteristics.

The workhorse flap to cover defects following infection, trauma and tumour excision in the anterior portion of the knee is still the medial gastrocnemius muscle flap. It provides good vascularized tissue that helps sterilize the recipient site, it is wide and bulky enough to cover a prosthesis and fill the dead space if needed, and can be harvested including muscle and skin to obtain a complete external coverage.

Patients with Haemophilia suffering from surgical complications as a wide wound dehiscence after surgical debridement related to an infection in some cases requires a medial thigh propeller flap to cover (Fig. **1**).

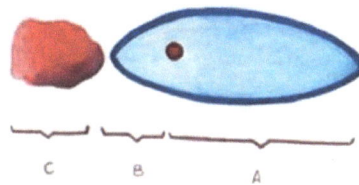

Fig. (1). Schematic diagram of propeller flap.

According to the haemathologists' consultation, prior to surgery, it is useful in such cases the infusion of missing factor. Tourniquet is necessary in order to obtain a bloodless field, reducing blood loss during surgery. For the medial thigh septocutaneous flap, the dominant pedicle is topically located at the apex of the femoral triangle approximately 6-8cm below the inguinal ligament and is bordered medially by the adductor longus and laterally by the sartorius. A perforator-based propeller flap designed on two perforators raising from the deep femoral artery is prepared (Fig. **2**).

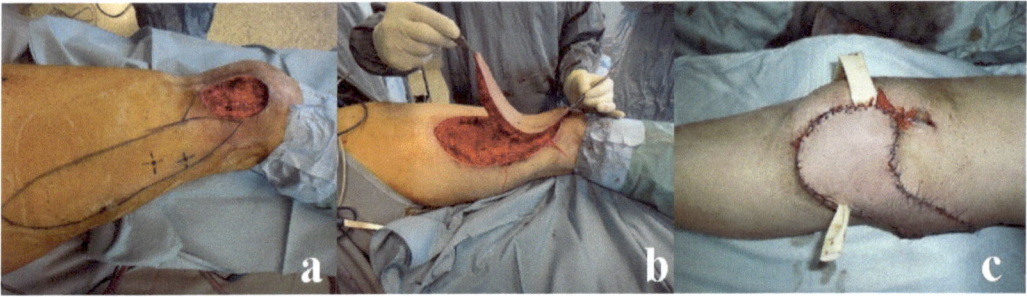

Fig. (2). Medial tight propeller flap designed for wound dehiscence after surgical debridement because of implant infection (a). Harvesting of the flap with his two perforators (b). Insetting of the flap covering the defect (c).

Preoperatively, an US with Colour or Power Doppler is used to map the location of musculocutaneous perforators and, according to the preoperative flap design, a preliminary explorative incision is made. Skin is carefully elevated until perforators are correctly identified. Its pedicle is then dissected in order to obtain the desired arc of rotation of the skin paddle without any pedicle kinking. A sufficient blood supply is guarantee during dissection. The flap is then rotated to cover soft tissues defect (Fig. **3**).

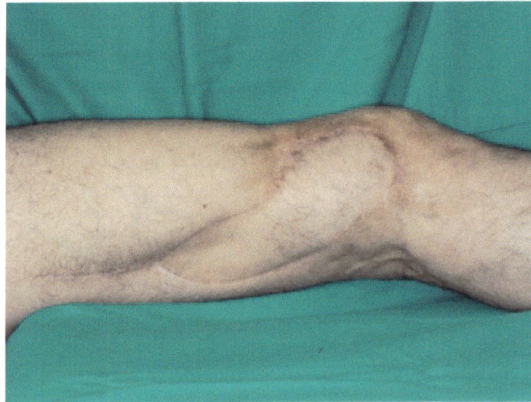

Fig. (3). Postoperative aspect after three months.

Propeller flaps have been extensively used for soft tissue reconstruction in almost all anatomical districts [36, 92]. They can be raised virtually everywhere a suitable perforator is available, and they usually follow simple principles. The eccentric location of the pedicle and the possibility to rotate the flap up to 180 degrees allow for a great coverage potential of small-to-medium-sized defects according to the principle of 'repair like with like'. The morbidity at the donor site is usually minimal. Any axial artery of an anatomical region (source artery) gives perforators able to supply skin flaps. Unfortunately, the medial gastrocnaemius flap may not easily reach the upper portion of the knee. In addition, the conventional musculocutaneous flap, raised along with the skin extension over the medial gastrocnaemius, is quite bulky and the cutaneous portion being attached to the underlying muscle cannot be freely and independently placed to increase the surface of the flap. As mentioned before, propeller flaps are proved to be safe and reliable, but sometimes *chimaeric* flaps (*e.g.* propeller flap based on medial sural artery perforator with classical medial gastrocnemius muscle flap) are necessary to cover the whole soft tissue defect (Fig. **4**) [93]. Patients suffering for bleeding disorders require a preoperative planning that includes haemathologist's consultation in order to avoid bleeding problems intrinsically connected to coagulation factors deficiency.

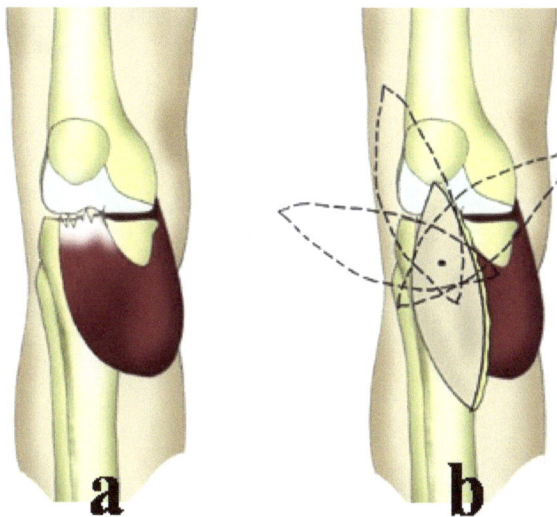

Fig. (4). Conventional medial gastrocnemius is ideal for coverage of tibial tuberosity but it is not adequate in case of larger defects involving the patella (a). A propeller fasciocutaneous flap may be designed based on a single perforator raising from the medial sural artery and rotated in any direction (b).

Tourniquet must be applied in order to obtain a bloodless field, reducing blood loss during surgery. The skin perforator is ideally located in the centre of the skin paddle but according to the principles of propeller flaps [94], it is more conveniently located in the proximity of either the distal or the proximal pole in order to increase the arc of rotation. Preoperatively, an US with Colour or Power Doppler is used to map the location of musculocutaneous perforators and, according to the preoperative flap design, a preliminary explorative incision is made. Skin is carefully elevated in a subfascial plane until perforators are identified (Figs. **5** and **6**). Once identified, the pedicle is then dissected to obtain an adequate arc of rotation, avoiding vessel kinking.

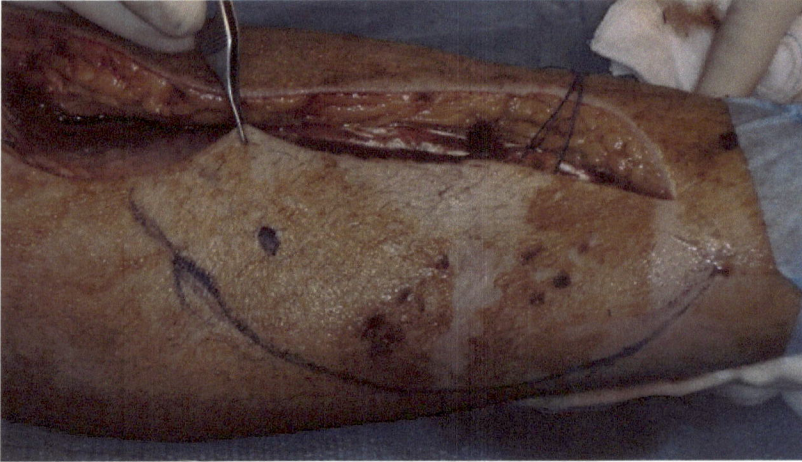

Fig. (5). Preoperative US investigation identifies the best perforator that is marked on the skin.

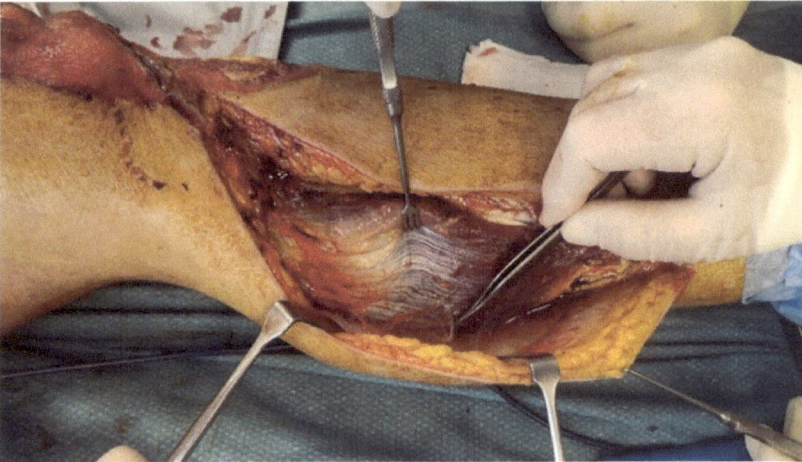

Fig. (6). A straightforward dissection in the sub-fascial plane allows for a direct visualization of the best perforator.

A sufficient blood supply is guaranteed during dissection. Flap is then rotated to cover soft tissues defect. The skin is elevated in a subfascial plane until the perforators are identified. All perforators identified during the dissection are spared until the dominant one is precisely located. Once the main perforator is identified and chosen, the flap design and skin incision are completed. Adequate vascularization of the skin paddle is then assessed. Intramuscular dissection of the perforator is performed in order to obtain the desired arc of rotation of the skin paddle without any pedicle kinking. The skin paddle is secured to the underlying muscle to avoid shearing before raising the conventional muscle flap. When the muscle flap is completely raised and the muscle belly securely sutured into the recipient site, sutures of the skin paddle can then be removed and the skin oriented in the desired direction (Figs. **7** and **8**).

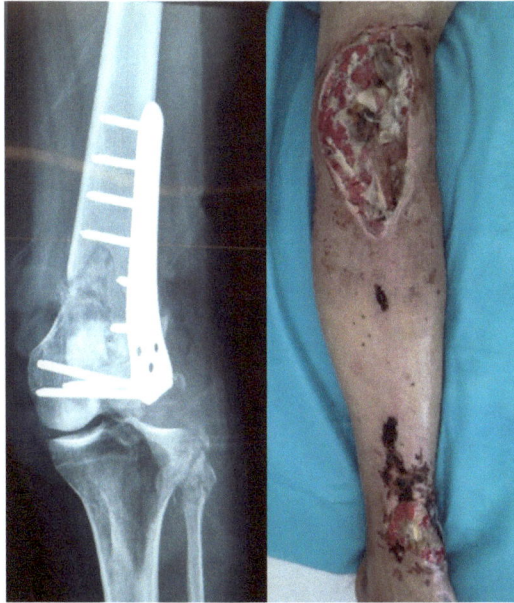

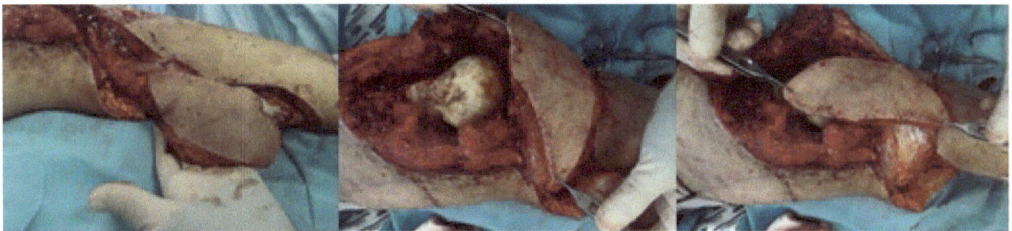

Figs. (7 and 8). Example of chimaeric flap for soft tissues reconstruction in a 46-year-old patient affected by VII factor deficiency. Preoperative clinical and radiographic aspects (above). The lateral condyle of the femur has been avulsed by the trauma. Large soft tissue defect, infected exposure of the knee joint, exposure of the hardware and bone necrosis. The miocutaneous flap is elevated and transferred into the recipient site. The skin paddle is then rotated upward to cover the cement spacer, which replaces the distal femur.

In conclusion, chimaeric flaps have proven to be versatile and highly reliable (Fig. **9**). Postoperative observation of the reconstructed area and flap donor site is critical and includes monitoring for vascular patency, bleeding tendency, haematoma formation, and tissue swelling.

Meticulous wound care and antisepsis measures have to be taken, particularly during the first 72 hours, and prophylactic antibiotics, covering also anaerobic bacteria, are mandatory.

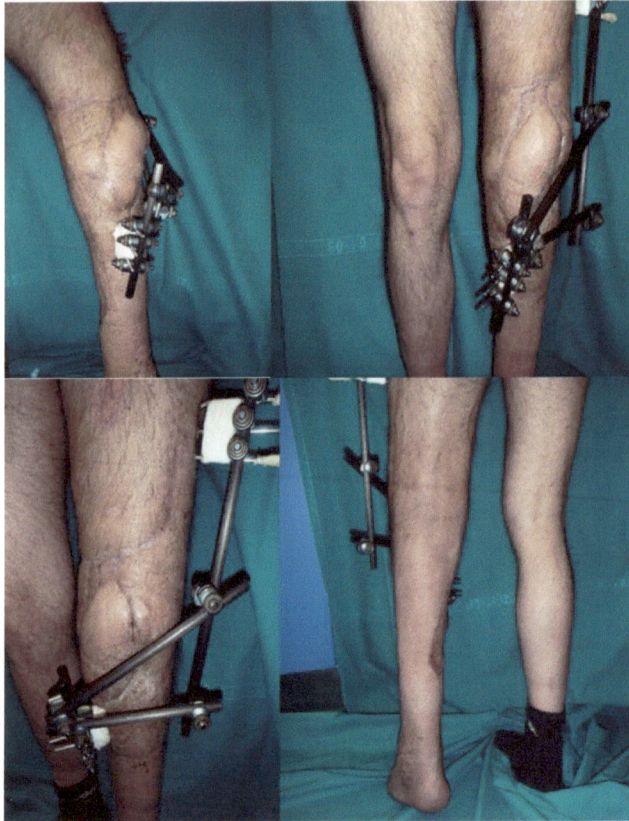

Fig. (9). Clinical outcomes at 3 months follow-up.

LATISSIMUS DORSI FREE FLAP FOR LIMB SALVAGE

Experience in reconstruction for limb savage increased the demand for new options to obtain better functionally and aesthetically results [95]. Since reconstructions became safer and more reliable, new suitable options to reconstruct wider defects have been proposed.

Deep muscle ablation, after trauma or oncological resections, requires reconstructive strategies sufficiently efficient to restore muscular function and to cover loss of soft tissues. Following the above mentioned like-to-like principles, free muscular flaps are widely used to replace loss of muscles and they can be also used to replace tissues in poorly vascularized areas (diabetic ulcers, osteomyelitis, and radiotherapy-induced necrosis (Fig. **10**).

Firstly introduced in the '70s, free flaps can reasonably be harvested if a suitable neurovascular bundle is present at the recipient site to permit microvascular anastomoses with donor tissue.

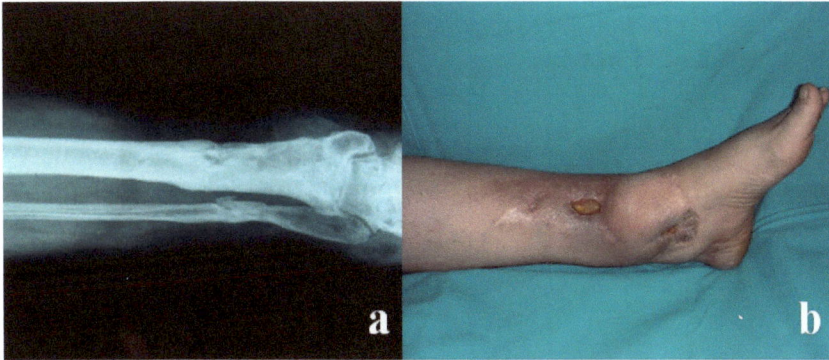

Fig. (10). X-rays showing an osteomyelitis of the distal right leg (a). Attempt to cover a skin ulcer by using a sural flap and others two ulcers of the right distal leg (b).

Anatomical Considerations

Latissimus dorsi origins from iliac crest inferiorly and posteriorly from the thoracolumbar fascia. It functions as humeral adductor, allowing its internal rotation. Innervated by the thoracodorsal nerve, part of brachial plexus, it comes along with the thoracodorsal artery.

Latissimus dorsi is supplied by the subscapular artery that originates from the axillary artery and sends a circumflex scapular branch and a serratus branch prior to enter into the muscle.

Subscapular artery, usually accompanied by a single vena comitans, has a calibre usually from 2 to 5 mms and a pedicle up to 15cm can be obtained by a careful dissection. Its vena comitans is usually slightly larger. Further vascular supply is guarantee by perforators derived from lumbar arteries and thoracic intercostal arteries but these vascular sources cannot be used for microsurgery because of their small dimension.

Surgical Technique

There are few papers in literature describing microsurgery techniques in patients affected by Haemophilia.

Essential elements for such type of surgery in patients with haematologic disorders include several aspects as:

- Careful evaluation of past medical history, preoperative medical condition and possible complications after surgery
- Multidisciplinary approach
- Meticulous surgical technique

By following this regimen, haemophilic patients can safely undergo free tissue transfers with reliable outcomes.

In order to avoid potentially fatal postoperative complications, monitoring is strictly mandatory, but overcorrection of bleeding predisposition may lead to hypercoagulation. Preoperative haematologic consultation must be provided and deficient factors must be replaced and maintained through all intraoperative and postoperative period (Figs. **11** and **12**).

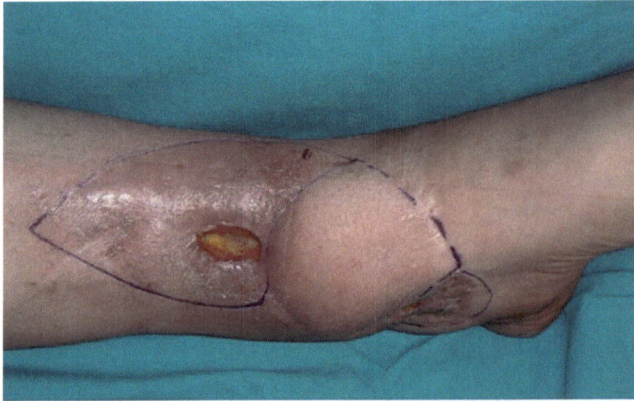

Fig. (11). Preoperative design of ulcer excisions preserving the sural flap.

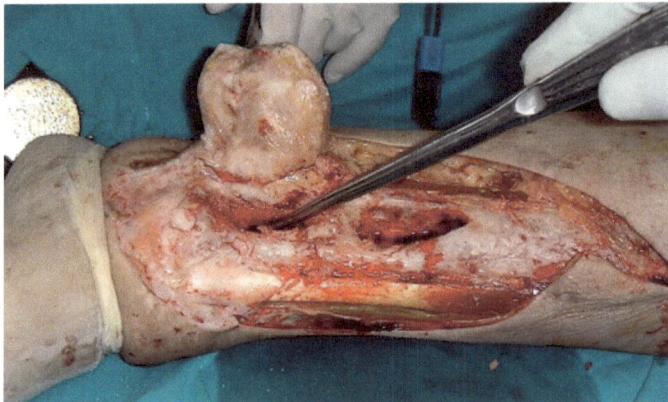

Fig. (12). Intraoperative surgical debridement of the ulcer and sural flap salvage showing its good vascularization.

The patient is placed in a lateral decubitus and, in order to prevent impingement of brachial plexus by the clavicle, a pad should be placed between the shoulder and the neck on the other side. To allow free movements the ipsilateral arm is included in the operating field, draped together with the lateral thorax, shoulder, axilla and back.

To reduce the surgery time, it is possible to choose the muscle of the same side of the affected leg in order to harvest the flap simultaneously.

It is useful to mark with a pen the lateral margin of the latissimus.

The incision is made from the posterior axillary fold, extended inferiorly and medially over the muscle. It is also possible to harvest a skin paddle within the muscle, a hand probe Doppler could be used to find the perforator of the skin paddle. For muscle exposure the skin flaps are raised superficially. The inferior angle of the scapula corresponds at the superior side of the latissums. With this technique it is easy to find the serratus instead of harvesting the flap from distal to proximal that could lead to serratus elevation. The dissection should not be done underneath the serratus, then the pocket is dissected.

The flap dissection goes below the inferior angle of the scapula to elevate the superior side of the latissimus. This is an easy plane of dissection and it goes directly through the midline with the division of the muscle near midline of the back. The dissection proceeds then inferiorly with the division of the medial muscle insertion. Finally, the superior edge of the muscle is elevated.

Attention must be paid in the inferior portion of the muscle.

With the release of medial and inferior muscle, the flap harvesting goes underneath the muscle toward the axilla where the plane is thinner and easily for the dissection. The harvesting should include the entire muscle and its tendon insertion into the homerus.

The division between the vascular pedicle of the latissimus and the serratus become clear reaching the axilla (Fig. **13**).

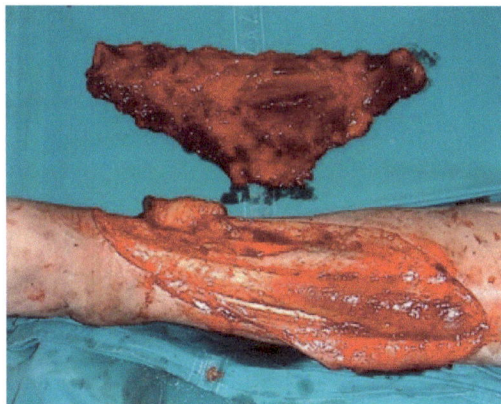

Fig. (13). Latissimus dorsi muscular free flap harvested to cover the defect.

The harvesting of the flap is complete with his pedicle attached. The wound is closed at the end of the surgery with a good thickness. At the end of surgery, the wound closure is performed in a loose fashion to allow for drainage; otherwise one or two suction drains are placed (Fig. **14**).

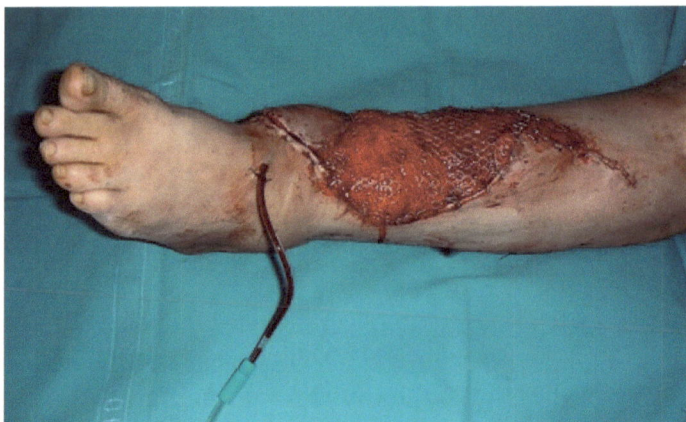

Fig. (14). Mashed skin-graft was used to cover the latissimus dorsi free flap.

The recipient site has to be prepared before the ligation of the neurovascular bundle to reduce the time of ischemia.

The extent of resection and approach depends on the size and eventually on the site of the defect. Once complete, the flap goes to the recipient site. The proximal tendon of the latissimus dorsi can be either sutured to the residual muscle stump or directly anchored to the bone. The use of few stitches allows flap position, then microvascular anastomoses are needed. For a less denervation period, the nerve repair is done as soon as possible.

Sutures of the vascular pedicle are usually done by the use of a microscope, using a coupler for vein anastomosis and nylon 9/0 for the artery. Haemostasis has been one of the main roles of this surgery: it is crucial to avoid bleedings after surgery. Failure of the flap could be reached by not treating the coagulopathy that can cause bleeding from both the reconstructed area and the donor site. Because of the peculiar coagulative status of haemophilic patients, the plastic surgeon has to pay attention to the meticulous haemostasis during any surgical procedure, using suture ligations and electrocauterization. A new session of careful haemostasis at the end of reconstruction is also mandatory. Blood pressure has to be taken under control from anaesthesiologists, avoiding hypotension which can hidden potential bleeding sources. The postoperative monitoring of flap circulation is done by US Doppler.

Haematologic evaluation is done every day in the postoperative period. Reconstructed limbs are immobilized for 4 weeks after surgery. A gentle passive mobilization of the leg can start and later electric stimulation, muscle strengthening, and assisted gait activity are generally allowed (Fig. **15**). Patients must be screened by electromyography (EMG) and periodic magnetic resonance imaging (MRI) to evaluate the perfusion of flaps and their function.

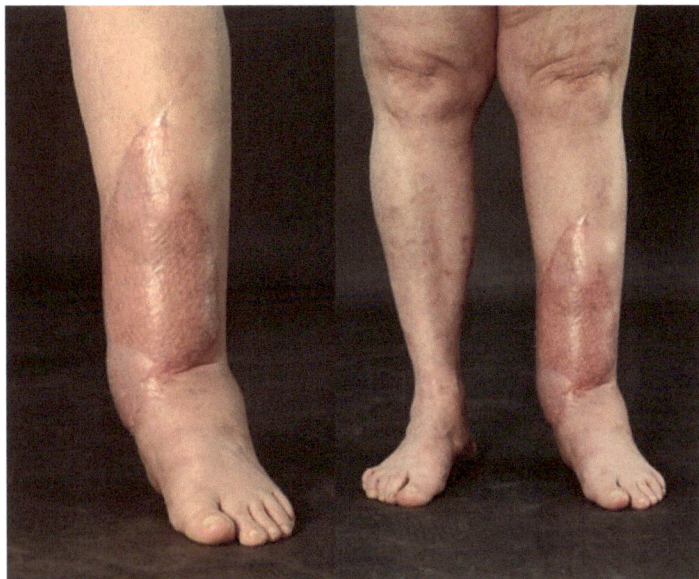

Fig. (15). Postoperative pictures after 6 months.

The functional evaluation may be performed by the 30-point Musculoskeletal Tumor Society Rating Score (MTSRS) [96], and muscle strength assessed using a manual test adapted by Doi *et al* [97].

CONCLUDING REMARKS

Several reconstructive options are available for soft tissue defects in Haemophilia particularly after failed joint replacements. Propeller pedicled flaps are easily harvested, but surrounding healthy tissues are required. In case that local flaps cannot be harvested, free flaps are a well-known solution allowing large fasciocutaneous and musculocutaneous reconstructions. New surgical approaches and a stronger knowledge of microsurgical techniques may improve the outcome in such challenging patients. In order to achieve better outcomes with fewer complications, a close monitoring of patient's coagulative aspects and postoperative haematoma in adherence to strict perioperative surgical protocols is a crucial point.

CONFLICT OF INTEREST

The authors confirm that they have no conflict of interest to declare for this publication.

ACKNOWLEDGEMENTS

Declared none.

REFERENCES

[1] McGregor IA, Jackson IT. The groin flap. Br J Plast Surg 1972; 25(1): 3-16.
[http://dx.doi.org/10.1016/S0007-1226(72)80003-1] [PMID: 4550433]

[2] McCraw JB, Furlow LT Jr. The dorsalis pedis arterialized flap. A clinical study. Plast Reconstr Surg 1975; 55(2): 177-85.
[http://dx.doi.org/10.1097/00006534-197502000-00007] [PMID: 1090947]

[3] Torii S, Namiki Y, Hayashi Y, Wong AC. Reverse-flow peroneal island flap for the reconstruction of leg and foot. Eur J Plast Surg 1988; 11: 26-31.
[http://dx.doi.org/10.1007/BF00294487]

[4] Liu K, Li Z, Lin Y, Cao Y. The reverse-flow posterior tibial artery island flap: anatomic study and 72 clinical cases. Plast Reconstr Surg 1990; 86(2): 312-6.
[http://dx.doi.org/10.1097/00006534-199008000-00019] [PMID: 2367580]

[5] Wee JT. Reconstruction of the lower leg and foot with the reverse-pedicled anterior tibial flap: preliminary report of a new fasciocutaneous flap. Br J Plast Surg 1986; 39(3): 327-37.
[http://dx.doi.org/10.1016/0007-1226(86)90042-1] [PMID: 3730678]

[6] Koshima I, Itoh S, Nanba Y, Tsutsui T, Takahashi Y. Medial and lateral malleolar perforator flaps for repair of defects around the ankle. Ann Plast Surg 2003; 51(6): 579-83.
[http://dx.doi.org/10.1097/01.sap.0000095654.07024.65] [PMID: 14646653]

[7] Ger R. The operative treatment of the advanced stasis ulcer. A preliminary communication. Am J Surg 1966; 111(5): 659-63.
[http://dx.doi.org/10.1016/0002-9610(66)90036-5] [PMID: 5327672]

[8] Orticochea M. The musculo-cutaneous flap method: an immediate and heroic substitute for the method of delay. Br J Plast Surg 1972; 25(2): 106-10.
[http://dx.doi.org/10.1016/S0007-1226(72)80029-8] [PMID: 4553998]

[9] Ger R. The technique of muscle transposition in the operative treatment of traumatic and ulcerative lesions of the leg. J Trauma 1971; 11(6): 502-10.
[http://dx.doi.org/10.1097/00005373-197106000-00007] [PMID: 4932138]

[10] Quaba O, Quaba AA. Pedicled perforator flaps for the lower limb. Semin Plast Surg 2006; 20: 103-11.
[http://dx.doi.org/10.1055/s-2006-941717]

[11] Hallock GG. Lower extremity muscle perforator flaps for lower extremity reconstruction. Plast Reconstr Surg 2004; 114(5): 1123-30.
[http://dx.doi.org/10.1097/01.PRS.0000135847.49178.F2] [PMID: 15457022]

[12] Kamath BJ, Joshua TV, Pramod S. Perforator based flap coverage from the anterior and lateral compartment of the leg for medium sized traumatic pretibial soft tissue defects a simple solution for a complex problem. J Plast Reconstr Aesthet Surg 2006; 59(5): 515-20.
[http://dx.doi.org/10.1016/j.bjps.2005.09.032] [PMID: 16749197]

[13]   Jakubietz RG, Jakubietz MG, Gruenert JG, Kloss DF. The 180-degree perforator-based propeller flap for soft tissue coverage of the distal, lower extremity: a new method to achieve reliable coverage of the distal lower extremity with a local, fasciocutaneous perforator flap. Ann Plast Surg 2007; 59(6): 667-71.
       [http://dx.doi.org/10.1097/SAP.0b013e31803c9b66] [PMID: 18046150]

[14]   Pontén B. The fasciocutaneous flap: its use in soft tissue defects of the lower leg. Br J Plast Surg 1981; 34(2): 215-20.
       [http://dx.doi.org/10.1016/S0007-1226(81)80097-5] [PMID: 7236984]

[15]   Haertsch P. The surgical plane in the leg. Br J Plast Surg 1981; 34(4): 464-9.
       [http://dx.doi.org/10.1016/0007-1226(81)90060-6] [PMID: 7296153]

[16]   Barclay TL, Cardoso E, Sharpe DT, Crockett DJ. Repair of lower leg injuries with fascio-cutaneous flaps. Br J Plast Surg 1982; 35(2): 127-32.
       [http://dx.doi.org/10.1016/0007-1226(82)90148-5] [PMID: 7044458]

[17]   Cormack GC, Lamberty BG. Fasciocutaneous vessels. Their distribution on the trunk and limbs, and their clinical application in tissue transfer. Anat Clin 1984; 6(2): 121-31.
       [http://dx.doi.org/10.1007/BF01773164] [PMID: 6388596]

[18]   Manchot C. The cutaneous arteries of the human body. New York: Springer-Verlag 1983.
       [http://dx.doi.org/10.1007/978-1-4613-8221-8]

[19]   Salmon M, Taylor GI, Tempest M. Arteries of the skin. London: Churchill Livingstone 1988.

[20]   Taylor GI, Palmer JH. The vascular territories (angiosomes) of the body: experimental study and clinical applications. Br J Plast Surg 1987; 40(2): 113-41.
       [http://dx.doi.org/10.1016/0007-1226(87)90185-8] [PMID: 3567445]

[21]   Taylor GI, Pan WR. Angiosomes of the leg: anatomic study and clinical implications. Plast Reconstr Surg 1998; 102(3): 599-616.
       [http://dx.doi.org/10.1097/00006534-199809010-00001] [PMID: 9727424]

[22]   Koshima I, Soeda S. Inferior epigastric artery skin flaps without rectus abdominis muscle. Br J Plast Surg 1989; 42(6): 645-8.
       [http://dx.doi.org/10.1016/0007-1226(89)90075-1] [PMID: 2605399]

[23]   Kroll SS, Rosenfield L. Perforator-based flaps for low posterior midline defects. Plast Reconstr Surg 1988; 81(4): 561-6.
       [http://dx.doi.org/10.1097/00006534-198804000-00012] [PMID: 3279442]

[24]   Song YG, Chen GZ, Song YL. The free thigh flap: a new free flap concept based on the septocutaneous artery. Br J Plast Surg 1984; 37(2): 149-59.
       [http://dx.doi.org/10.1016/0007-1226(84)90002-X] [PMID: 6713155]

[25]   Koshima I, Kawada S, Etoh H, Kawamura S, Moriguchi T, Sonoh H. Flow-through anterior thigh flaps for one-stage reconstruction of soft-tissue defects and revascularization of ischemic extremities. Plast Reconstr Surg 1995; 95(2): 252-60.
       [http://dx.doi.org/10.1097/00006534-199502000-00004] [PMID: 7824604]

[26]   Koshima I, Urushibara K, Inagawa K, Moriguchi T. Free tensor fasciae latae perforator flap for the reconstruction of defects in the extremities. Plast Reconstr Surg 2001; 107(7): 1759-65.
       [http://dx.doi.org/10.1097/00006534-200106000-00018] [PMID: 11391196]

[27]   Koshima I, Nanba Y, Tsutsui T, Takahashi Y, Itoh S. Perforator flaps in lower extremity reconstruction. Handchir Mikrochir Plast Chir 2002; 34(4): 251-6.
       [http://dx.doi.org/10.1055/s-2002-36291] [PMID: 12491184]

[28]   Angrigiani C, Grilli D, Siebert J. Latissimus dorsi musculocutaneous flap without muscle. Plast Reconstr Surg 1995; 96(7): 1608-14.
       [http://dx.doi.org/10.1097/00006534-199512000-00014] [PMID: 7480280]

[29]   Koshima I, Saisho H, Kawada S, Hamanaka T, Umeda N, Moriguchi T. Flow-through thin latissimus dorsi perforator flap for repair of soft-tissue defects in the legs. Plast Reconstr Surg 1999; 103(5): 1483-90.
        [http://dx.doi.org/10.1097/00006534-199904020-00021] [PMID: 10190449]

[30]   Kim JT, Koo BS, Kim SK. The thin latissimus dorsi perforator-based free flap for resurfacing. Plast Reconstr Surg 2001; 107(2): 374-82.
        [http://dx.doi.org/10.1097/00006534-200102000-00012] [PMID: 11214052]

[31]   Hallock GG, Sano K. The medial sural MEDIAL GASTROCNEMIUS perforator free flap: an ideal prone position skin flap. Ann Plast Surg 2004; 52(2): 184-7.
        [http://dx.doi.org/10.1097/01.sap.0000095438.33962.31] [PMID: 14745270]

[32]   Geddes CR, Tang M, Yang D. Anatomy of the integument of the lower extremity. In: Blondeel PN, Morris SF, Hallock GG, Eds. Perforator flaps: anatomy, technique & clinical applications. St. Louis: Quality Medical Publishing, Inc. 2006; pp. 541-78.

[33]   Saint-Cyr M, Schaverien M, Arbique G, Hatef D, Brown SA, Rohrich RJ. Three- and four-dimensional computed tomographic angiography and venography for the investigation of the vascular anatomy and perfusion of perforator flaps. Plast Reconstr Surg 2008; 121(3): 772-80.
        [http://dx.doi.org/10.1097/01.prs.0000299338.97612.90] [PMID: 18317127]

[34]   Schaverien M, Saint-Cyr M. Perforators of the lower leg: analysis of perforator locations and clinical application for pedicled perforator flaps. Plast Reconstr Surg 2008; 122(1): 161-70.
        [http://dx.doi.org/10.1097/PRS.0b013e3181774386] [PMID: 18594401]

[35]   Saint-Cyr M, Wong C, Schaverien M, Mojallal A, Rohrich RJ. The perforasome theory: vascular anatomy and clinical implications. Plast Reconstr Surg 2009; 124(5): 1529-44.
        [http://dx.doi.org/10.1097/PRS.0b013e3181b98a6c] [PMID: 20009839]

[36]   Lecours C, Saint-Cyr M, Wong C, *et al.* Freestyle pedicle perforator flaps: clinical results and vascular anatomy. Plast Reconstr Surg 2010; 126(5): 1589-603.
        [http://dx.doi.org/10.1097/PRS.0b013e3181f02ee3] [PMID: 21042115]

[37]   Rubino C, Coscia V, Cavazzuti AM, Canu V. Haemodynamic enhancement in perforator flaps: the inversion phenomenon and its clinical significance. A study of the relation of blood velocity and flow between pedicle and perforator vessels in perforator flaps. J Plast Reconstr Aesthet Surg 2006; 59(6): 636-43.
        [http://dx.doi.org/10.1016/j.bjps.2005.07.010] [PMID: 16817260]

[38]   Georgescu AV, Matei I, Ardelean F, Capota I. Microsurgical nonmicrovascular flaps in forearm and hand reconstruction. Microsurgery 2007; 27(5): 384-94.
        [http://dx.doi.org/10.1002/micr.20376] [PMID: 17557279]

[39]   Parrett BM, Talbot SG, Pribaz JJ, Lee BT. A review of local and regional flaps for distal leg reconstruction. J Reconstr Microsurg 2009; 25(7): 445-55.
        [http://dx.doi.org/10.1055/s-0029-1223847] [PMID: 19593730]

[40]   El-Sabbagh AH. Skin perforator flaps: an algorithm for leg reconstruction. J Reconstr Microsurg 2011; 27(9): 511-23.
        [http://dx.doi.org/10.1055/s-0031-1284238] [PMID: 21796584]

[41]   Lee BT, Lin SJ, Bar-Meir ED, Borud LJ, Upton J. Pedicled perforator flaps: a new principle in reconstructive surgery. Plast Reconstr Surg 2010; 125(1): 201-8.
        [http://dx.doi.org/10.1097/PRS.0b013e3181c2a4c9] [PMID: 20048613]

[42]   Hyakusoku H, Yamamoto T, Fumiiri M. The propeller flap method. Br J Plast Surg 1991; 44(1): 53-4.
        [http://dx.doi.org/10.1016/0007-1226(91)90179-N] [PMID: 1993239]

[43]   Hallock GG. The propeller flap version of the adductor muscle perforator flap for coverage of ischial or trochanteric pressure sores. Ann Plast Surg 2006; 56(5): 540-2.
        [http://dx.doi.org/10.1097/01.sap.0000210512.81988.2b] [PMID: 16641632]

[44]   Pignatti M, Ogawa R, Hallock GG, *et al.* The Tokyo consensus on propeller flaps. Plast Reconstr Surg 2011; 127(2): 716-22.
[http://dx.doi.org/10.1097/PRS.0b013e3181fed6b2] [PMID: 21285776]

[45]   Teo TC. Perforator local flaps in lower limb reconstruction. Cir Plast Iberlatinamer 2006; 32: 15-6.

[46]   Whetzel TP, Barnard MA, Stokes RB. Arterial fasciocutaneous vascular territories of the lower leg. Plast Reconstr Surg 1997; 100(5): 1172-83.
[http://dx.doi.org/10.1097/00006534-199710000-00016] [PMID: 9326779]

[47]   Carriquiry C, Aparecida Costa M, Vasconez LO. An anatomic study of the septocutaneous vessels of the leg. Plast Reconstr Surg 1985; 76(3): 354-63.
[http://dx.doi.org/10.1097/00006534-198509000-00003] [PMID: 3898166]

[48]   Yoshimura M, Shimada T, Hosokawa M. The vasculature of the peroneal tissue transfer. Plast Reconstr Surg 1990; 85(6): 917-21.
[http://dx.doi.org/10.1097/00006534-199006000-00012] [PMID: 2349296]

[49]   Hwang WY, Chen SZ, Han LY, Chang TS. Medial leg skin flap: vascular anatomy and clinical applications. Ann Plast Surg 1985; 15(6): 489-91.
[http://dx.doi.org/10.1097/00000637-198512000-00006] [PMID: 3880198]

[50]   Koshima I, Moriguchi T, Ohta S, Hamanaka T, Inoue T, Ikeda A. The vasculature and clinical application of the posterior tibial perforator-based flap. Plast Reconstr Surg 1992; 90(4): 643-9.
[http://dx.doi.org/10.1097/00006534-199210000-00014] [PMID: 1410001]

[51]   Heitmann C, Khan FN, Levin LS. Vasculature of the peroneal artery: an anatomic study focused on the perforator vessels. J Reconstr Microsurg 2003; 19(3): 157-62.
[http://dx.doi.org/10.1055/s-2003-39828] [PMID: 12806576]

[52]   Masia J, Moscatiello F, Pons G, Fernandez M, Lopez S, Serret P. Our experience in lower limb reconstruction with perforator flaps. Ann Plast Surg 2007; 58(5): 507-12.
[http://dx.doi.org/10.1097/01.sap.0000239841.47088.a5] [PMID: 17452834]

[53]   Tos P, Innocenti M, Artiaco S, *et al.* Perforator-based propeller flaps treating loss of substance in the lower limb. J Orthop Traumatol 2011; 12(2): 93-9.
[http://dx.doi.org/10.1007/s10195-011-0136-0] [PMID: 21544548]

[54]   Jiga LP, Barac S, Taranu G, *et al.* The versatility of propeller flaps for lower limb reconstruction in patients with peripheral arterial obstructive disease: initial experience. Ann Plast Surg 2010; 64(2): 193-7.
[http://dx.doi.org/10.1097/SAP.0b013e3181a72f8c] [PMID: 20098106]

[55]   Pignatti M, Pasqualini M, Governa M, Bruti M, Rigotti G. Propeller flaps for leg reconstruction. J Plast Reconstr Aesthet Surg 2008; 61(7): 777-83.
[http://dx.doi.org/10.1016/j.bjps.2007.10.077] [PMID: 18450531]

[56]   Rad AN, Singh NK, Rosson GD. Peroneal artery perforator-based propeller flap reconstruction of the lateral distal lower extremity after tumor extirpation: case report and literature review. Microsurgery 2008; 28(8): 663-70.
[http://dx.doi.org/10.1002/micr.20557] [PMID: 18846577]

[57]   Niranjan NS, Price RD, Govilkar P. Fascial feeder and perforator-based V-Y advancement flaps in the reconstruction of lower limb defects. Br J Plast Surg 2000; 53(8): 679-89.
[http://dx.doi.org/10.1054/bjps.2000.3428] [PMID: 11090325]

[58]   Wong CH, Cui F, Tan BK, *et al.* Nonlinear finite element simulations to elucidate the determinants of perforator patency in propeller flaps. Ann Plast Surg 2007; 59(6): 672-8.
[http://dx.doi.org/10.1097/SAP.0b013e31803df4e9] [PMID: 18046151]

[59]   Taylor GI, Doyle M, McCarten G. The Doppler probe for planning flaps: anatomical study and clinical applications. Br J Plast Surg 1990; 43(1): 1-16.
[http://dx.doi.org/10.1016/0007-1226(90)90039-3] [PMID: 2178717]

[60]   Morris SF, Taylor GI. Predicting the survival of experimental skin flaps with a knowledge of the vascular architecture. Plast Reconstr Surg 1993; 92(7): 1352-61.
[PMID: 8248411]

[61]   Dhar SC, Taylor GI. The delay phenomenon: the story unfolds. Plast Reconstr Surg 1999; 104(7): 2079-91.
[http://dx.doi.org/10.1097/00006534-199912000-00021] [PMID: 11149772]

[62]   Bhattacharya V, Deshpande SB, Watts RK, Reddy GR, Singh SK, Goyal S. Measurement of perfusion pressure of perforators and its correlation with their internal diameter. Br J Plast Surg 2005; 58(6): 759-64.
[http://dx.doi.org/10.1016/j.bjps.2005.04.039] [PMID: 16040015]

[63]   Panse NS, Bhatt YC, Tandale MS. What is safe limit of the perforator flap in lower extremity reconstruction ? Do we have answers yet? Plast Surg Int 2011; 2011: 349-57.

[64]   Blondeel PN, Beyens G, Verhaeghe R, *et al.* Doppler flowmetry in the planning of perforator flaps. Br J Plast Surg 1998; 51(3): 202-9.
[http://dx.doi.org/10.1016/S0007-1226(98)80010-6] [PMID: 9664879]

[65]   Yu P, Youssef A. Efficacy of the handheld Doppler in preoperative identification of the cutaneous perforators in the anterolateral thigh flap. Plast Reconstr Surg 2006; 118(4): 928-33.
[http://dx.doi.org/10.1097/01.prs.0000232216.34854.63] [PMID: 16980853]

[66]   Khan UD, Miller JG. Reliability of handheld Doppler in planning local perforator-based flaps for extremities. Aesthetic Plast Surg 2007; 31(5): 521-5.
[http://dx.doi.org/10.1007/s00266-007-0072-9] [PMID: 17659407]

[67]   McCraw JB, Myers B, Shanklin KD. The value of fluorescein in predicting the viability of arterialized flaps. Plast Reconstr Surg 1977; 60(5): 710-9.
[http://dx.doi.org/10.1097/00006534-197711000-00006] [PMID: 335416]

[68]   Morykwas MJ, Hills H, Argenta LC. The safety of intravenous fluorescein administration. Ann Plast Surg 1991; 26(6): 551-3.
[http://dx.doi.org/10.1097/00000637-199106000-00009] [PMID: 1883161]

[69]   Eren S, Rübben A, Krein R, Larkin G, Hettich R. Assessment of microcirculation of an axial skin flap using indocyanine green fluorescence angiography. Plast Reconstr Surg 1995; 96(7): 1636-49.
[http://dx.doi.org/10.1097/00006534-199512000-00018] [PMID: 7480284]

[70]   Holm C, Mayr M, Höfter E, Becker A, Pfeiffer UJ, Mühlbauer W. Intraoperative evaluation of skin-flap viability using laser-induced fluorescence of indocyanine green. Br J Plast Surg 2002; 55(8): 635-44.
[http://dx.doi.org/10.1054/bjps.2002.3969] [PMID: 12550116]

[71]   Matsui A, Lee BT, Winer JH, Vooght CS, Laurence RG, Frangioni JV. Real-time intraoperative near-infrared fluorescence angiography for perforator identification and flap design. Plast Reconstr Surg 2009; 123(3): 125e-7e.
[http://dx.doi.org/10.1097/PRS.0b013e31819a3617] [PMID: 19319038]

[72]   Mehrotra S. Perforator-plus flaps: a new concept in traditional flap design. Plast Reconstr Surg 2007; 119(2): 590-8.
[http://dx.doi.org/10.1097/01.prs.0000239570.18647.83] [PMID: 17230095]

[73]   Parrett BM, Winograd JM, Lin SJ, Borud LJ, Taghinia A, Lee BT. The posterior tibial artery perforator flap: an alternative to free-flap closure in the comorbid patient. J Reconstr Microsurg 2009; 25(2): 105-9.
[http://dx.doi.org/10.1055/s-0028-1090616] [PMID: 18924067]

[74]   Saint-Cyr M, Schaverien M, Rohrich RJ. Preexpanded second intercostal space internal mammary artery pedicle perforator flap: case report and anatomical study. Plast Reconstr Surg 2009; 123(6): 1659-64.
[http://dx.doi.org/10.1097/PRS.0b013e3181a64eb0] [PMID: 19483563]

[75]   Asko-Seljavaara S. Free style free flaps. Seventh Congress of the International Society of Reconstructive Microsurgery. 1983 Jun 19–30; New York, NY.

[76]   Saint-Cyr M, Schaverien MV, Rohrich RJ. Perforator flaps: history, controversies, physiology, anatomy, and use in reconstruction. Plast Reconstr Surg 2009; 123(4): 132e-45e.
[http://dx.doi.org/10.1097/PRS.0b013e31819f2c6a] [PMID: 19337067]

[77]   Quaba AA, Davison PM. The distally-based dorsal hand flap. Br J Plast Surg 1990; 43(1): 28-39.
[http://dx.doi.org/10.1016/0007-1226(90)90042-X] [PMID: 2310896]

[78]   Mardini S, Tsai FC, Wei FC. The thigh as a model for free style free flaps. Clin Plast Surg 2003; 30(3): 473-80.
[http://dx.doi.org/10.1016/S0094-1298(03)00047-6] [PMID: 12916602]

[79]   Wei FC, Mardini S. Free-style free flaps. Plast Reconstr Surg 2004; 114(4): 910-6.
[http://dx.doi.org/10.1097/01.PRS.0000133171.65075.81] [PMID: 15468398]

[80]   Wallace CG, Kao HK, Jeng SF, Wei FC. Free-style flaps: a further step forward for perforator flap surgery. Plast Reconstr Surg 2009; 124(6) (Suppl.): e419-26.
[http://dx.doi.org/10.1097/PRS.0b013e3181bcf189] [PMID: 19952709]

[81]   Yildirim S, Taylan G, Aköz T. Freestyle perforator-based V-Y advancement flap for reconstruction of soft tissue defects at various anatomic regions. Ann Plast Surg 2007; 58(5): 501-6.
[http://dx.doi.org/10.1097/01.sap.0000247953.36082.f4] [PMID: 17452833]

[82]   DArpa S, Cordova A, Pirrello R, Moschella F. Free style facial artery perforator flap for one stage reconstruction of the nasal ala. J Plast Reconstr Aesthet Surg 2009; 62(1): 36-42.
[http://dx.doi.org/10.1016/j.bjps.2008.06.057] [PMID: 18945660]

[83]   DArpa S, Cordova A, Pignatti M, Moschella F. Freestyle pedicled perforator flaps: safety, prevention of complications, and management based on 85 consecutive cases. Plast Reconstr Surg 2011; 128(4): 892-906.
[http://dx.doi.org/10.1097/PRS.0b013e3182268c83] [PMID: 21921765]

[84]   Georgescu AV, Capota I, Matei I, *et al.* The place of local/regional perforator flaps in complex traumas of the forearm. J Hand Microsurg 2009; 1(1): 25-31.
[http://dx.doi.org/10.1007/s12593-009-0007-6] [PMID: 23129928]

[85]   Matei I, Georgescu A, Chiroiu B, Capota I, Ardelean F. Harvesting of forearm perforator flaps based on intraoperative vascular exploration: clinical experiences and literature review. Microsurgery 2008; 28(5): 321-30.
[http://dx.doi.org/10.1002/micr.20497] [PMID: 18537174]

[86]   Lee GK. Invited discussion: Harvesting of forearm perforator flaps based on intraoperative vascular exploration: clinical experiences and literature review. Microsurgery 2008; 28(5): 331-2.
[http://dx.doi.org/10.1002/micr.20498] [PMID: 18537175]

[87]   Innocenti M, Menichini G, Baldrighi C, Delcroix L, Vignini L, Tos P. Are there risk factors for complications of perforator-based propeller flaps for lower-extremity reconstruction? Clin Orthop Relat Res 2014; 472(7): 2276-86.
[http://dx.doi.org/10.1007/s11999-014-3537-6] [PMID: 24706021]

[88]   Tang M, Mao Y, Almutairi K, Morris SF. Three-dimensional analysis of perforators of the posterior leg. Plast Reconstr Surg 2009; 123(6): 1729-38.
[http://dx.doi.org/10.1097/PRS.0b013e3181a3f376] [PMID: 19483572]

[89] Zhang X, Wang X, Wen S, *et al.* Posterior tibial artery-based multilobar combined flap free transfer for repair of complex soft tissue defects. Microsurgery 2008; 28(8): 643-9.
[http://dx.doi.org/10.1002/micr.20529] [PMID: 18846571]

[90] Beppu M, Hanel DP, Johnston GH, Carmo JM, Tsai TM. The osteocutaneous fibula flap: an anatomic study. J Reconstr Microsurg 1992; 8(3): 215-23.
[http://dx.doi.org/10.1055/s-2007-1006703] [PMID: 1629801]

[91] Wei FC, Chen HC, Chuang CC, Noordhoff MS. Fibular osteoseptocutaneous flap: anatomic study and clinical application. Plast Reconstr Surg 1986; 78(2): 191-200.
[http://dx.doi.org/10.1097/00006534-198608000-00008] [PMID: 3523559]

[92] Gir P, Cheng A, Oni G, Mojallal A, Saint-Cyr M. Pedicled-perforator (propeller) flaps in lower extremity defects: a systematic review. J Reconstr Microsurg 2012; 28(9): 595-601.
[http://dx.doi.org/10.1055/s-0032-1315786] [PMID: 22715046]

[93] Innocenti M, Cardin-Langlois E, Menichini G, Baldrighi C. Gastrocnaemius-propeller extended miocutanous flap: a new chimaeric flap for soft tissue reconstruction of the knee. J Plast Reconstr Aesthet Surg 2014; 67(2): 244-51.
[http://dx.doi.org/10.1016/j.bjps.2013.10.011] [PMID: 24211051]

[94] Teo TC. The propeller flap concept. Clin Plast Surg 2010; 37: 615-26.

[95] http://www.microsurgeon.org/latissimus Copyright 2001-2015 Rudolf Buntic- Rudy Buntic, MD

[96] Enneking WF, Dunham W, Gebhardt MC, Malawar M, Pritchard DJ. A system for the functional evaluation of reconstructive procedures after surgical treatment of tumors of the musculoskeletal system. Clin Orthop Relat Res 1993; (286): 241-6.
[PMID: 8425352]

[97] Doi K. Management of total paralysis of the brachial plexus by the double free-muscle transfer technique. J Hand Surg Eur Vol 2008; 33(3): 240-51.
[http://dx.doi.org/10.1177/1753193408090140] [PMID: 18562352]

CHAPTER 19

Haematological Care in Patients with Haemophilia and Inhibitors Candidate to Orthopaedic Surgery

Giuseppe Tagariello[1,*], Marco Basso[2], Alberto Ricciardi[3] and Paolo Radossi[1]

[1] *Transfusion Service, Haemophilia Centre and Hematology, Castelfranco Veneto, Treviso, Italy*

[2] *Pharmacology and Hematology, Castelfranco Veneto, Treviso, Italy*

[3] *Orthopedics, Castelfranco Veneto General Hospital, Castelfranco Veneto, Treviso, Italy*

Abstract: A standard replacement treatment by FVIII or FIX concentrates is in most cases ineffective in haemophilic patients with inhibitors. To overcome this problem, the so-called bypassing agents (BPAs) have been introduced in the market and patients may be efficaciously treated also in the orthopaedic setting. However not all patients with inhibitors need to be treated at the same manner. In a proportion of patients a standard replacement therapy by FVIII and FIX concentrates may be useful for the postoperative period or just for a part of it. Ancillary therapy by tranexamic acid may significantly contribute to the bleeding control while anti-thrombotic drugs seem unnecessary differently from non haemophilic patients. Brand new drugs are now being studied representing a potential actual revolution in the treatment of patients with haemophilia and inhibitors.

Keywords: Haemophilia, Inhibitors, Orthopaedic surgery.

INTRODUCTION

During the last decades, joint replacement has become the gold standard for end stage haemophilic arthropathy. One of the limitation or concern about approaching a surgical procedure in a proportion of haemophiliacs is the presence of "inhibitors", that prevent the efficacy of the standard replacement treatment by FVIII or FIX concentrates (see Chapters 2 and 3).

Significantly more severe arthropathies have been reported in patients with inhibitors [1] and the burden of orthopedic implications on the impact on QoL is more severe in haemophilic patients who have developed inhibitors than in those without inhibitors [2]. This justifies such type of surgery in those patients to

---

[*] **Corresponding author: Giuseppe Tagariello,** Castelfranco General Hospital, Castelfranco Veneto, Treviso, Italy; Tel: 0039 0423 732341; E-mail: giuseppe.tagariello@ulssasolo.ven.it

Christian Carulli (Ed.)

restore an articular function and improve their quality of life, otherwise very compromised.

Until recent years, major surgery in such patients was seldom performed due to the inefficacy of standard replacement by FVIII or FIX concentrates. Fortunately patients with inhibitors may now be treated by efficacious therapies using the so-called "bypassing" agents (BPAs) [3, 4].

The treatment by BPAs pones further concerns related to the high costs as stated by the COCIS study where it was demonstrated that the management of inhibitor patients was significantly more expensive when compared to the use of rFVIIa either in orthopedic surgery or in severe bleeding episodes [5].

In this chapter we would like to address the medical approach in this sub group of patients with inhibitors candidate to major orthopaedic surgery.

CURRENT CONCEPTS

In the last two decades many surgeries have been performed worldwide mostly using recombinant activated FVII (rFVIIa, Novoseven, Novonordisk, Denmark). More recently also activated prothrombin complex concentrates (aPCC, FEIBA, Baxter Healthcare, Vienna, Austria) have demonstrated good clinical effects. Moreover, both agents have been tested in a sequential manner with positive outcomes [3, 4].

In the recent past, There was a greater concern in planning surgery in patients with inhibitors. The reason was related to the dramatic severity of the arthropathy needing difficult and long reconstructions and the higher risk of bleeding. This strategy was then associated to severe sequelae given the slow but inexorable joint deterioration related to the haemophilic arthropathy in such patients: the late the surgical procedure, the more challenging intraoperative theatre, and the worst the clinical outcome.

To date, nearly 400 procedures using rFVIIa have been reported [3], and more than 200 using aPCC [4]. The first experience of major surgery in patients with inhibitors with BPAs was reported in 1989 by Ula Hedner [6]. Since then the introduction of activated recombinant factor VIIa has allowed a safer elective surgery in subjects with inhibitors. Several pitfalls associated with its use have been however reported: the short half-life, necessitating frequent intravenous injections, and its very high costs. In fact, the administration of rFVIIa is recommended by bolus injection (BI) at short intervals of two hours at the dosage of 90-120ng/kg/bw for the first 24-48 hours after surgery. Progressively, the intervals may become longer and doses reduced. A possible option to avoid such these aspects may be the use of rFVIIa in continuous infusion (CI) as this way of administration may warrant the same efficacy saving nearly 30% of the product and consequently reducing costs. This approach has been efficaciously tested in several centers, including our institution [7 - 10].

A prerequisite for CI is the stability of the product and the safety of the diluted drug. This has been clearly demonstrated for rFVIIa in previous reports and CI has already been shown to be effective [7, 8]. CI with coagulative factors has demonstrated to provide further advantages: it avoids peaks and troughs; it is cheaper due to lower usage of clotting factor; finally, in the specific case of rFVIIa, it may avoid too frequent administrations. Other advantages are the possibility to associate the antiphibrinolitic drug (tranexamic acid), and to prevent an anamnestic response to FVIII or FIX, which may occur with the other alternative treatments.

Major orthopaedic surgery in Haemophilia is represented mostly by Total Knee Arthroplasty (TKA) and Total Hip Arthroplasty (THA), as mentioned in Chapters 11 and 12. In our personal experience we have reported a THA in two patients with severe Haemophilia A and high titre inhibitors to FVIII using rFVIIa therapy by CI. In one case a failure was reported because of recurrent bleedings, while in the second patient the procedure was successful. Of noting that the total amount of rFVIIa administrated was similar in the two patients (9.93 mg kg^{-1}and 9.32 mg kg^{-1}, respectively), but the way of administration was substantially different. The first patient received the therapy for a longer period, but with a lower dosage, while the second was treated intensively for 12 days only. In both subjects, the level of plasma FVII:C was for most of the time above 10 U mL^{-1} (Figs. **1a & 1b**), which was at that time considered to be the target for optimal rFVIIa efficacy. In our opinion, the crucial point is to obtain a full haemostatic control during the early perioperative phase. For this reason, we usually used high amounts of rFVIIa at the beginning of the operation in the second patient [10]. Starting from this experience we do recommend a maintenance of the FVII:C level well above 10 U mL-1, particularly if there is a significant involvement of soft tissues as usually for standard THA. Saline infusions are useful to avoid local thrombophlebitis at the site of the vascular access. Furthermore tranexamic acid administration seems to produce a better result if given by CI, helping the bleeding control without thrombogenic effects.

In 2003 we have described for the first time a simultaneous THA and TKA in a haemophiliac with inhibitors. The amount of rFVIIa concentrate used (8.57 mg) was similar to that normally used for a single joint replacement. Also in this case the use of continuous infusions allowed an easier administration, and further contributed to the reduction of related costs [11].

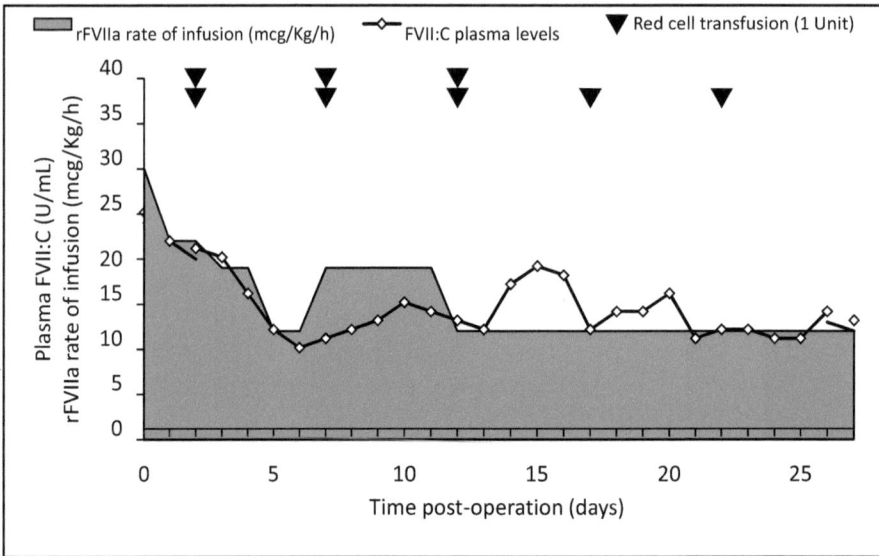

Fig. (1a). Levels of plasma FVII:C and amount of rFVIIa administered in the first patient of two undergoing a THA. The peak of FVII was 24 U mL-1 following the bolus injection, and the trough is 8 U mL-1 in the 8th day. The total amount of rFVIIa administered was 9.93 mg kg-1, and the duration of CI was 29 days. Black arrows show blood transfusions (two bags).

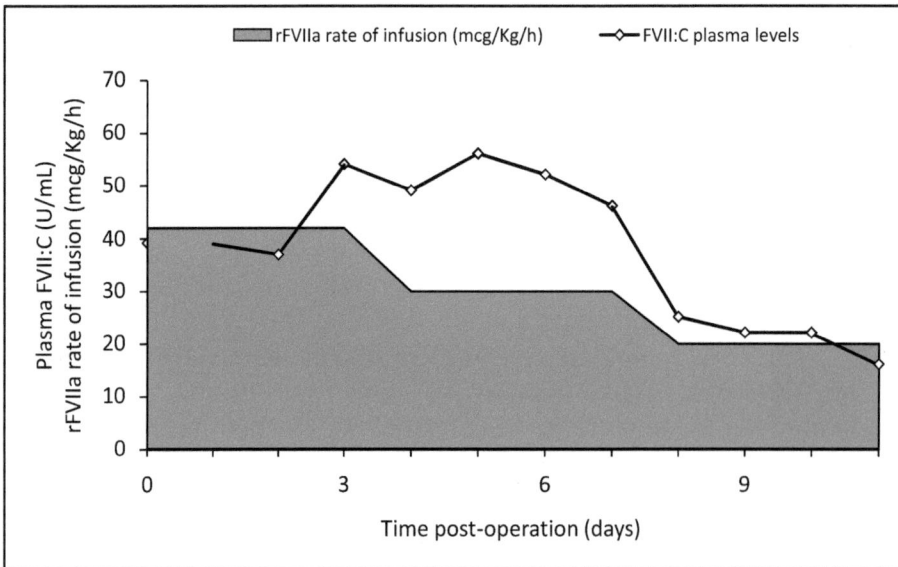

Fig. (1b). Levels of plasma FVII:C and amount of rFVIIa administered in the second patient undergoing a THA. The peak of FVII was 56 U mL-1 in the 7th day when possibly the haemostatic need becomes weaker. The total amount of rFVIIa administered was 9.32 mg kg-1, and the duration of CI was 12 days. No blood transfusion was necessary.

As mentioned in Chapter 14, given the very young age of haemophilic patients and their comorbidities, a failure of a previous knee or hip implant may realize for several reasons. One of the most common mechanism of failure is represented by a deep infection.

The revision of an infected TKA is routinely performed in a two-stage procedure. The first step consists in the removal of the failed implant, and the positioning of an antibiotic-loaded cemented spacer. The second procedure consists in the removal of the spacer, and the final implant of a knee prosthesis with a higher constraint (see Chapter 15). We have described the first revision of an infected knee prosthesis by a one-stage procedure in a haemophilic patient with inhibitors. The use of rFVIIa by bolus injection during surgery and the CI for the postoperative period were effective in controlling the haemostasis of the patient. The amount of rFVIIa for surgery was actually less than the amount previously used for patients undergoing single-joint replacements [12]. The ten-year follow-up is now confirming that such kind of surgery may be possible and safe in selected cases.

Although the general experience in surgical operations is longer for rFVIIa with respect to other drugs, an interest on agents like aPCC is arising by several clinical studies. This drug is effective and safe when used for nonsurgical haemostatic control in haemophilic patients with high inhibitor titers [13, 14]. Experiences with a perioperative use of aPCC is to date still limited, but resulted in good bleeding control in minor and major surgery [15]. In a recent paper by Negrier *et al*, a multicentric collection of surgical experiences with aPCC (SURF study) showed to be an effective strategy for the management of haemophilic patients with inhibitors undergoing surgery [16]. The dosage of aPCC was prescribed at the discretion of physicians in accordance with the approved product characteristics or in line with the current literature. General dosing recommendations for aPCC were provided: 50–100 U kg^{-1} were administered at intervals of 6–12 h during or after surgery, taking care not to exceed the maximum daily dose of 200 U.

Thirty-five surgical procedures were performed in 24 patients across 19 centres where outcome measures comprised aPCC infusion details, type of surgery, assessment of haemostatic efficacy, adverse events (AEs), and blood loss evaluation.

Among the surgical procedures, 37.1% (13 of 35) were characterized by a severe risk, 25.7% (9 of 35) moderate risk, and 37.1% (13 of 35) mild risk. Historical inhibitor titres were from 19 BU mL^{-1} to 8000 BU mL^{-1}, with a median value of 333 BU. Among patients with Haemophilia A, the longest exposure to FEIBA was 28 days, with a cumulative aPCC dose of 241 000 U.

The conclusion of the SURF study documents the safety and efficacy of aPCC for surgery in haemophiliacs with inhibitors [16]. However, no experience is reported for aPCC in CI.

More recently an increasing number of reports of both minor and major surgical procedures dealt with the possible combination of aPCC and rFVIIa.

In order to optimize the bleeding management and to reduce such risks the United Kingdom Haemophilia Centre Doctors Organization (UKHCDO) guidelines [17] and the Canadian expert consensus document [18] have been released suggesting that both agents may be used to cover major surgeries. This hybrid regimen combines the advantages of the dosing flexibility of rFVIIa in the immediate postoperative period with the less frequent dosing of aPCC in the later stages. The result is clear in terms of cost-effectiveness of the regimen with rFVIIa alone, reduction of the dosing frequency, and possibly a less pressure on nursing staff [19].

However, not all patients with inhibitors need to be treated only by BPAs as some subject is not completely unresponsive to the standard treatment. This subgroup of patients, identified as "low responders" (stable low titer or high responders with transient low titer), may be treated by a standard replacement therapy with FVIII or FIX: the difference consists in the need of a larger amount of concentrates for the entire surgical period (low responders) or for a partial period (high responders with low titer). (Figs. **2** and **3**) show the strategy for the treatment of different inhibitor states, and the formula to calculate the amount of FVIII when BU are <5.

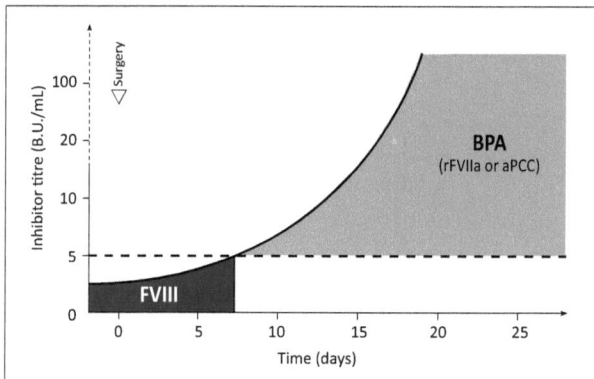

Fig. (2a). "Theoretical" trend of the treatment in a high responder patient with low titer inhibitors (BU < 5) at the time of surgery. FVIII administration at the beginning represents a "booster" dose and within 5-7 days the inhibitor titer increased, so BPAs were necessary. This approach allows the best result from the hemostatic point of view, and at the same time may contribute to costs reduction.

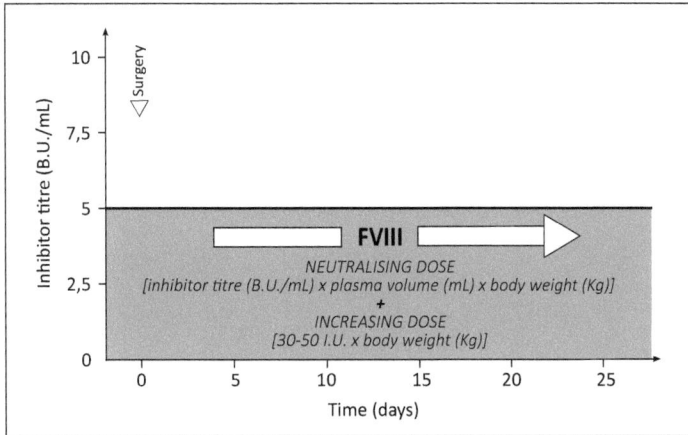

Fig. (2b). Treatment in a "stable" low responder patient with low titer inhibitors (BU < 5) at the time of surgery. This approach allowed a treatment using higher amounts of FVIII (neutralizing dose + increasing dose) calculated according to the formula reported into the graphic. This is the best result from the hemostatic point of view, reducing related costs as BPAs were not used.

Antifibrinolytic Treatment

Tranexamic acid (TXA) is a synthetic derivative of the amino acid lysine that exerts its antifibrinolytic effect through a reversible blockade of lysine binding sites on plasminogen molecules. The process of fibrin breakdown begins when plasminogen, a glycoprotein proenzyme produced by the liver, binds to stands of fibrin.

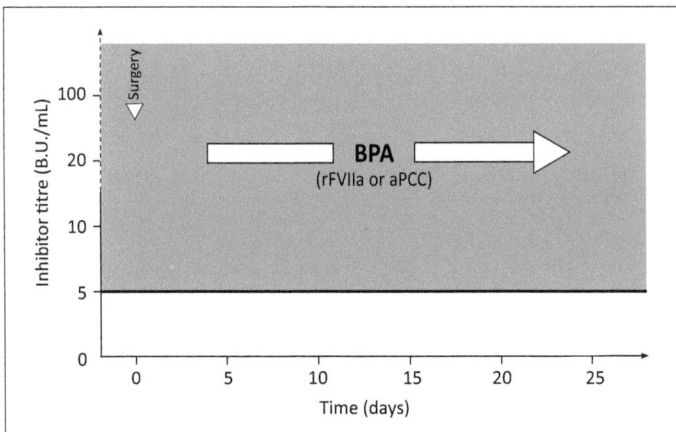

Fig. (3). Treatment in a "stable" high responder patient with a high titer inhibitors (BU > 5) at the time of surgery. This patient needed BPAs for the entire pre- and post-surgical period.

Although TXA has been used for many years in case of bleedings, only recently was evaluated in a systematic manner in the setting of non-haemophilic patients undergoing elective and emergency surgery [20].

From this systematic review and meta-analysis on 104 clinical trials, the conclusions were that TXA was able to reduce blood loss and blood transfusions in about one-third independently by the type of surgery. A crucial point seems to be the timing of administration and in most of the trials the key point is that TXA should be administered immediately before the beginning of surgery. In patients with Haemophilia its use is further supported by the demonstration that *in vitro* TXA at varying concentrations of FVIII or recombinant FVIIa improves the clot stability to levels that were not significantly different from controls. These results support the concept that a more efficient, reliable, and cost effective treatment may be obtained if TXA is combined with factor concentrates to treat haemophiliacs [21]. However, TXA is extensively used as an adjunct in Haemophilia care. Unfortunately, the clinical use results as entirely empirical and only a limited controlled experience exists on the effect of TXA administered in combination with BPAs both in patients with Haemophilia and healthy controls. Five healthy volunteers and 6 Haemophilia inhibitor patients were enrolled in a prospective crossover study [22] and the results showed that combination of aPCC or rFVIIa with TXA normalizes the clot stability in haemophilic patients with inhibitors as compared to healthy controls treated with TXA.

The conclusions of this study suggests that the adjunct use of TXA and BPAs may be a safe and effective method to improve the haemostatic response in Haemophilia A patients with inhibitors as compared to standard therapy with BPAs alone.

Historically, TXA administration in patients treated by aPCC was contraindicated because of the high risk of venous thromboembolism (VTE). In the SURF study the concomitant use of fibrinolytic inhibitors was reported and even if recommended, there was no evidence to indicate that the use of TXA contributed to the development of VTE [22].

Pharmacologic Anti-thrombotic Prophylaxis in Patients with Haemophilia?

VTE is a recognized complication after joint replacement surgery, and a prophylaxis is routinely used in patients without bleeding disorders. However, for patients with Haemophilia, the pharmacologic prophylaxis is highly variable and controversial because of the inherent bleeding risk.

A recent review analysed 42 consecutive patients with Haemophilia A or B undergoing 71 hip or knee replacements, was compared to the literature in order to estimate the incidence of VTE after THA and TKA in the haemophilic population [23].

All patients used compression stockings for up to 6 weeks after surgery; additionally, 6 cases (10.5%; 57 with available data) used sequential intermittent compression devices, and 2 (2.8%) received a low-molecular-weight heparin regimen postoperatively. One patient (1.4%) receiving low-molecular-weight heparin had a symptomatic, lower-extremity VTE ten days after the hip replacement for a traumatic proximal femur fracture. None of the remainders (70 patients) reported any symptomatic VTE within 3 months after surgery. Analysis of pooled data from published series of haemophilic patients undergoing a joint replacement showed an estimated incidence of symptomatic VTE of 0.5%. The conclusion was that in patients with Haemophilia, joint replacement surgery can be performed safely without a routinary VTE prophylaxis, and without an increasing risk of thromboembolic events [23].

FUTURE HOPES

Although the possibility of new rFVIIa variants with a prolonged activity is now under investigation, a new haematologic treatment for patients with inhibitors, employing a bi-specific antibody to factors IXa and X, has been recently presented [24]. These scientists produced a bispecific FVIII mimics antibody against the FIXa/FX complex named ACE910. This antibody has demonstrated haemostatic effects on ongoing and spontaneous joint bleedings, and a phase 1 study was then initiated. Furthermore, in the experimental model, bleedings were remarkably decreased by weekly subcutaneous administrations. Moreover, it has been evaluated a prophylactic efficacy at a markedly reduced frequency of administrations as its long half-life is approximately 30 days.

CONCLUDING REMARKS

The landscape for major orthopaedic surgery in patients with Haemophilia and inhibitors is becoming safer than years ago. We have two excellent and efficacious drugs, rFVIIa and aPCC, able to control bleedings during and after surgery. They can be used alone or in combination. Another promising agent is now being studied, and possibly may definitely change not only the surgical setting but the whole approach to the treatment of patients with inhibitors.

To date, the management of patients with inhibitors undergoing orthopaedic surgery is based on a multidisciplinary approach taking into account that the best results, in terms of patients' satisfaction as well as optimization of resources, may be obtained only in selected centers with prolonged experience in this field, and by the close cooperation between haematologists and orthopaedic surgeons.

CONFLICT OF INTEREST

The authors confirm that they have no conflict of interest to declare for this publication.

ACKNOWLEDGEMENTS

We thank Lagev (Libera associazione genitori e emofilici del Veneto) and APE onlus (AVIS per il progresso ematologico) for supporting this work.

REFERENCES

[1]   Morfini M, Haya S, Tagariello G, *et al.* European study on orthopaedic status of haemophilia patients with inhibitors. Haemophilia 2007; 13(5): 606-12.

[2]   Scalone L, Mantovani LG, Mannucci PM, Gringeri A. Quality of life is associated to the orthopaedic status in haemophilic patients with inhibitors. Haemophilia 2006; 12(2): 154-62.
       [http://dx.doi.org/10.1111/j.1365-2516.2006.01204.x] [PMID: 16476090]

[3]   Valentino LA, Cooper DL, Goldstein B. Surgical experience with rFVIIa (NovoSeven) in congenital haemophilia A and B patients with inhibitors to factors VIII or IX. Haemophilia 2011; 17(4): 579-89.
       [http://dx.doi.org/10.1111/j.1365-2516.2010.02460.x] [PMID: 21294815]

[4]   Rangarajan S, Austin S, Goddard NJ, *et al.* Consensus recommendations for the use of FEIBA(®) in haemophilia A patients with inhibitors undergoing elective orthopaedic and non-orthopaedic surgery. Haemophilia 2013; 19(2): 294-303.
       [http://dx.doi.org/10.1111/hae.12028] [PMID: 22989234]

[5]   Gringeri A, Mantovani LG, Scalone L, Mannucci PM. Cost of care and quality of life for patients with hemophilia complicated by inhibitors: the COCIS Study Group. Blood 2003; 102(7): 2358-63.
       [http://dx.doi.org/10.1182/blood-2003-03-0941] [PMID: 12816859]

[6]   Hedner U, Glazer S, Pingel K, *et al.* Successful use of recombinant factor VIIa in patient with severe haemophilia A during synovectomy. Lancet 1988; 2(8621): 1193.
       [http://dx.doi.org/10.1016/S0140-6736(88)90259-0] [PMID: 2903400]

[7]   Schulman S, Bech Jensen M, Varon D, *et al.* Feasibility of using recombinant factor VIIa in continuous infusion. Thromb Haemost 1996; 75(3): 432-6.
       [PMID: 8701403]

[8]   Schulman S. Safety, efficacy and lessons from continuous infusion with rFVIIa. rFVIIa-CI Group. Haemophilia 1998; 4(4): 564-7.
       [http://dx.doi.org/10.1046/j.1365-2516.1998.440564.x] [PMID: 9873795]

[9]   Schulman S, dOiron R, Martinowitz U, *et al.* Experiences with continuous infusion of recombinant activated factor VII. Blood Coagul Fibrinolysis 1998; 9 (Suppl. 1): S97-S101.
       [PMID: 9819037]

[10]   Tagariello G, De Biasi E, Gajo GB, *et al.* Recombinant FVIIa (NovoSeven) continuous infusion and total hip replacement in patients with haemophilia and high titre of inhibitors to FVIII: experience of two cases. Haemophilia 2000; 6(5): 581-3.
       [http://dx.doi.org/10.1046/j.1365-2516.2000.00400.x] [PMID: 11012706]

[11]   Tagariello G, Bisson R, Radossi P, *et al.* Concurrent total hip and knee replacements in a patient with haemophilia with inhibitors using recombinant factor VIIa by continuous infusion. Haemophilia 2003; 9(6): 738-40.
       [http://dx.doi.org/10.1046/j.1351-8216.2003.00820.x] [PMID: 14750941]

[12]　Sartori R, Bisson R, Baars GW, *et al.* One-stage replacement of infected knee prosthesis in a patient with haemophilia A and high titre of inhibitors. Haemophilia 2008; 14(2): 375-7.
[http://dx.doi.org/10.1111/j.1365-2516.2007.01619.x] [PMID: 18179576]

[13]　Holme PA, Brosstad F, Tjønnfjord GE. Acquired haemophilia: management of bleeds and immune therapy to eradicate autoantibodies. Haemophilia 2005; 11(5): 510-5.
[http://dx.doi.org/10.1111/j.1365-2516.2005.01136.x] [PMID: 16128896]

[14]　Negrier C, Goudemand J, Sultan Y, Bertrand M, Rothschild C, Lauroua P. Multicenter retrospective study on the utilization of FEIBA in France in patients with factor VIII and factor IX inhibitors. French FEIBA Study Group. Factor Eight Bypassing Activity. Thromb Haemost 1997; 77(6): 1113-9.
[PMID: 9241742]

[15]　Tjønnfjord GE, Brinch L, Gedde-Dahl T, Brosstad FR. Activated prothrombin complex concentrate (FEIBA) treatment during surgery in patients with inhibitors to FVIII/IX. Haemophilia 2004; 10(2): 174-8.
[http://dx.doi.org/10.1046/j.1365-2516.2003.00857.x] [PMID: 14962207]

[16]　Négrier C, Lienhart A, Numerof R, *et al.* SURgical interventions with FEIBA (SURF): international registry of surgery in haemophilia patients with inhibitory antibodies. Haemophilia 2013; 19(3): e143-50.
[http://dx.doi.org/10.1111/hae.12080] [PMID: 23282031]

[17]　Collins PW, Chalmers E, Hart DP, *et al.* Diagnosis and treatment of factor VIII and IX inhibitors in congenital haemophilia Br J Haematol 4th. 2013; 160: 153-70.

[18]　Teitel JM, Carcao M, Lillicrap D, *et al.* Orthopaedic surgery in haemophilia patients with inhibitors: a practical guide to haemostatic, surgical and rehabilitative care. Haemophilia 2009; 15(1): 227-39.
[http://dx.doi.org/10.1111/j.1365-2516.2008.01840.x] [PMID: 18752535]

[19]　van Veen JJ, Maclean RM, Hampton KK, Hamer A, Makris M. Major surgery in severe haemophilia A with inhibitors using a recombinant factor VIIa and activated prothrombin complex concentrate hybrid regimen. Haemophilia 2014; 20(4): 587-92.
[http://dx.doi.org/10.1111/hae.12365] [PMID: 24517157]

[20]　Roberts I. Tranexamic acid in trauma: how should we use it? J Thromb Haemost 2015; 13 (Suppl. 1): S195-9.
[http://dx.doi.org/10.1111/jth.12878] [PMID: 26149023]

[21]　Rea CJ, Foley JH, Bevan DH, Sørensen B. An in-vitro assessment of tranexamic acid as an adjunct to rFVIII or rFVIIa treatment in haemophilia A. Ann Hematol 2014; 93(4): 683-92.
[http://dx.doi.org/10.1007/s00277-013-1921-z] [PMID: 24193375]

[22]　Tran HT, Sørensen B, Rea CJ, *et al.* Tranexamic acid as adjunct therapy to bypassing agents in haemophilia A patients with inhibitors. Haemophilia 2014; 20(3): 369-75.
[http://dx.doi.org/10.1111/hae.12318] [PMID: 24251535]

[23]　Perez Botero J, Spoon DB, Patnaik MS, Ashrani AA, Trousdale RT, Pruthi RK. Incidence of symptomatic venous thromboembolism in patients with hemophilia undergoing joint replacement surgery: a retrospective study. Thromb Res 2015; 135(1): 109-13.
[http://dx.doi.org/10.1016/j.thromres.2014.11.010] [PMID: 25434629]

[24]　Muto A, Yoshihashi K, Takeda M, *et al.* Anti-factor IXa/X bispecific antibody ACE910 prevents joint bleeds in a long-term primate model of acquired hemophilia A. Blood 2014; 124(20): 3165-71.
[http://dx.doi.org/10.1182/blood-2014-07-585737] [PMID: 25274508]

CHAPTER 20

Miscellaneous

Christian Carulli[1,*] and **Gianluigi Pasta[2]**

[1] *Orthopaedic Clinic, University of Florence, Florence, Italy*

[2] *Fondazione IRCCS Ca' Granda Ospedale Maggiore Policlinico, Milan, Italy*

Abstract: Haemophilia as other complex diseases deserves several peculiar orthopaedic conditions that may not be classified in specific routinary categories. A multidisciplinary approach and a full information of the patients may be useful to treat such usually difficult cases. An overview of unusual clinical settings regarding joints, bones, and muscles are reported. Finally, a brief summary of the gene therapies and novel approaches is presented.

Keywords: Antithrombin, Adeno-associated virus, Bilateral joint replacement, Gene therapy, Haemophilia, Haematoma, Iliopsoas, Periarticular ossifications, Pseudotumours, Simultaneous bilateral joint replacement, Surgical treatment.

INTRODUCTION

As for other complex diseases, Haemophilia offers several uncommon orthopaedic conditions that may involve joints, bones, and muscles, and not belonging to specific categories. Such conditions may be sometimes challenging and no help is usually found in literature. Thus, only a dedicated and experienced multidisciplinary team may decide with the patient to undergo a novel type of treatment.

Moreover, the future direction of the treatment of Haemophilia and its complications (as arthropathy and musculoskeletal alterations) will surely be its complete prevention. This goal will be achieved by novel approaches as gene therapy and non-factor solutions that in the last two decades have been studied by preclinical experiments and translational researches. Encouraging outcomes are emerging, confirming their theoretical validity.

The following is an overview of several rare conditions and their related treatment, and a brief summary of the gene and other novel therapies recently proposed.

* **Corresponding author Christian Carulli:** Orthopaedic Clinic, University of Florence, Florence, Italy; Tel: 0039 055 794 8200; Email: christian.carulli@unifi.it

JOINTS

Multiple Joint Replacements

Some decades ago, it was unimaginable to think about a simultaneous bilateral Total Knee or Total Hip Arthroplasty (TKA, THA) in patients affected by Osteoarthritis. Similarly, it was considered unsafe to perform a combined TKA and THA in such subjects. Later, multiple replacements have however become safe and feasible in selected cases given the gross improvements in surgical and anaesthesiologic techniques, tailored substitutive therapies, and closer perioperative care of patients [1 - 3]. Many osteoarthritic patients may be efficiently treated with rates of complications and functional outcomes similar to unilateral or staged procedures, but with lesser costs [3].

In Haemophilia, this type of experience has been faced in very few cases and in specific centers, but associated with a significant rate of complications and variable clinical results [4, 5]. Reichel and colleagues reported about 6 cases treated by a one-stage bilateral TKA: they finally suggested strict indications due to high risk of intra and postoperative complications [4]. Frauchiger and colleagues reported a single case of a simultaneous bilateral TKA in a 40-years old haemophilic patient with inhibitors who developed, after surgery, an aneurysm of the popliteal artery that requested a further surgical procedure [5].

A better knowledge of the coagulative profile of patients, a strong motivation showed by some subjects (asking the faster resolution for their orthopaedic problems), a rigorous selection of candidates to such procedures, and a full information about risks and benefits have led to the opportunity to perform multiple arthroplasties (Fig. **1**). Even if these procedures do not represent the rule and may be realized only in selected subjects, a step forward in the management of haemophilic patients has been made. Just few years ago, such attempts in rather larger series have been reported with better outcome [6, 7]. Mortazavi *et al* presented a series of 8 haemophiliacs safely undergoing bilateral TKAs with half the costs of a staged procedure [6]. Thès *et al* reported a cost-effectiveness analysis related to 5 patients candidate to a simultaneous bilateral TKA compared to 12 patients undergoing a staged bilateral TKA: similar outcomes but lesser costs were recorded for the bilateral cases [7]. In a single case, a simultaneous TKA and THA has been reported with clinical success in a haemophilic patient with high titer of inhibitors [8].

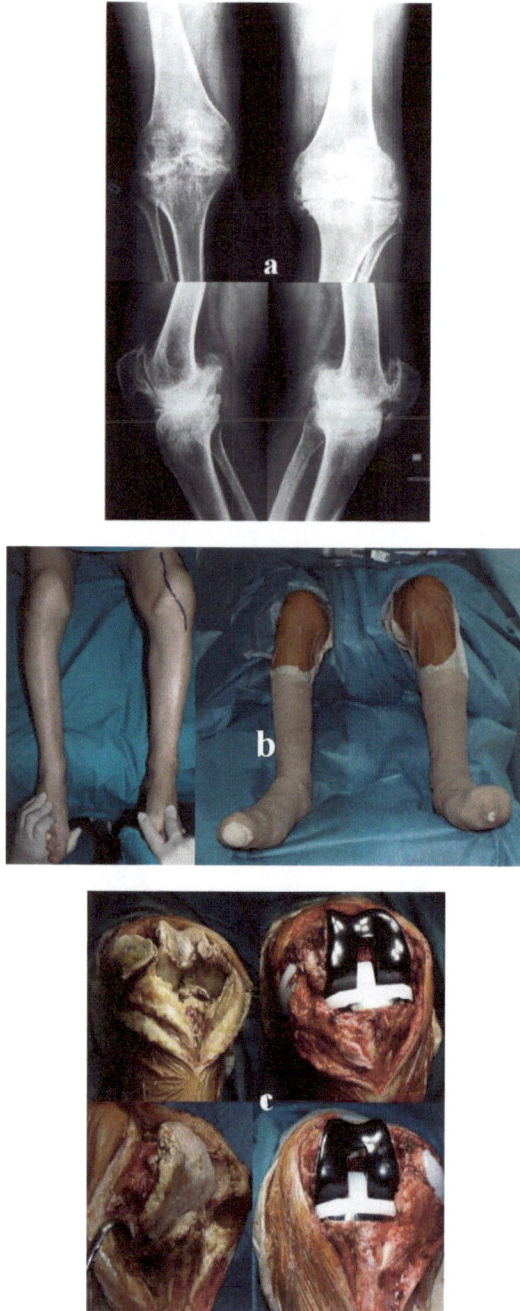

Fig. (1). Simultaneous bilateral TKA in a 51-years old haemophiliac affected by severe Haemophilia A. X-rays (a) and clinical (b) aspect of his knee (Petterson score 12 and 13). Intraoperative pictures before and after the implant of a modern high-tribologic properties TKA (c).

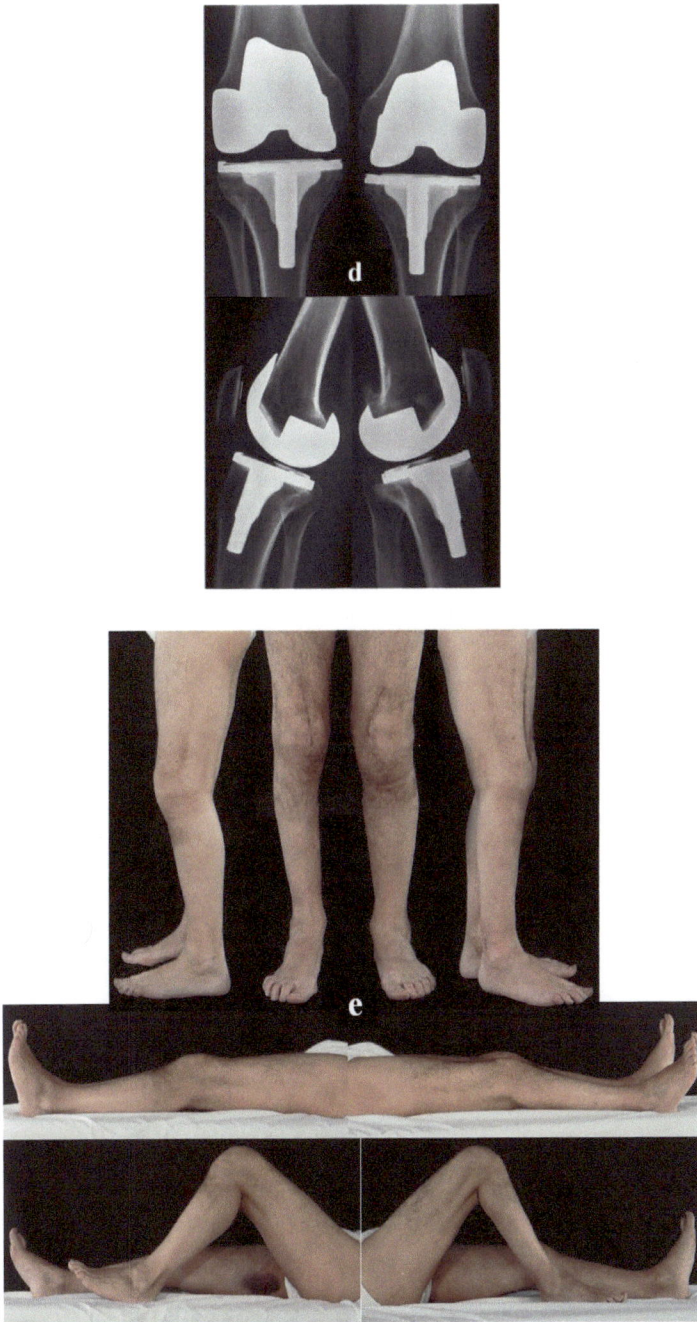

Fig. (1). (*continued*). Postoperative radiographs at 3.5 years (d). Clinical aspect and functional ability 5 years after surgery (e).

BONES

Subchondral Cyst

Subchondral cysts are usually related with the arthropathy. The first radiological sign of haemophilic arthropathy are represented by narrowing of the joint space and small abnormalities in the subchondral bone. Subchondral cysts develop later, and usually become multiple, irregularly distributed, and larger than cysts usually observed in non-haemophilic children or adolescents. These cysts may be connected and exposed in the joint accompanied by gross alterations of the subchondral bone. In some cases cyst enlargements result in osteolytic lesions that may provoke pathological fractures [9].

Surgery is usually indicated for subchondral cysts with a size greater than 15% of the area of the joint, especially in weight-bearing areas or in small cysts showing a progression on x-rays [10]. The primary purpose of the treatment is to avoid the collapse of the joint. Various treatment modalities have been described varying from the grafting with autologous or heterologous bone (Fig. **2**) to the filling with coralline hydroxyapatite by a percutaneous approach as recently proposed by Caviglia *et al* [10].

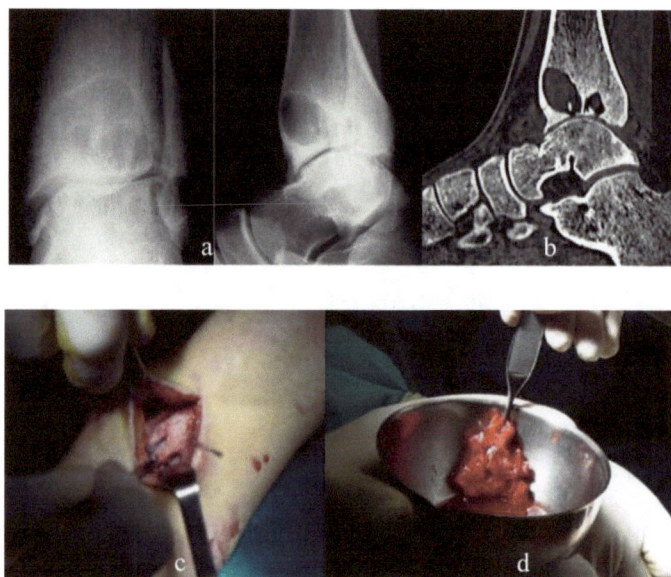

Fig. (2). X-rays (a) and MRI (b) of the ankle of a 20-years old haemophilic subject with severe Haemophila A complaining of ankle pain and functional impairment for one year. Intraoperative pictures (c, d).

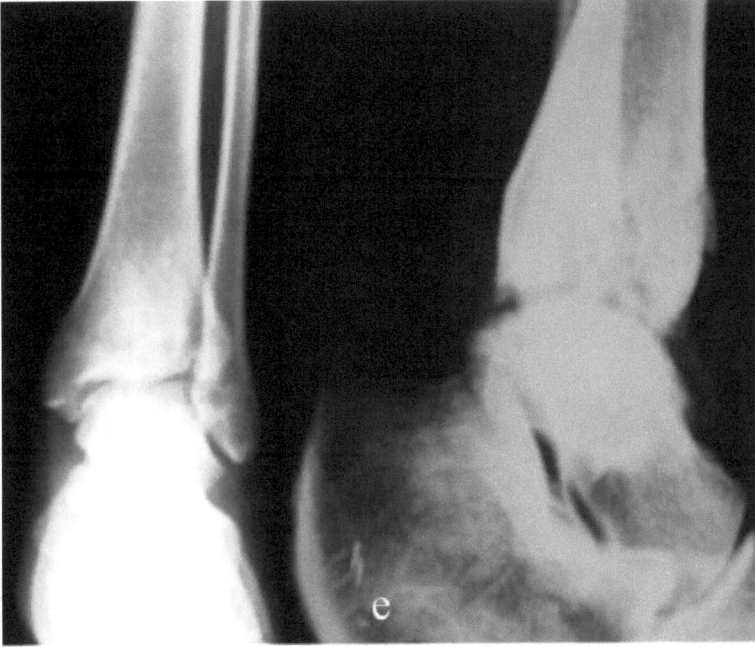

Fig. (2). (*continued*). Postoperative x-rays (e).

Pseudotumor

Pseudotumour is an uncommon complication in haemophilic patients. It is characterized by an encapsulated, chronic, slowly expanding haematoma. Many patients usually refer an injury prior to development of the pseudotumor [11].

Pseudotumors generally develop in soft tissues (often intramuscular), bones, or in the subperiosteal space. Bones as femur, pelvis, tibia, and hand are most frequently involved [12]. The diagnosis is not easy and almost 50% of cases are not diagnosed at time of initial presentation with a delay ranging from 6 weeks to 6 years [13]. There are many benign and malignant bone tumors that have similar aspect and features. A differential diagnosis is needed but may be demanding. Computer Tomography (CT) and Magnetic Resonance Imaging (MRI) are useful to evaluate the nature and extent of the pseudotumor in bones and soft tissues, defining the anatomic relationship between the mass and neurovascular structures (see Chapter 6) [12].

The treatment should be selected on a case-by-case manner to preserve anatomy and function. Conservative management, radiation therapy, or surgical resection are the available options (Fig. **3**).

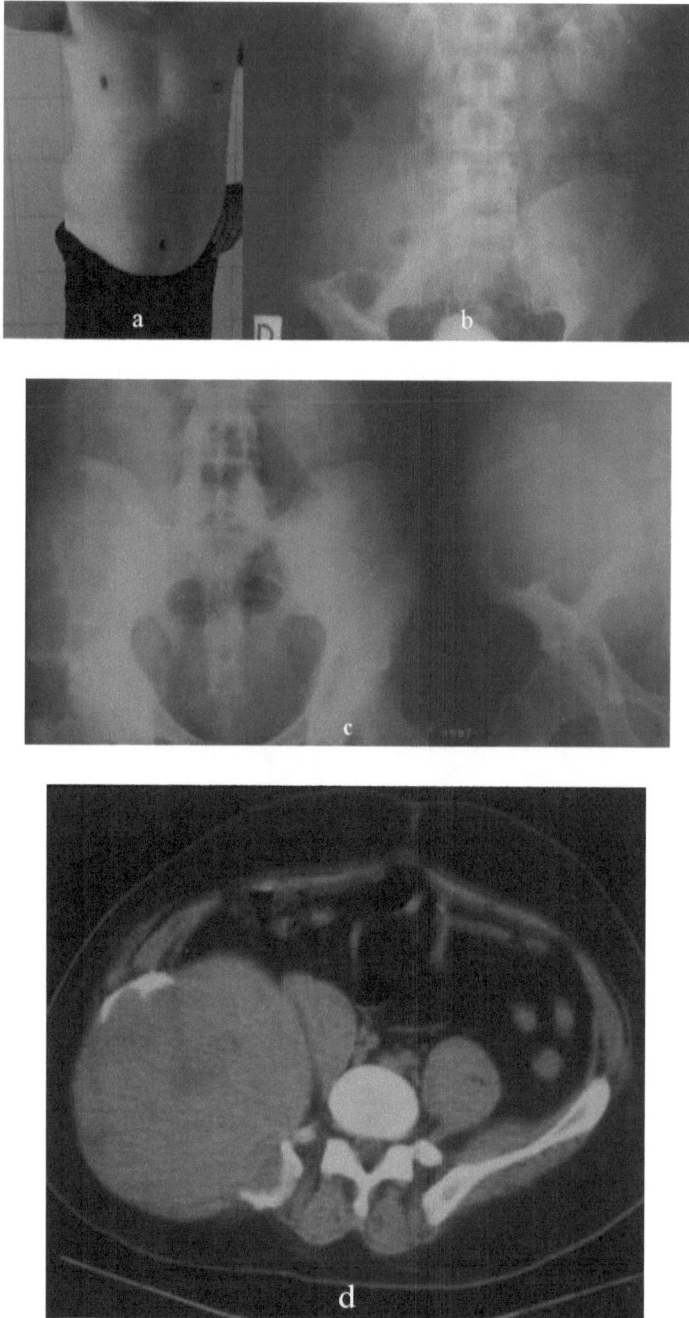

Fig. (3). Clinical presentation (a) and x-rays (b,c) of a right pelvic pseudotumor in a haemophilic subject affected by severe Haemophilia A. CT evaluation (d).

MUSCLES

Haematoma

Between 10% and 23% of bleedings in the musculoskeletal system of haemophilic patients occur in muscles [14]. The iliopsoas is probably the most frequently affected muscle. It classically presents with a painful flexion deformity of the hip. The clinical suspect of an iliopsoas haematoma could be difficult. Hip flexion contracture and a positive iliopsoas sign may indicate a haemorrhage into the hip joint, in the rectus femoral muscle, or even in the anterior abdominal wall. A correct diagnosis is fundamental in order to start with an early treatment. Primarily, an early enhanced correction of factor deficiency must be started until the full disappearance of the haematoma (Fig. **4**). If untreated, iliopsoas muscle bleeding can cause complications such as permanent nerve injury, myositis ossificans, pseudotumour, and even infection (abscess).

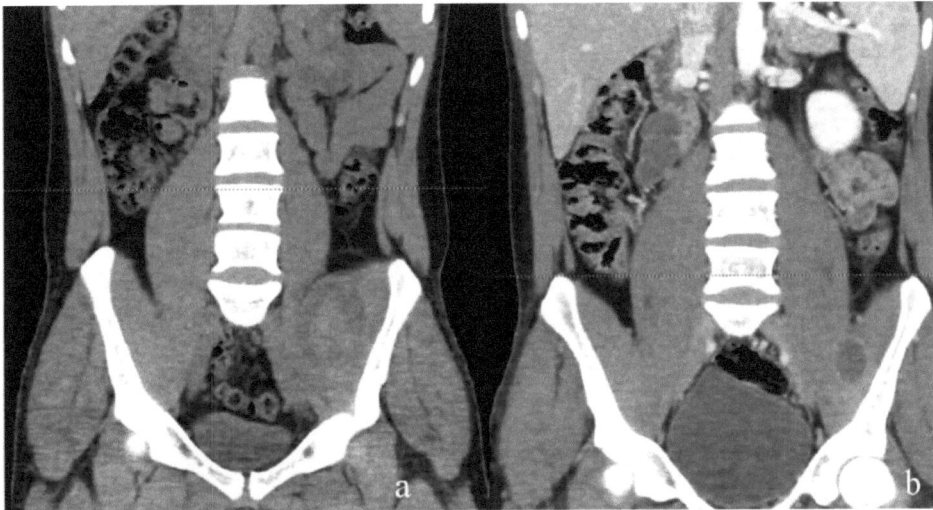

Fig. (4). CT evaluation of a right iliopsoas haematoma in a 25-years old haemophilic subject affected by mild Haemophilia B complaining for hip pain and functional impairment (a). CT assessment 1 month after conservative treatment and factor replacement therapy (b).

Ossifications

Heterotopic ossification is an uncommon complication characterized by formation of mature bone in the soft tissues, following several clinical settings, as posttraumatic conditions, joint replacement, neurological disorders and genetic pathologies. Muscles are typical sites of bleeding, particularly after bruises, strain or tears: ossification may develop, producing pain and functional impairment

(Fig. **5**). Posttraumatic muscular haematoma is a common complication of haemophilia, even if articular bleeding in target joints is certainly most frequent. However, muscle bleeding may present spontaneously: generally symptomatic and self-limiting, it may be reversible with immediate infusion of recombinant factor. Occasionally, muscle bleeding also in haemophilic patients may be complicated by bone formation: a rarely reported condition regarding the quadratus femoris muscle, described in few articles without specific diagnostic algorithm or precise therapeutic proposal [15, 16].

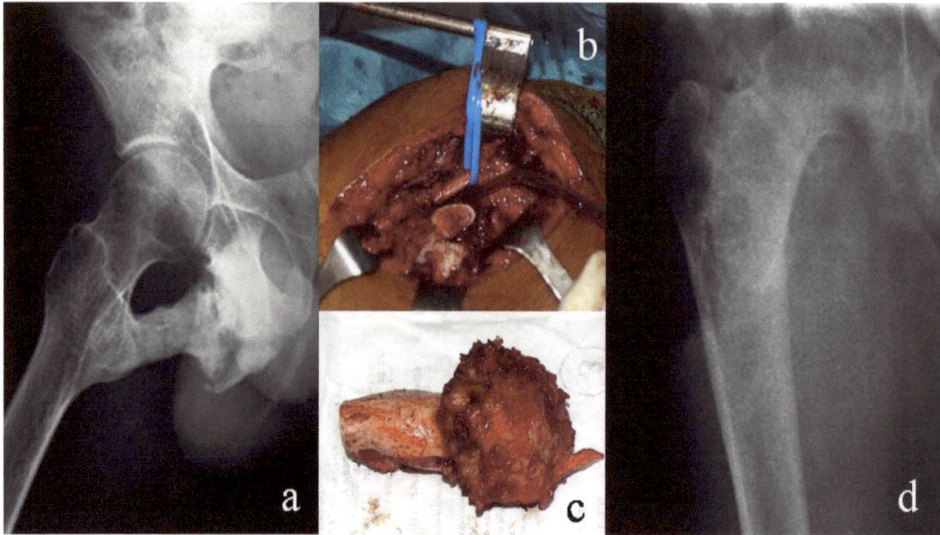

Fig. (5). X-rays of the right hip of a 24-years old haemophilic subject with severe Haemophilia A complaining for one year of buttock pain and functional impairment related to an ossification of its quadratus femuris (a). Intraoperative picture (b). Aspect of the removed *en bloc* ossification (c). Postoperative x-rays (d).

Some authors reported incomplete ossifications leading to groin or buttock pain with ROM limitation in young haemophilic subjects, with complete recovery by postural exercises and clinical follow-up [15, 17]. Others reported about subjects with mild or fair symptoms, treated only by observation and haematological prophylaxis [16]. Finally, others observed severe pain and functional impairment in haemophilic patients needing surgery to limit symptoms, without detailed description of the procedure [18, 19].

GENE THERAPIES

Gene transfer strategies represent the new frontier of therapy for haemophilic patients [20 - 22]. Two are the main pathways of such approach: the use of a viral/non-viral vectors to introduce transgenes into pluripotent cells, and the use of integrating or non-integrating viral vectors to introduce transgenes into long-living, non-dividing cells [23, 24].

Preliminary but encouraging results have been obtained by several phase I studies [25 - 30].

In a study dermal fibroblasts harvested by patients affected by Haemophilia A were grown in culture and transfected with plasmids containing human FVIII gene. These cloned fibroblast cells were then isolated and injected into the omentum of 12 haemophiliacs by laparoscopy. Transitory elevations of FVIII levels were recorded in 7 out of nine patients [26, 27]. In another experiment, dermal fibroblasts isolated from 2 patients affected by Haemophilia B were transfected by human FIX gene-modified retroviruses and injected under their skin: also for these patients transient modifications of FIX levels were recorded [25].

Another study consisted in the use of retroviruses carrying human FVIII genes intravenously injected in 13 Haemophilia A subjects: 9 out of 13 patients had a transient elevation of FVIII levels [28]. Even if all reported studies showed high tolerability of the procedures, cases of oncogenic transformation (leukemia) were recorded [29, 30].

Given such risks, alternative studies with Adeno-associated virus (AAV), derived from a single-stranded DNA of parvovirus, were proposed. An attempt to increase the level of FIX were made in 8 haemophilic patients by intramuscular injections of recombinant AAV expressing human FIX: no increase of FIX was detected [31, 32].

Two Haemophilia B patients were treated by intravenous catheterization of recombinant AAV loaded with FIX gene through the hepatic artery: a transient elevation of FIX was recorded and at the same time the detection of an immune response against AAV capsid antigen was found [33].

To avoid or induce a lower immune response, an attempt was made by the use of a codon-optimized version of human FIX, a synthetic liver-specific promoter, and a double-stranded AAV vector-mediated gene transfer in 10 Haemophilia B subjects: an elevation of FIX levels was found with a mean follow-up of 3.2 years [34, 35], and 4 patients stopped their prophylaxis due to the permanent increase of FIX and the dramatic reduction of bleeding rates. Four subjects showed on the other hand an increase of transaminases resolved by a simple steroid administration. This seems to date the future pathway for gene therapy in Haemophilia B: several phase I and II studies are still open to obtain other outcomes and further clinical informations [23].

Haemophilia A still lacks of similar advanced studies, given the too large sequence of the factor VIII gene to be packaged into a AAV vector [23]. Recently, a group of scientists found a way to use AAV vectors in mice and primates affected by Haemophilia A [36]. A codon-optimized human factor VIII (in which its 226 amino acid B-domain spacer has been replaced by a 17 amino acid peptide with 6 glycosylation of triplets from the B-domain) was used by intravenous administration obtaining high levels of FVIII expression.

To date, 11 phase I or II gene therapy clinical trials have been made on haemophilic human subjects, and 6 of them are currently ongoing [22].

NOVEL THERAPIES

Several preclinical or phase I trials are planned or now being developed with novel approaches to Haemophilia [23, 37 - 45].

ACE910 is a bispecific monoclonal antibody to factors IXa and X mimicking factor VIII cofactor activity by binding FIXa and FX simultaneously [38]. Recent studies consisting in the weekly prophylactic injection of such substance in Haemophilia patients with and without inhibitors resulted in a significant reduction of the number of bleedings [39].

TFPI is a single-chain peptide able to inhibit factors Xa, VIIA, and tissue factor (TF) thus downregulating the coagulative cascade [40]. The blockage of TFPI by aptamers or monoclonal antibodies may increase the factor Xa and thrombin release as in some recent clinical phase I studies [40 - 43].

Finally, Antithrombin is a glycoprotein inhibiting several proteins of the coagulation, mainly thrombin and FXa. ALN-AT3 is a RNA interface therapeutic able to suppress the hepatic production of Antithrombin. In a preclinical study, the subcutaneous administration of ALN-AT3 in mice and primates showed the reduction of production of Antithrombin in a dose-dependent and reversible fashion [44]. This drug is now under investigation in trials involving human subjects.

CONCLUDING REMARKS

Peculiar orthopaedic conditions regarding joints, bones, and muscles are reported in Haemophilia deserving difficult diagnosis and empiric treatments. The importance of a close cooperation between multidisciplinary figures and a detailed informed consent are critical for a correct approach of such challenging cases.

Gene therapies and novel strategies involving monoclonal antibodies and RNA-derived substances represent the actual future direction of the prevention of all complications related to Haemophilia and its induced bleedings.

CONFLICT OF INTEREST

The authors confirm that they have no conflict of interest to declare for this publication.

ACKNOWLEDGEMENTS

Declared none.

REFERENCES

[1]   Restrepo C, Parvizi J, Dietrich T, Einhorn TA. Safety of simultaneous bilateral total knee arthroplasty. A meta-analysis. J Bone Joint Surg Am 2007; 89(6): 1220-6.
       [http://dx.doi.org/10.2106/00004623-200706000-00009] [PMID: 17545424]

[2]   Pavone V, Johnson T, Saulog PS, Sculco TP, Bottner F. Perioperative morbidity in bilateral one-stage total knee replacements. Clin Orthop Relat Res 2004; (421): 155-61.
       [http://dx.doi.org/10.1097/01.blo.0000126309.72205.f7] [PMID: 15123941]

[3]   Noble J, Goodall JR, Noble DJ. Simultaneous bilateral total knee replacement: a persistent controversy. Knee 2009; 16(6): 420-6.
       [http://dx.doi.org/10.1016/j.knee.2009.04.009] [PMID: 19464899]

[4]   Reichel H, Birke A, Wolf HH. [Knee endoprosthesis implantation in hemophiliac arthropathy: results, problems and complications]. Z Orthop Ihre Grenzgeb 2001; 139(2): 120-6.
       [http://dx.doi.org/10.1055/s-2001-15042] [PMID: 11386100]

[5]   Frauchiger LH, Harstall R, Kajahn J, Anderson S, Eggli S. Bilateral total knee arthroplasty in a patient with hemophilia A, high inhibitor titre and aneurysm spurium of the popliteal artery. A case report. Swiss Med Wkly 2010; 140: w13094.
       [PMID: 20734280]

[6]   Mortazavi SM, Haghpanah B, Ebrahiminasab MM, Baghdadi T, Hantooshzadeh R, Toogeh G. Simultaneous bilateral total knee arthroplasty in patients with haemophilia: a safe and cost-effective procedure? Haemophilia 2015. Epub ahead of print
       [PMID: 26536858]

[7]   Thès A, Molina V, Lambert T. Simultaneous bilateral total knee arthroplasty in severe hemophilia: a retrospective cost-effectiveness analysis. Orthop Traumatol Surg Res 2015; 101(2): 147-50.
       [http://dx.doi.org/10.1016/j.otsr.2014.12.010] [PMID: 25687369]

[8]   Tagariello G, Bisson R, Radossi P, *et al.* Concurrent total hip and knee replacements in a patient with haemophilia with inhibitors using recombinant factor VIIa by continuous infusion. Haemophilia 2003; 9(6): 738-40.
       [http://dx.doi.org/10.1046/j.1351-8216.2003.00820.x] [PMID: 14750941]

[9]   Caviglia HA, Galatro G, Nuova P. Intraosseous and subchondral cysts. In: Caviglia HA, Solimeno LP, Eds. Orthopedic surgery in patients with hemophilia. Springer 2008; pp. 235-40.
       [http://dx.doi.org/10.1007/978-88-470-0854-0_32]

[10]   Caviglia H, Galatro G, Cambiaggi G, Landro ME, Candela M, Neme D. Treatment of subchondral cysts in patients with haemophilia. Haemophilia 2015. Epub ahead of print
       [PMID: 26634632]

[11] Jaovisidha S, Ryu KN, Hodler J, Schweitzer ME, Sartoris DJ, Resnick D. Hemophilic pseudotumor: spectrum of MR findings. Skeletal Radiol 1997; 26(8): 468-74.
[http://dx.doi.org/10.1007/s002560050268] [PMID: 9297751]

[12] Stafford JM, James TT, Allen AM, Dixon LR. Hemophilic pseudotumor: radiologic-pathologic correlation. Radiographics 2003; 23(4): 852-6.
[http://dx.doi.org/10.1148/rg.234025154] [PMID: 12853660]

[13] Lim MY, Nielsen B, Ma A, Key NS. Clinical features and management of haemophilic pseudotumours: a single US centre experience over a 30-year period. Haemophilia 2014; 20(1): e58-62.
[http://dx.doi.org/10.1111/hae.12295] [PMID: 24354486]

[14] De la Corte-Rodriguez H, Rodriguez-Merchan EC. Treatment of muscle haematomas in haemophiliacs with special emphasis on percutaneous drainage. Blood Coagul Fibrinolysis 2014; 25(8): 787-94.
[http://dx.doi.org/10.1097/MBC.0000000000000159] [PMID: 24914744]

[15] Heim MD, Strauss S, Horoszowski H. Peripelvic new bone formation following straddle injuries in hemophiliac patients: report of two cases. J Trauma 1979; 19(11): 846-7.
[http://dx.doi.org/10.1097/00005373-197911000-00010] [PMID: 117117]

[16] Rodriguez-Merchan EC, Goddard NJ. Muscular bleeding, soft-tissue haematomas and pseudotumors. In: Rodriguez-Merchan EC, Goddard NJ, Lee CA, Eds. Musculoskeletal Aspects of Haemophilia. Oxford: Blackwell Science Ltd 2000; pp. 85-91.
[http://dx.doi.org/10.1002/9780470693872.ch13]

[17] Aydogdu S, Memis A, Kavakli K, Balkan C. The pelvi-femoral incomplete bone bridge in a patient with mild haemophilia. Haemophilia 2001; 7(2): 224-6.
[http://dx.doi.org/10.1046/j.1365-2516.2001.00496.x] [PMID: 11260284]

[18] Massey GV, Kuhn JG, Nogi J, et al. The spectrum of myositis ossiticans in haemophilia. Haemophilia 2004; 10(2): 189-93.
[http://dx.doi.org/10.1046/j.1365-2516.2003.00854.x] [PMID: 14962211]

[19] Kalenderer O, Bozoglan M, Agus H. Heterotopic ossification in quadratus femoris muscle in a haemophilic patient. Haemophilia 2012; 18(1): e13-4.
[http://dx.doi.org/10.1111/j.1365-2516.2011.02637.x] [PMID: 21883706]

[20] Lheriteau E, Davidoff AM, Nathwani AC. Haemophilia gene therapy: Progress and challenges. Blood Rev 2015; 29(5): 321-8.
[http://dx.doi.org/10.1016/j.blre.2015.03.002] [PMID: 26049173]

[21] Knobe K, Berntorp E. New treatments in hemophilia: insights for the clinician. Ther Adv Hematol 2012; 3(3): 165-75.
[http://dx.doi.org/10.1177/2040620712440007] [PMID: 23556123]

[22] Spencer HT, Riley BE, Doering CB. State of the art: gene therapy of haemophilia. Haemophilia 2016; 22 (Suppl. 5): 66-71.
[http://dx.doi.org/10.1111/hae.13011] [PMID: 27405679]

[23] Kumar R, Dunn A, Carcao M. Changing paradigm of Hemophilia management: extended half-life factor concentrates and gene therapy. Semin Thromb Hemost 2016; 42(1): 18-29.
[http://dx.doi.org/10.1055/s-0035-1568877] [PMID: 26771678]

[24] Ward P, Walsh CE. Current and future prospects for hemophilia gene therapy. Expert Rev Hematol 2016; 9(7): 649-59. Epub ahead of print
[http://dx.doi.org/10.1080/17474086.2016.1182859] [PMID: 27153210]

[25] Qiu X, Lu D, Zhou J, et al. Implantation of autologous skin fibroblast genetically modified to secrete clotting factor IX partially corrects the hemorrhagic tendencies in two hemophilia B patients. Chin Med J (Engl) 1996; 109(11): 832-9.
[PMID: 9275366]

[26]   Roth DA, Tawa NE Jr, OBrien JM, Treco DA, Selden RF. Nonviral transfer of the gene encoding coagulation factor VIII in patients with severe hemophilia A. N Engl J Med 2001; 344(23): 1735-42. [http://dx.doi.org/10.1056/NEJM200106073442301] [PMID: 11396439]

[27]   Roth DA, Tawa NE, Proper J, *et al.* Implantation of non-viral *ex vivo* genetically modified autologous dermal fibroblasts that express B-domain deleted human factor VIII in 12 severe hemophilia A study subjects. Blood 2002; 100: 116a-7a.

[28]   Powell JS, Ragni MV, White GC II, *et al.* Phase 1 trial of FVIII gene transfer for severe hemophilia A using a retroviral construct administered by peripheral intravenous infusion. Blood 2003; 102(6): 2038-45. [http://dx.doi.org/10.1182/blood-2003-01-0167] [PMID: 12763932]

[29]   Hacein-Bey-Abina S, von Kalle C, Schmidt M, *et al.* A serious adverse event after successful gene therapy for X-linked severe combined immunodeficiency. N Engl J Med 2003; 348(3): 255-6. [http://dx.doi.org/10.1056/NEJM200301163480314] [PMID: 12529469]

[30]   Gansbacher B. Report of a second serious adverse event in a clinical trial of gene therapy for X-linked severe combined immune deficiency (X-SCID). J Gene Med 2003; 5(3): 261-2. [http://dx.doi.org/10.1002/jgm.390] [PMID: 12666192]

[31]   Kay MA. Evidence for gene transfer and expression of factor IX in Haemophilia B patients treated with severe hemophilia B patients treated with an AAV vector. Nat Genet 2000; 24: 257-61. [http://dx.doi.org/10.1038/73464] [PMID: 10700178]

[32]   Manno CS, Chew AJ, Hutchison S, *et al.* AAV-mediated factor IX gene transfer to skeletal muscle in patients with severe hemophilia B. Blood 2003; 101(8): 2963-72. [http://dx.doi.org/10.1182/blood-2002-10-3296] [PMID: 12515715]

[33]   High KA, Manno CS, Sabatino DE, *et al.* Immune responses to AAV and to factor IX in a phase I study of AAV-mediated, liver-directed gene transfer for Hemophilia B. Blood 2003; 102: 154a-5a.

[34]   Nathwani AC, Tuddenham EG, Rangarajan S, *et al.* Adenovirus-associated virus vector-mediated gene transfer in hemophilia B. N Engl J Med 2011; 365(25): 2357-65. [http://dx.doi.org/10.1056/NEJMoa1108046] [PMID: 22149959]

[35]   Nathwani AC, Reiss UM, Tuddenham EG, *et al.* Long-term safety and efficacy of factor IX gene therapy in hemophilia B. N Engl J Med 2014; 371(21): 1994-2004. [http://dx.doi.org/10.1056/NEJMoa1407309] [PMID: 25409372]

[36]   McIntosh J, Lenting PJ, Rosales C, *et al.* Therapeutic levels of FVIII following a single peripheral vein administration of rAAV vector encoding a novel human factor VIII variant. Blood 2013; 121(17): 3335-44. [http://dx.doi.org/10.1182/blood-2012-10-462200] [PMID: 23426947]

[37]   Oldenburg J, Albert T. Novel products for haemostasis - current status. Haemophilia 2014; 20 (Suppl. 4): 23-8. [http://dx.doi.org/10.1111/hae.12428] [PMID: 24762271]

[38]   Lillicrap D. A complex substitute: antibody therapy for hemophilia. Nat Med 2012; 18(10): 1460-1. [http://dx.doi.org/10.1038/nm.2959] [PMID: 23042345]

[39]   Shima M, Hanabusa H, Taki M, *et al.* Long-term safety and prophylactic efficacy of once-weekly subcutaneous administration of ACE910, in Japanese Hemophilia A patients with and without FVIII inhibitors: interim results of the extension study of a phase I study. J Thromb Haemost 2015; 13: 6-7.

[40]   Hilden I, Lauritzen B, Sørensen BB, *et al.* Hemostatic effect of a monoclonal antibody mAb 2021 blocking the interaction between FXa and TFPI in a rabbit hemophilia model. Blood 2012; 119(24): 5871-8. [http://dx.doi.org/10.1182/blood-2012-01-401620] [PMID: 22563084]

[41]   Gissel M, Orfeo T, Foley JH, Butenas S. Effect of BAX499 aptamer on tissue factor pathway inhibitor function and thrombin generation in models of hemophilia. Thromb Res 2012; 130(6): 948-55.
[http://dx.doi.org/10.1016/j.thromres.2012.08.299] [PMID: 22951415]

[42]   Gu JM, Ho E, Zhao XY, *et al.* Pharmacodynamics and pharmacokinetics of TFPI-neutralizing antibody (BAY1093884) in cyno-molgus monkeys and prediction of human dose. J Thromb Haemost 2015; 13: 7-7.

[43]   Waters Ek, Sigh J, Ezban M, Hilden I. Thrombin generation is increased in plasma from healthy males who have received concizumab, an antibody against tissue factor pathway inhibitor (Explorer TM2). J Thromb Haemost 2015; 13: 7-7.

[44]   Kumar R, Chan AK, Dawson JE, Forman-Kay JD, Kahr WH, Williams S. Clinical presentation and molecular basis of congenital antithrombin deficiency in children: a cohort study. Br J Haematol 2014; 166(1): 130-9.
[http://dx.doi.org/10.1111/bjh.12842] [PMID: 24684277]

[45]   Sehgal A, Barros S, Ivanciu L, *et al.* An RNAi therapeutic targeting antithrombin to rebalance the coagulation system and promote hemostasis in hemophilia. Nat Med 2015; 21(5): 492-7.
[http://dx.doi.org/10.1038/nm.3847] [PMID: 25849132]

CHAPTER 21

Final Considerations

Giorgia Saccullo[1,*] and **Michael Makris**[1,2]

[1] *Sheffield Haemophilia and Thrombosis Centre, Royal Hallamshire Hospital, Glossop Road, Sheffield, UK*

[2] *Department of Infection Immunity and Cardiovascular Disease, University of Sheffield, UK*

INTRODUCTION

Despite significant improvements in Haemophilia care, joint disease remains an issue for many patients. Most bleeding episodes occur in the musculoskeletal system and recurrent joint bleeds result in progressive joint damage leading to haemophilic arthropathy. Early identification and treatment of musculoskeletal bleeding episodes is crucial to prevent dysfunction. The routine use of prophylactic clotting factor concentrate has resulted in significant improvement in the quality of life and life expectancy of haemophilic individuals.

PATHOGENESIS OF JOINT DISEASE

The severity of bleeding experienced by persons with Haemophilia is generally correlated with the baseline clotting factor level, although considerable heterogeneity in bleeding pattern exists [1, 2]. Approximately 80-90% of bleeding episodes in Haemophilia occur in the musculoskeletal system [3]. Joint bleeding is associated with acute pain, swelling, tenderness and reduced mobility, resulting primarily from the intraarticular presence of blood, which is degraded and gradually resorbed by the synovial tissue [4].

The ability of the synovium to resorb the blood is compromised by rebleeding into the same joint, which results in synovitis and more bleeding [5 - 7]. The development of progressive joint destruction includes several processes involving the joint synovium, cartilage and bone. Furthermore, prolonged exposure of cartilage to blood in a target joint causes cartilage damage with bone remodelling occuring as joint disease progresses. Each of these aspects contributes to the development of the progressive degenerative arthropathy. To prevent the development of chronic synovitis, degenerative arthritis and haemophilic

* **Corresponding author Giorgia Saccullo:** Sheffield Haemophilia and Thrombosis Centre, Royal Hallamshire Hospital, Glossop Road, Sheffield, UK; Tel: +44 1142268843; Email: giorgia.saccullo@sth.nhs.uk

Christian Carulli (Ed.)

arthropathy, this cycle of recurrent joint bleeds needs to be broken. Evidence from research into the pathophysiology of Osteoarthritis and Rheumatoid arthritis, aspects of which resemble haemophilic arthropathy, suggests that several mediators in blood, including iron, cytokines and pro-angiogenic factors, may be involved in the initiation of the synovial changes [5, 6]. However, the mechanisms of cartilage and bone destruction after bleeding remain undefined, and more research is needed to fully elucidate the pathogenesis of haemophilic arthropathy. A more detailed account of the molecular aspects of the pathogenesis of haemophilic arthropathy is given by Melchiorre and colleagues in chapter 1 of this book.

Interestingly Melchiorre *et al* also propose that there are molecular explanations for the less severe arthropathy that has been reported in Haemophilia B. This issue was first reported by a group of Italian Haemophilia treaters led by Tagariello in 2009 [8]. Despite initial scepticism among the Haemophilia community this has now been confirmed by a number of other studies. The underlying reason for the milder arthropathy in Haemophilia B appears to be the less frequent presence of null mutations in Haemophilia B [9]. Thus in contrast to Haemophilia A, Haemophilia B patients appear to express some residual factor that is below the sensitivity of the current laboratory tests to detect.

THE MULTIDISCIPLINARY TEAM APPROACH

Increasingly it is recognized that the management of all patients with Haemophilia and those with haemophilic arthropathy in particular require the services of the multidisciplinary team. The different roles of the members of the team in the management of haemophilic arthropathy are outlined at the start of this book by a haematologist (chapter 2), a nurse (chapter 5), a laboratory technician/scientist (chapter 4), a physical therapist (chapter 9) as well as the orthopedic surgeons whose role is obviously critical as addressed by the majority of the remaining chapters.

The value of the physical therapist in the multidisciplinary team in managing arthropathy is critical and so obvious to any Haemophilia treater, that we remain surprised by the many Haemophilia centres in Europe which lack specialized physiotherapy. The value of the physical therapist is well described in chapters 9 and 16. The first explains the role of physical therapy in the treatment of acute bleeds as well as in the management of chronic arthropathy. It is unfortunately common for clinicians to treat arthropathy with increasing doses of concentrate rather than using physical therapy and appropriate analgesia.

The role of post-operative physical therapy and rehabilitation are outlined in considerable detail in chapter 16 by Pasquetti and colleagues. Although they largely tackle Total Knee and Total Hip replacement, it is likely that their recommendations will be appropriate in the management of other joint replacements which are less frequently tackled. The described management is detailed and clearly gained through years of experience. This is an area where randomized studies are very difficult to do and Haemophilia centres with very experienced physical therapists are very fortunate in managing in having these facilities to manage these patients.

CLINICAL EVALUATION OF THE HAEMOPHILIC JOINT

The first assessment by clinician of structural and functional joint damage is through physical joint assessment. The main tools commonly used are the Gilbert score [10] and more recently the HJHS 2.1 [11]. The HJHS has several advantages over the Gilbert Score: it is more sensitive to the smaller and earlier signs of joint changes, is better designed for use in children, and has undergone rigorous reliability and validation testing [11 - 13]. However, the data on the application of HJHS refers to a population of children with or without mild joint impairment, usually on prophylaxis. Consequently, further studies in adults and in patients with advanced joint disease are needed for the validation of this tool in these setting.

Because of the possibility of sub-clinical microhemorrhage, imaging continues to be required for the exhaustive evaluation of joint status, besides being an important complementary tool for the evaluation of complications, diagnostic confirmation and therapeutic follow-up of haemophilic arthropathy.

IMAGING THE STATE OF JOINTS

Any clinician managing patients with Haemophilia needs to know the status of the joints even if a patient does not complain of any problems. Traditionally this involved x-rays which have the limitation of exposure of patients to radiation and only show abnormalities when arthropathy is well established. Roselli and colleagues in chapter 6 report on the historical value of conventional radiological investigation and describe the radiological scoring systems of Arnold-Hilgartner and Pettersson. Whilst the Pettersson score is the more widely used one of the two, it has fallen out of favour and its value remains for research studies.

Over the last decade the use of ultrasound has been shown to be valuable in detecting early arthropathy but the major advance has been the realization that members of the Haemophilia team can use this technique. In chapter 7, Melchiorre and Matucci-Cerinic in a highly illustrated chapter take the reader through the way haemophilic joints can be systematically assessed using this technique. The details of the most widely used HEAD-US protocol [14] are explained and any clinician, especially someone without direct experience, will find this very valuable. We believe that this technique has great promise but it is important to appreciate that it relies on the expertise of the operator.

Undoubtedly the most accurate assessment of the haemophilic joint is with the use of MRI and scoring systems for this have been developed. This technique however is time consuming, expensive and for very young children requires sedation. The practical aspects of MRI examination in Haemophilia are eloquently described by Roselli and colleagues in chapter 6. Our view is that the MRI scoring systems will remain research tools, whilst MRI of specific joints when an abnormality is suspected will become the main investigation to assess the haemophilic joint in the future.

THE OPERATIVE MANAGEMENT OF HAEMOPHILIC ARTHRO-PATHY

As expected the largest part of this book deals with the invasive management of haemophilic arthropathy. Radio and chemo-synovectomy are addressed in chapter 8 and these techniques are of considerable value where synovitis is prominent. As expected they are much more widely used in underdeveloped countries where primary prophylaxis is not widely developed.

Most chapters deal with the orthopaedic management of specific joints. Although technical in nature, all of these chapters are highly illustrated with operative images and we believe that all members of the Haemophilia team will be enlightened if they consult the relevant chapter prior to managing their patients who are undergoing the relevant procedure.

The complications of orthopaedic surgery are described in chapter 17 by Solimeno and colleagues from the Milan group, a centre with some of the largest haemophilic orthopaedic experience in the world. As expected the issues of bleeding and infection receive the most attention. We were interested to see that they do not recommend thromboprophylaxis except in selected cases. We note with interest that there are different professional groups in the Haemophilia community that believe and do not believe in the value of thromboprophylaxis after orthopaedic surgery in Haemophilia. It should be possible to conduct a multicenter randomized trial to investigate the value of thromboprophylaxis in this group of patients in the future but this will require international collaboration.

THE MANAGEMENT OF INHIBITOR PATIENTS

The development of allo-antibodies to FVIII is the most important complication of Haemophilia care today because it transforms the lives of patients for the worse. The management of acute bleeding is with rFVIIa (NovoSeven) or activated prothrombin complex concentrate (FEIBA). A recent Cochrane review concluded that these two products are equally efficacious with some patients preferring one and others the other [15].

The management of surgery in patients with inhibitors is the most complex and challenging that a Haemophilia treater will encounter. Because in Italy major orthopaedic surgery in these patients is concentrated in the centres of Florence, Milan and Castelfranco Veneto, a lot of expertise has been accumulated by these centres. Tagariello and colleagues in chapter 19 describe their experience in conducting surgery in inhibitor patients and compare it to that in the literature. This group pioneered the simultaneous surgery on two joints which results in significant financial savings. In the Sheffield Haemophilia centre in the UK, major orthopaedic surgery is carried out using a hybrid regimen where for the first 4 days NovoSeven is used and the last 6 days FEIBA is preferred due to its longer mode of action [16]. The most important point to make is that surgery in inhibitor patients is not for the inexperienced or understaffed Haemophilia centre and should be concentrated in centres of expertise. Tagariello *et al* (chapter 19) also tackle two very controversial issues in this field which are the use of tranexamic acid and thromboprophylaxis. Whilst most centres use tranexamic acid with NovoSeven, this tends to be avoided in patients on FEIBA, although this has been challenged recently. Thromboprophylaxis, however, tends to be avoided in patients with inhibitors undergoing major orthopaedic surgery.

THE FUTURE

A person with Haemophilia born today in a country with ready availability of clotting factor concentrate can look forward to a bright future with very limited morbidity and significantly less arthropathy than older individuals. The use of prophylaxis has changed the landscape and it is now possible to live with less than 2-3 bleeds per year.

We are now in a very unusual time in the field of Haemophilia with over 20 different products or therapies currently in development. The new therapies can be divided into 3 main groups:

Extended Half Life Products

A whole series of products are about to be introduced in Europe which have 1.5-1.7x longer half life for FVIII and 3.0-5.0x longer for FIX. This prolongation in half life is achieved by the pegylation or addition of the Fc or albumin to the recombinant FVIII or FIX molecule.

Non-Substitutive Products

Three new technologies are promising to revolutionise the treatment of haemophilia. The first is the development of a bispecific antibody against FIXa and FX which juxtaposes the molecules leading to FXa generation (17). The result is a subcutaneous injection once a week generating an equivalent of 10% baseline FVIII. The second is siRNA against antithrombin which suppresses the production of antithrombin and leads to higher thrombin levels, allowing once a month subcutaneous injection as prophylaxis in Haemophilia. The third approach is through tissue factor pathway antibodies which also allow subcutaneous administration to improve thrombin generation.

Gene Therapy and Gene Editing

Although gene therapy has been on the horizon for more than 20 years, real progress has been achieved in the last five years with now at least 10 companies having gene therapy programs in Haemophilia A or B. The Haemophilia B gene therapy trial at the Royal Free Hospital in London has shown that it is possible to safely use gene therapy for the long term production of FIX.

In the last couple of years another promising technique of gene editing using Clustered Regularly-Interspaced Short Palindromic Repeats (CRISPR) has seen an explosion of therapeutic capabilities in animals and trials in Haemophilia are about to commence.

All the above new therapies are likely to lead to higher trough levels in patients. Based on current therapies prophylaxis has proven to be highly successful when achieving a trough FVIII level of a minimum of 1%. It is likely that this level does not prevent all clinical bleeds and certainly does not prevent microbleeds which are possibly the cause of ankle arthropathy in patients on current levels of prophylaxis. With the new therapies, however, it is feasible that severe haemophilic patients can have trough levels of 5-10% which is likely to eliminate all bleeds. It is hoped that these levels of treatment will truly abolish the development of haemophilic arthropathy. Until such times we will have a cohort of adults with established arthropathy and children with possible microbleeds who will need joint monitoring, physiotherapy and ultimately joint replacement.

This book offers a state of the art account of the status of investigation and management of haemophilic arthropathy and will be of great value to all members of the Haemophilia multidisciplinary team.

CONFLICT OF INTEREST

The authors confirm that they have no conflict of interest to declare for this publication.

ACKNOWLEDGEMENTS

This work is supported by a grant to Dr G Saccullo from the NovoNordisk Access to Insight initiative.

REFERENCES

[1]   van Dijk K, Fischer K, van der Bom JG, Grobbee DE, van den Berg HM. Variability in clinical phenotype of severe haemophilia: the role of the first joint bleed. Haemophilia 2005; 11(5): 438-43.
        [http://dx.doi.org/10.1111/j.1365-2516.2005.01124.x] [PMID: 16128885]

[2]   Carcao MD, van den Berg HM, Ljung R, Mancuso ME. Correlation between phenotype and genotype in a large unselected cohort of children with severe hemophilia A. Blood 2013; 121(19): 3946-3952, S1.
        [http://dx.doi.org/10.1182/blood-2012-11-469403] [PMID: 23482934]

[3]   Srivastava A, Brewer AK, Mauser-Bunschoten EP, *et al.* Guidelines for the management of hemophilia. Haemophilia 2013; 19(1): e1-e47.
        [http://dx.doi.org/10.1111/j.1365-2516.2012.02909.x] [PMID: 22776238]

[4]   Mulder K, Llinás A. The target joint. Haemophilia 2004; 10 (Suppl. 4): 152-6.
        [http://dx.doi.org/10.1111/j.1365-2516.2004.00976.x] [PMID: 15479389]

[5]   Luck JV Jr, Silva M, Rodriguez-Merchan EC, Ghalambor N, Zahiri CA, Finn RS. Hemophilic arthropathy. J Am Acad Orthop Surg 2004; 12(4): 234-45.
        [http://dx.doi.org/10.5435/00124635-200407000-00004] [PMID: 15473675]

[6]   Roosendaal G, Lafeber FP. Pathogenesis of haemophilic arthropathy. Haemophilia 2006; 12 (Suppl. 3): 117-21.
        [http://dx.doi.org/10.1111/j.1365-2516.2006.01268.x] [PMID: 16684006]

[7]   Valentino LA. Blood-induced joint disease: the pathophysiology of hemophilic arthropathy. J Thromb Haemost 2010; 8(9): 1895-902.
        [http://dx.doi.org/10.1111/j.1538-7836.2010.03962.x] [PMID: 20586922]

[8]   Tagariello G, Iorio A, Santagostino E, *et al.* Comparison of the rates of joint arthroplasty in patients with severe factor VIII and IX deficiency: an index of different clinical severity of the 2 coagulation disorders. Blood 2009; 114(4): 779-84.
        [http://dx.doi.org/10.1182/blood-2009-01-195313] [PMID: 19357395]

[9]   Santagostino E, Mancuso ME, Tripodi A, *et al.* Severe hemophilia with mild bleeding phenotype: molecular characterization and global coagulation profile. J Thromb Haemost 2010; 8(4): 737-43.
        [http://dx.doi.org/10.1111/j.1538-7836.2010.03767.x] [PMID: 20102490]

[10]   Gilbert MS. Prophylaxis: musculoskeletal evaluation. Semin Hematol 1993; 30(3) (Suppl. 2): 3-6.
        [PMID: 8367740]

[11]   Hilliard P, Funk S, Zourikian N, *et al.* van den Berg, Feldman BM. Haemophilia joint halth score reliability study. Haemophilia 2006; 12: 518-25.
        [http://dx.doi.org/10.1111/j.1365-2516.2006.01312.x] [PMID: 16919083]

[12]   Feldman BM, Funk SM, Bergstrom BM, *et al.* Validation of a new pediatric joint scoring system from the International Hemophilia Prophylaxis Study Group: validity of the hemophilia joint health score. Arthritis Care Res (Hoboken) 2011; 63(2): 223-30.
[http://dx.doi.org/10.1002/acr.20353] [PMID: 20862683]

[13]   Sun J, Hilliard PE, Feldman BM, *et al.* Blanchette *VS*, Luke KH, Poon MC. Chinese hemophilia joint health score 2.1 reliability study. Haemophilia 2014; 20(3): 435-40.
[http://dx.doi.org/10.1111/hae.12330] [PMID: 24330460]

[14]   Martinoli C, Della Casa Alberighi O, Di Minno G, *et al.* Development and definition of a simplified scanning procedure and scoring method for Haemophilia Early Arthropathy Detection with Ultrasound (HEAD-US). Thromb Haemost 2013; 109(6): 1170-9.
[http://dx.doi.org/10.1160/TH12-11-0874] [PMID: 23571706]

[15]   Matino D, Makris M, Dwan K, DAmico R, Iorio A. Recombinant factor VIIa concentrate *versus* plasma-derived concentrates for treating acute bleeding episodes in people with haemophilia and inhibitors. Cochrane Database Syst Rev 2015; 12(12): CD004449.
[PMID: 26677005]

[16]   van Veen JJ, Maclean RM, Hampton KK, Hamer A, Makris M. Major surgery in severe haemophilia A with inhibitors using a recombinant factor VIIa and activated prothrombin complex concentrate hybrid regimen. Haemophilia 2014; 20(4): 587-92.
[http://dx.doi.org/10.1111/hae.12365] [PMID: 24517157]

[17]   Makris M. Hemophilia A treatment: disruptive technology ahead. Blood 2016; 127(13): 1623-4.
[http://dx.doi.org/10.1182/blood-2016-01-691469] [PMID: 27034415]

SUBJECT INDEX

A

Achilles tendon 101, 127, 171, 174, 175
Active flexion 216, 223, 224
   exercises 216, 223
Advanced ankle arthropathy 172
Adverse events (AEs) 65, 269
Alloantibodies 25, 33, 52
Aluminum hydroxide gel 30
American orthopaedic foot and ankle society
   (AOFAS) 177
Amino acids 26, 31
Anaesthesia 140, 141, 149, 163
Analgesic effects 130
Anastomoses 240, 241, 245
Anatomical districts 243, 244, 248
Ankle and subtalar joints 176, 177
Ankle arthrodesis 176, 177
Ankle arthroplasty 178, 196
Ankle distraction 171, 174, 176
Ankle haemophilic arthropathy 171
Ankle replacements 112, 140, 171, 173, 207
   total 171, 173
Ankylosed patellofemoral 151
Ankyloses 8, 70, 72, 73, 86
Anteroposterior 172, 224
Antibodies 34, 36, 49, 52, 53, 273, 286, 287
   monoclonal 286, 287
Anticoagulant 45
Antifibrinolytic agents 35
Antithrombin 276, 286, 296
Apoptosis 1, 4
Arnold-Hilgartner classification 74, 76, 148,
   149
Arteries 115, 241, 243, 245, 246, 253, 256,
   277
   anterior tibial 243, 245, 246
   popliteal 245, 277
   subscapular 253
Arthrodesis 173, 177, 178
Arthrodiastasis 171, 174, 178
Arthrolysis 138, 140
Arthropathies, mild 138, 142

Arthropathy 1, 7, 8, 25, 37, 86, 70, 71, 72, 73,
   74, 76, 77, 78, 83, 85, 90, 92, 97, 103,
   110, 111, 112, 114, 116, 122, 126, 128,
   129, 140, 141, 148, 149, 150, 151, 162,
   171, 178, 181, 182, 185, 199, 207, 213,
   214, 221, 229, 265, 266, 276, 280, 292,
   293, 295, 296
   chronic 129, 292
   haemophilia 213
   severe 37, 86, 116, 140, 148, 151, 185, 199,
      265, 292
Arthroplasty 147, 198, 199, 233
Arthroscopic debridement 171, 173, 174, 178,
   184
Arthroscopy in haemophilic subjects 138
Aseptic failure 199, 202
Aseptic loosenings 165
Associated infectious disease 113, 156

B

Bethesda unit (BU) 34, 53, 54, 55, 269, 270,
   271
Bilateral joint replacement 276
Biochemical markers 7, 8
Bleeding disorders, inherited 25, 28, 59
Bleeding episodes 34, 37, 62, 97, 214, 235,
   291
Bleeding management 147, 148, 155, 157
   appropriate 147, 157
   modern 148, 155
Bleedings, posttraumatic 91, 92
Blood pressure 64, 65, 256
Blood products 85, 89
Blood transfusions 148, 268, 272
Body weight (BW) 14, 16, 18, 19, 20, 32, 271
Bolus injection (BI) 266, 268, 269
Bone erosion 70, 72, 83, 89, 90, 103, 106
Bone grafts 153, 203, 205, 207
   heterologous 203, 205
Bone marrow oedema 83, 90
Bone remodelling 6, 74, 103, 106
Bone resorption 6, 199

total amount of 267, 268

use of 266, 267, 269

Rheumatoid arthritis 111, 138, 149, 191, 199, 232, 292

Rifampicine 110, 112, 113, 114, 116, 174

S

Septic arthritis 199, 200, 233, 234

Short-tau inversion recovery (STIR) 78, 81, 84, 85

Signal intensity 81, 82, 85, 88, 89, 90

  characteristic low 81, 82

  low 82, 85, 88

Signal noise ratio (SNR) 83

Signals, diffuse hyperechoic 103

Simultaneous bilateral joint replacement 276

Simultaneous bilateral TKA 277, 278

Skin incision 188, 234, 250

Skin paddle 248, 249, 250, 251, 255

Soft tissues defect 248, 250

Stages of evolution 87, 88

Stems 164, 166, 167

  modern short 164, 166, 167

  standard 166, 167

Stiff elbow 181

Stiffness 124, 156, 164, 199, 213, 214

  joint 213, 214

Subtalar arthrodesis 174, 176

Surgery 18, 27, 29, 35, 37, 46, 48, 61, 65, 66, 71, 86, 111, 112, 115, 116, 138, 140, 141, 148, 149, 151, 155, 156, 162, 163, 164, 165, 167, 168, 171, 173, 177, 181, 186, 196, 197, 198, 200, 201, 203, 204, 207, 213, 214, 215, 216, 217, 222, 223, 224, 229, 230, 231, 232, 234, 235, 236, 240, 247, 249, 253, 256, 257, 265, 266, 269, 270, 271, 272, 273, 277, 279, 280, 284, 295

  aggressive 138

  arthroscopic 231

  complex 181

  delay 116

  dental 65

  emergency 272

  invasive 115, 142

  multiple 207

oncologic 115, 204

performing 230

plan 86

planning 266

reconstructive 207

salvage 196, 204

simultaneous 295

undergoing 48, 66, 198, 269

Surgery isometric contractions 217

Surgery pain 222

Surgical approaches 150, 163, 184, 204, 207

Surgical procedures 35, 111, 177, 181, 189, 196, 205, 207, 256, 265, 266, 269, 277

Surgical technique 140, 149, 155, 163, 186, 214, 232, 246, 253

Surgical treatment 70, 90, 115, 147, 171, 174, 276

Synovectomy 37, 138, 139, 140, 141, 142, 171, 173, 174, 181, 184, 190

  arthroscopic 142, 171, 174, 175, 178

  chemical 171, 173, 174, 181

Synovial hyperplasia 78, 79

Synovial hyperthrophy 103, 105

Synovial membrane 1, 2, 5, 78, 81, 82

Synovial tissue 3, 4, 7, 8, 71, 81, 85, 99, 100, 111, 113, 115, 148, 162, 173, 182, 221, 291

Synoviocytes 6

Synoviorthesis 110, 113, 184

  chemical 110, 113

Synovitis 1, 3, 81, 97, 98, 113, 115, 129, 141, 152, 171, 173, 174, 178, 182, 183, 184, 291, 294

  chronic 113, 115, 129, 141, 152, 173, 174, 184, 291

  perpetuate 97

T

Target cells 36

Tetracyclines 113

Therapeutic modalities for haemophilia 28

Thrombin 35, 44, 286

  small amounts of 44

Thromboplastin 46

Thromboprophylaxis 294, 295

  value of 294

www.ingramcontent.com/pod-product-compliance
Lightning Source LLC
Chambersburg PA
CBHW041725210326

41598CB00008B/779